# COMMUNICATION
# PROBLEMS IN
# AUTISM

# CURRENT ISSUES IN AUTISM
## Series Editors: Eric Schopler and Gary B. Mesibov

*University of North Carolina School of Medicine*
*Chapel Hill, North Carolina*

AUTISM IN ADOLESCENTS AND ADULTS
Edited by Eric Schopler and Gary B. Mesibov

THE EFFECTS OF AUTISM ON THE FAMILY
Edited by Eric Schopler and Gary B. Mesibov

COMMUNICATION PROBLEMS IN AUTISM
Edited by Eric Schopler and Gary B. Mesibov

# COMMUNICATION PROBLEMS IN AUTISM

Edited by
## Eric Schopler
and
## Gary B. Mesibov

*University of North Carolina School of Medicine*
*Chapel Hill, North Carolina*

PLENUM PRESS • NEW YORK AND LONDON

Library of Congress Cataloging in Publication Data

Main entry under title:

Communication problems in autism.

  (Current issues in autism)
  Based on the fourth annual TEACCH conference, held in 1983.
  Includes bibliographies and index.
  1. Autistic children — Language — Congresses. 2. Interpersonal communication — Congresses. 3. Sign language — Congresses. I. Schopler, Eric. II. Mesibov, Gary B. III. University of North Carolina at Chapel Hill. Dept. of Psychiatry. Division TEACCH. IV. Series. [DNLM: 1. Autism — congresses. 2. Communication — congresses. WM 203.5 C7339 1983]
  RJ506.A9C666  1985                      618.92′8982                      85-3416
  ISBN 0-306-41859-2

©1985 Plenum Press, New York
A Division of Plenum Publishing Corporation
233 Spring Street, New York, N.Y. 10013

Printed in the United States of America

To the autistic children of North Carolina

# Contributors

CHRISTIANE A. M. BALTAXE, Department of Psychiatry and Biobehavioral Sciences, University of California, School of Medicine, Los Angeles, California 90024

THOMAS D. BOYLE, Rutgers University, Piscataway, New Jersey 08854

EDWARD G. CARR, Department of Psychology and Suffolk Child Development Center, State University of New York at Stony Brook, Stony Brook, New York 11794-2500

M. J. DEMETRAS, Early Childhood Language Research Laboratory, Department of Speech and Hearing Sciences, University of Arizona, Tucson, Arizona 85721

SANDRA L. HARRIS, Rutgers University, Piscataway, New Jersey 08854

BEATE HERMELIN, Medical Research Council, Institute of Education, 2 Taviton Street, London WC1, England

D. ELISE LINDSTEDT, Department of Speech Pathology and Audiology, University of Denver, Denver, Colorado 80208

CATHERINE LORD, Department of Pediatrics, University of Alberta, Glenrose Hospital, Edmonton, Alberta T5G 0B7, Canada

PAULA MENYUK, Boston University, School of Education, Boston, Massachusetts 02215

GARY B. MESIBOV, Division TEACCH, University of North Carolina, Chapel Hill, North Carolina 27514

NEIL O'CONNOR, Medical Research Council, Institute of Education, 2 Taviton Street, London WC1, England.

J. GREGORY OLLEY, Division TEACCH, University of North Carolina, Chapel Hill, North Carolina 27514

BARRY M. PRIZANT, Speech and Language Department, Emma Pendleton Bradley Hospital, 1011 Veterans Memorial Parkway, East Providence, Rhode Island 02915

KATHLEEN QUILL, Boston University, School of Education, Boston, Massachusetts 02215

ERIC SCHOPLER, Division TEACCH, University of North Carolina, Chapel Hill, North Carolina 27514

ADRIANA L. SCHULER, Department of Special Education, San Francisco State University, San Francisco, California 94132

JAMES Q. SIMMONS III, Department of Psychiatry and Biobehavioral Sciences, University of California, School of Medicine, Los Angeles, California 90024

LYNN S. SNYDER, Department of Speech Pathology and Audiology, University of Denver, Denver, Colorado 80208

LINDA SWISHER, Early Childhood Language Research Laboratory, Department of Speech and Hearing Sciences, University of Arizona, Tucson, Arizona 85721

HELEN TAGER-FLUSBERG, Department of Psychology, University of Massachusetts, Boston, Massachusetts 02125

LINDA R. WATSON, Division TEACCH, University of North Carolina, Chapel Hill, North Carolina 27514

RONNIE B. WILBUR, Department of Audiology and Speech Sciences, Purdue University, West Lafayette, Indiana 47907

# Preface

The North Carolina State Legislature's mandate to Division TEACCH has three major components. First, to provide the most up-to-date and cost-effective services possible for families with autistic or similar language-impaired children; second, to conduct research aimed toward the better understanding of such devastating disorders; and third, to provide training for the professionals needed to pursue these goals. One element in achieving these aims is to hold annual conferences on topics of special importance to the understanding and treatment of autism and similar disorders.

In addition to training professionals and parents on the most recent developments in each conference topic, we are publishing a series, *Current Issues in Autism,* based on these conferences. These books are not, however, simply the published proceedings of the conference papers. Instead, some chapters are expanded conference presentations, whereas others come from national and international experts whose work is beyond the scope of the conference, but essential in our attempt at comprehensive coverage of the conference theme. These volumes are intended to provide the most current knowledge and professional practice available to us at the time.

This volume is the culmination of our fourth annual TEACCH Conference, held in 1983, which concerned communication problems in autism. Although researchers and clinicians have been interested in the communication problems inherent in autism ever since the syndrome was first identified, some recent developments in the field make this topic especially timely. Most of the contributing authors express in their chapters the view that we are on the threshold of major changes in the conceptualization of the most useful research and treatment for the severe and challenging communication problems of these puzzling youngsters. These include the emphasis on communication skills, rather than language, and on the special utility of psycholinguistic theory toward that end.

This volume provides a historical overview of communication problems in autism, thus placing in context the most current data, perspectives, and directions. Although we were not able to include all the important work being done in this area, we believe the information in this volume will be most useful to all professionals and parents concerned with understanding and helping people with autism.

ERIC SCHOPLER
GARY B. MESIBOV

# Acknowledgments

No undertaking of this scope can be accomplished without the cooperation of numerous people. It is our pleasure to acknowledge our many sources of assistance. First, our thanks to Cindy Fesmire who was instrumental in organizing the conference that was the starting point for this book. Our secretarial and typing needs were met competently and cheerfully by Deborah Carr and Sandy Troth. Judy Davis has been invaluable in providing editorial assistance, strengthening individual chapters, organizing our efforts, and managing the project with great skill and ease. Judy's work has been significant in each volume of this series. We thank Dr. Linda Watson whose expertise clarified many points for us, and we would also like to thank our many other colleagues in the TEACCH program whose thoughtful, stimulating, and persistent efforts at helping these severely handicapped youngsters have provided many insights and helpful ideas. Finally, the help of our colleague, Dr. Catherine Lord, has been invaluable. Dr. Lord is one of the most knowledgeable experts on both normal language development and the communication problems in autism. Her suggestions, ideas, and input have influenced both this project and our thinking about this important topic over a period of years.

Most importantly, this book, as well as all our efforts in the TEACCH program, would not have materialized without the assistance of the families of autistic people in North Carolina, the state legislature, and the support of the Department of Psychiatry of the University of North Carolina School of Medicine at Chapel Hill. These families continue to impress upon us the difficulty of their plight and the heroism of their struggle. We are indeed fortunate to live in a state where the legislative and university structures have been committed to the study and amelioration of this complex handicap.

E. S.
G. B. M.

# Contents

Chapter 3
BEHAVIORAL APPROACHES TO
LANGUAGE AND COMMUNICATION                                           37

Edward G. Carr

Chapter 3A
CONTRIBUTION OF BEHAVIORAL APPROACHES
TO THE LANGUAGE AND COMMUNICATION
OF PERSONS WITH AUTISM                                               59

Catherine Lord

Chapter 4
PSYCHOLINGUISTIC APPROACHES TO
LANGUAGE AND COMMUNICATION IN AUTISM                                 69

Helen Tager-Flusberg

Chapter 10
PARENTS AS LANGUAGE TRAINERS OF
CHILDREN WITH AUTISM                                                     207

Sandra L. Harris and Thomas D. Boyle

Chapter 11
SIGN LANGUAGE AND AUTISM                                                 229

Ronnie B. Wilbur

PART V: GENERAL ISSUES

Chapter 12
AUTISM AND THE COMPREHENSION OF LANGUAGE                  257

Catherine Lord

Chapter 13
LOGICO-AFFECTIVE STATES AND
NONVERBAL LANGUAGE                                              283

B. Hermelin and N. O'Connor

Chapter 14
SOCIAL ASPECTS OF COMMUNICATION
IN CHILDREN WITH AUTISM                                         311

J. Gregory Olley

I

# Introduction

# Introduction to Communication Problems in Autism

## ERIC SCHOPLER and GARY B. MESIBOV

### OVERVIEW

Although autism is frequently described as a low-incidence disorder (Rutter & Schopler, 1978), the syndrome has attracted a growing cadre of researchers, clinicians, and teachers. This attraction can be attributed to autism's devastating effect on families, the unusual and puzzling behaviors it produces, and its overlap with most other childhood disorders because it involves multiple problems with language, social relationships, emotional adjustment, conceptualization, hyperactivity, and learning. This growing interest has resulted in a better understanding and treatment of autistic people than has ever been available in the past. However, the proliferation of articles, books, treatment programs, and media coverage has also brought increased confusion and misconceptions. There is the problem of staying up to date with the increasing amount of information from both the professional and popular literature along with the difficulty in distinguishing sound research from that which is careless or pointless. A related concern is how to distinguish new treatment or educational methods that are effective from primarily self-promoting exaggerations that offer only false hope.

For two reasons, these problems are especially difficult in the area of communication. First, communication deficits are a central symptom of the autism syndrome. Second, communication problems are intertwined with the social and cognitive difficulties that also characterize the autism syndrome. For these

ERIC SCHOPLER and GARY B. MESIBOV • Division TEACCH, University of North Carolina, Chapel Hill, North Carolina 27514.

reasons, communication problems have attracted an especially impressive amount of interest. The purpose of this book is to assist the reader in sorting through the literature on language and communication in autism for the most relevant, verifiable, and potentially useful evidence accumulated to date. We have tried to do this by establishing certain criteria for manuscripts to appear in this volume. Before inviting a contribution, we have asked to what extent the new knowledge, theories, or treatment programs are based on empirical data, some established rules of evidence, or rationality. Although we were not able to include all the work being done in this area, these chapters have been carefully judged by these criteria, resulting in a volume we consider relevant, up to date, and useful.

## HISTORICAL PERSPECTIVE

Before describing some of the important developments and exciting new perspectives that appear in this book, we would like to outline briefly some historical trends in the areas of autism and communication so that the reader can place the current research and practice in an appropriate context. Any historical consideration of the autism syndrome must begin with Kanner (1943) and his original series of 11 autistic children. In addition to the severe and early onset of problems in social relationships, repetitive behaviors, rituals, and intellectual peak skills, Kanner viewed autism as a problem of communication and useful language. Research has changed key elements of Kanner's definition (Schopler, 1983) with data showing that cold and rejecting upper-middle-class mothers cannot make their children autistic with deviant child-rearing practices and, also, that most autistic children do not have normal intellectual potential. However, the problems of communication and functional language that Kanner observed have never been disputed. In fact, some of his early descriptions are still among the clearest for describing the language difficulties of these puzzling children.

The amount of attention Kanner (1946) devoted to this symptom suggests that he saw language problems as central to autism and probably the most interesting of its symptoms. In describing his first autistic patients, the aspects of language he referred to most frequently were echolalia (of particular fascination for Kanner), substitutions, literalness, repetitions, and pronoun reversals. Kanner also noted that a large percentage of the sample had little or no communicative ability. When those who spoke were able to complete sentences, they seemed "parrot-like," echolalic in their repetitions of words they had previously heard. Kanner did note that a large percentage of the children who had language showed significant improvement over time.

Kanner's language- and cognitive-oriented explanation of the autism syndrome received further support from studies (Eisenberg & Kanner, 1956; Kanner, 1971) that followed up on Kanner's original sample. Of the 63 cases in the follow-up study, Eisenberg and Kanner (1956) described those with good adjustments and those with poor adjustments. One of the most important distinguishing characteristics between those who made poor adjustments and those who made good adjustments was the presence of useful speech by 5 years of age. Therefore, there was already corroborative evidence for autism as a language and cognitive disability in the late 1950s.

Unfortunately, the evidence for a language-based disorder was generally overlooked because of the predominance of psychodynamic theories in the 1950s and 1960s. These theorists viewed autism as a function of cold, rejecting middle-class mothers who could not communicate with their children, thus causing a voluntary withdrawal. Despite Kanner's emphasis on the language problem, autism was generally viewed as an emotional and interpersonal problem. Language training was systematically ignored or avoided and replaced by individual psychotherapy or play therapy.

A good example of how psychodynamic theory caused many researchers to overlook linguistic aspects of the disorder can be found with the issue of pronoun reversals. Kanner (1946) accounted for pronoun reversals by noting the absence of spontaneous sentence formation in autistic children and their frequent use of echolalia instead. This formulation was later confirmed by Bartak and Rutter (1974) when they showed experimentally that autistic children did not avoid any pronoun, but instead echoed the last pronoun to end a sentence. In other words, autistic children frequently respond by repeating what they hear last and therefore do not always change pronouns appropriately. Kanner observed that as language develops, children learn more grammatical rules and develop the ability to use them so that pronoun reversals become less common.

Others, however, chose to reject this interpretation of pronoun reversals for psychoanalytic explanations. For example, Despert (1951) saw this as a manifestation of a child's inability to separate himself or herself from others. Bettelheim (1967) devoted the better part of a book to promoting the notion that pronoun reversal represents a child's lack of identity and the rejection of his or her own existence. These explanations precluded a more careful analysis of the linguistic problems involved. Echolalia was viewed in much the same way. Different psychoanalytic interpretations of echolalia were advanced, suggesting that children understood a great deal more than they let on and were somehow holding back what they knew.

The popular press supported the psychodynamic interpretations of the 1950s and 1960s. Successful treatment was presented as resulting from therapists reaching autistic people by breaking through their autistic shell to find a normally functioning person. Although these explanations and interpretations might seem unscientific and old fashioned today, examples still persist, such as the Tinbergens' (1983) recent book asserting that autistic children are anxious and thereby suppress their communication with others.

Although psychodynamic theories were in vogue during the 1950s and 1960s, there was ample precedent for a more language-based explanation of the disorder for those who were interested. Kanner's earlier work has already been described. In addition, the French physician Itard worked with the first autistic boy reported in the literature back in the 1700s (Lane, 1976). Itard's child, Victor, was described as a feral child raised in the wilderness by animals. In developing Victor's language, Itard tried different methods of teaching communication, including pictures, sensory training, behavior modification, and symbols similar to signing. By developing communication techniques through direct trial and error, Itard hit on some procedures that are still quite effective today.

Itard's and Kanner's language-based approach was resumed in the early 1960s, when several studies appeared in the literature on the language of autistic children (Cunningham & Dixon, 1961; Wolff & Chess, 1965). However, it was the events of the mid- to late-1960s that primarily triggered the revolution in thinking of autism as a language and cognitive disorder rather than an emotional disorder. Most important of these was the publication of Rimland's (1964) book, *Infantile Autism,* which proposed a cognitive model for understanding autistic behaviors. Rimland's work was widely acclaimed and established an important frame of reference for Hermelin and O'Connor's (1970) series of studies by suggesting that autism represented a cognitive disability in interpreting stimuli meaningfully. In addition, Schopler (1971) and Schopler and Reichler (1971) were demonstrating that parents are not the cause of an emotional disorder, but are instead the child's most important asset for remediation of this cognitive disability. At the same time, follow-up studies (DeMyer *et al.,* 1973; Lockyer & Rutter, 1970; Rutter, Greenfeld, & Lockyer, 1967) were all pointing to a cognitive, linguistic disorder as the main problem in autism.

Although the 1960s represented a major change in the conceptualization of autism, not much work was reported on language remediation. Most of the established forms of speech therapy, emphasizing articulation, were not especially appropriate for autistic children. The main intervention approach was behavior modification (Lovaas, 1977), and operant conditioning techniques were widely regarded as the main hope for improving autistic children's communication.

The 1970s saw a new trend emphasizing language remediation. Following the acceptance of the cognitive and linguistic bases of autistic behaviors, the implications of this discovery and how it affected specific remediation efforts were reviewed, and many new intervention approaches were developed, based on the growing understanding of normal language acquisition and increasing clinical experience with autistic children.

The 1980s might represent still another crossroads in how we view the language of autistic people and its implications for remediation. The past decade has seen a virtual explosion of research on the language and communication processes, some of which have important implications for the teaching of those with severe communication handicaps. Most of the important trends that will influence this work are contained in this book and we would like to briefly highlight them here.

## CURRENT TRENDS

### Communicative Use of Language

The reader of this book will immediately be impressed by the change in emphasis toward the teaching of communication skills to autistic children. Virtually every theoretical perspective, and every professional discipline, has highlighted the necessity for shifting from teaching language skills to teaching communication skills. This new emphasis is more than a semantic shift. It means that there will be far less emphasis on simply increasing vocabularies, less one-to-one teaching of specific words. There will be, instead, more emphasis on tying communication training to a child's specific interests and activities and more emphasis on alternative communication systems such as signing, gesturing, picture cards, or any other system meaningful to a child. The important concept behind this shift in emphasis is that we must teach autistic children language that enhances useful communication for them. Moreover, it places an added emphasis on accepting autism as a chronic developmental disability, in which the unique language impairment of each child must be assessed, accepted, and shaped toward the child's optimum communication potential. If the 1970s represented a shift from speech and operant therapies to language therapy, the 1980s will move us from language therapy to communication training.

This shift can be seen in nearly every theoretical orientation represented in this volume. Carr (Chapter 3) suggests that behaviorists might need to change their focus from a discrete-trial teaching format to incidental teaching if they are to promote the communicative use of language. In Chapter 9, Watson discusses the TEACCH curriculum, which is based on psycholinguistic theory and which emphasizes communication as opposed to language skills to give the highest priority to improving the child's communication skills in everyday situations. Snyder and Lindstedt (Chapter 2) point out that the constructivist theories of child language development, based on Piagetian principles, stress the need for meaningful language training carried out where the child is learning, in preference to a therapy room or other artificial environment.

It should also be noted that arguments for communication training in natural environments are not restricted to any specific discipline or language system. Psychologists, as well as speech pathologists, see this need for a change in the ways we teach both verbal language and signing (Wilbur, Chapter 11). As this trend continues, we should see much more training in such natural environments as classrooms or group homes and a greater focus on integrating communication training with other daily activities.

## Echolalia as a Form of Communication

Among the most exciting of the new ideas in communication is the connecting of echolalia with the communication process. Two of the major researchers in this area, Schuler and Prizant, have contributed an admirable overview of this work (Chapter 8). Although Kanner (1943) meticulously described many types of echolalia and speculated on its probable function and what it told us about autism, this work was not pursued through much of the following four decades. Instead, echolalia was seen as a self-stimulatory behavior to be eliminated so that more appropriate forms of language could be acquired.

The present decade promises to alter our view of echolalia dramatically. Schuler and Prizant describe echolalia as a form of communication and a precursor to the development of more meaningful language. Their work will focus more attention on the communicative nature of echolalia and how it evolves into other forms of language. In addition, the scheme outlined by Schuler and Prizant for analyzing the different types of echolalia should prove quite useful in these efforts.

## Increased Application of Normal Language and Development Research

As mentioned earlier, much of the research on language and autism in the 1970s involved looking very carefully at normal language development. This research has been most useful for those working with autisic people because it provides a framework for better understanding language processes in these youngsters. In addition, intensive research efforts for over a decade have enabled us to delineate more carefully the differences between autistic and nonautistic children in their development of language. Several chapters in this book deal specifically with the recent knowledge gained about these language differences.

Tager-Flusberg (Chapter 4) argues convincingly that autistic people generally do attempt to communicate and that their basic problem is not simply disinterest. For higher functioning autistic people, the main problem seems to be their pragmatic deficits, whereas lower, nonverbal autistic people never learn to segment sounds into meaningful units. Syntax, according to Tager-Flusberg, is also more of a problem for autistic youngsters than for nonhandicapped children. However, here the inability of autistic people to integrate large amounts of information may be the crucial factor. For syntactic rules that are independent of other factors (for example, word order), Tager-Flusberg notes that autistic children perform similarly to normal children in the development of these rules. Linguistic features related to semantic, environmental, or conceptual factors, however, present greater difficulties for autistic children in comparison with other groups.

Swisher and Demetras (Chapter 7) agree that autistic children definitely have the desire to communicate. They identify two aspects of language that differentiate autistic from normal children and also from children with mental retardation or specific language impairments. The first is the weak cognitive underpinnings of their language. Autistic children often produce a string of words that are syntactically correct, but simply echo what someone else has said. Wing (1976) referred to this as a "store of phrases." The other factor that differentiates autistic children from others is that their utterances frequently do not fit a given context. Children of similar developmental levels are able to convey considerably more information because one can often understand their meanings from a given context. This mismatch between the content and context makes communication with autistic people more difficult.

Menyuk and Quill (Chapter 6) discuss the development of meaning for nonhandicapped and autistic children. They describe the semantic and relational problems that characterize autistic children and their language development. Autistic children have difficulty analyzing the composition of words, sentences, or conversations and do not seem to be able to decode information to the level of single words or units. Although they can develop some strategies to improve their comprehension, their classifications are limited and so are their analytic skills. This results in rigid approaches to interpreting sentence meanings. Among the most capable of the autistic population, discourse still poses considerable difficulties because of the multiple levels on which it occurs.

Although studies on prosody reviewed by Baltaxe and Simmons (Chapter 5) also point to some important developmental trends, this area has not yet generated the same amount of research interest as the work concerning pragmatics and syntax has. However, it does appear that autistic children have trouble with assigning stresses to appropriate words and with other prosodic characteristics of language.

In summary, the research comparing autistic children with nonhandicapped controls at the same approximate developmental level has led us to a more sophisticated understanding of the language process in autistic children. It is no longer sufficient to say that such children are simply delayed in all areas. Rather, they seem to have the greatest difficulty with linguistic concepts that must be integrated into a context, with those that have a certain meaning, and with the process of breaking down sentences or phrases into their component parts. Their inability to integrate and recombine units of information results in a rigidity that is characteristic of their language and their behavior in general.

## RELATING SOCIAL DEFICITS TO LANGUAGE PROBLEMS

Although social deficits have been among the most obvious of autistic people's difficulties and were noted by Kanner (1943), they have received surprisingly little research attention over the years. Those few investigators who examined these deficits have looked at social behavior as a separate difficulty, rather than as a part of the other problems found in autism. More recently, however, Rutter (1983) has suggested that social deficits are part of the cognitive and language problem of autistic people and can only be understood in that context. Rutter claimed that autistic people have general difficulties in processing cognitive information and especially information that carries emotional or social meanings.

The relationships among social problems and other difficulties experienced by autistic people promise to be a growing area of inquiry. Several chapters in this book deal with this, especially those by Lord (Chapter 12), Hermelin and O'Connor (Chapter 13), and Olley (Chapter 14). Olley gives a fine overview of the relationships between language and social problems in autism. He begins by outlining difficulties in reciprocal interaction, one of the most basic and most enduring problems experienced by these children (Rutter, 1983). He then discusses assessment instruments designed to identify these factors and intervention techniques that change either antecedent factors or consequences to help facilitate more effective language development.

Lord (Chapter 12) examines the crucial issue of comprehension. The inability to imitate (and otherwise extract meanings from social interactions) is detailed and described as one of the autistic person's most pressing deficits. According to Lord, comprehension deficits in autistic people result from their inability to understand social meanings, plus their difficulties with abstracting rules. Lord presents some excellent suggestions for dealing with these problems, as well as a fine overview and integration of the relevant literature.

Hermelin and O'Connor (Chapter 13) present fascinating insights and observations about the social problems of autism. These difficulties involve a complex combination of communicative and social functions, which these authors review with great understanding. They begin by examining the language problems of autistic people and especially their difficulties in pragmatics (language and its interactive role between speaker and listener). The problem of interactive communication and reciprocal behavior arises repeatedly and is clearly a crucial aspect of the autism syndrome. Hermelin and O'Connor also present a series of intriguing experiments on nonverbal communication and the ability to extract nonverbal meanings. These experiments provide fresh and interesting insights into why autistic people neither make nor understand nonverbal communications as well as other communications and will surely suggest many hypotheses for investigators to pursue in the years ahead.

## NEW TRENDS IN APPLICATIONS

Because most of the contributors to this volume are also involved in direct clinical work with autistic people, specific suggestions for intervention and remediation receive considerable attention in this book. Two general suggestions recur throughout.

The first concerns the need to provide language training in a naturalistic context and to make this training as meaningful as possible. This means that language training should be done in a setting in which a child generally spends a considerable percentage of his or her time. Snyder and Lindstedt (Chapter 2) state that both theorists of nativism and of constructionism make this recommendation in general. Wilbur (Chapter 11) views this as equally important with sign language and Lord (Chapter 12) makes the point for comprehension as well. In addition, Olley (Chapter 14), in his discussion of social aspects of communication, emphasizes the need for training in one's natural environment.

The second general suggestion is that a thorough developmental assessment is mandatory before teaching language to autistic people. This point is emphasized in the TEACCH curriculum (Watson, Chapter 9) and also by Swisher and Demetras (Chapter 7) and by Lord (Chapter 12). Swisher makes the compelling argument that the language of autistic people is generally quite misleading in that their language abilities are so inconsistent from one language domain to another. They seem to store the semantic structure of an utterance without the meaning accompanying it. A knowledge of general developmental levels is necessary to assess the actual level of the autistic person's language.

Swisher and Demetras (Chapter 7) also make several other interesting points. The uneven developmental levels in the language of autistic people put them at risk for starting language intervention programs too early. One must be very sure that they are ready for language training and at what level; this can only be done where their developmental levels are known. Swisher and Demetras especially warn researchers against emphasizing picture identification too strongly as an assessment procedure. This technique overestimates most autistic children's language ability. Tests of comprehension would appear to be much more appropriate (see Lord, Chapter 12). Repeated observations and language samples in a variety of settings are suggested as more appropriate assessment strategies.

Harris and Boyle (Chapter 10) present some excellent suggestions for parent training. These include necessary skills (behavior shaping, reinforcement, prompting and fading, structured teaching) and methods for teaching (media, videotapes, written manuals, direct instructions, group training). The Harris and Boyle training technique involves information and instruction in a model that combines hands-on experience with didactic presentations and a most crucial posttraining consultation program.

Wilbur (Chapter 11) discusses one of the most talked about areas of language training for autistic people, the use of sign language. She suggests that autistic persons whose communicative abilities are deficient or whose speech is inadequate to the requirements of their communicative abilities are good candidates for learning these techniques. Wilbur describes sign language as also useful for establishing self-direction, maintaining a line of thought, and aiding memory. As with the other authors in the book, she suggests that language training, even with signs, should be done in context, and especially should involve the child's interests. Teachers of sign language should be especially fluent with this medium and "grammatically well-formed sentences are a luxury that the early communicator, autistic or not, can ill afford" (p. 28).

Finally, Lord (Chapter 12) presents interesting and important suggestions in the area of comprehension. Prior to Lord's excellent analysis, comprehension has been viewed by many as a crucial skill for autistic people, but there had been few ideas about how to develop it. Lord suggests modifying language so that it describes the task a child is doing when it is being done. In addition, behaviors should be taught through repetitive demonstrations with appropriate language added afterwards. As with many other authors in this volume, Lord emphasizes the need to make language meaningful, functional, and interesting to the individual child. In these ways, language development will be facilitated in general and comprehension will be promoted in particular.

## SUMMARY

Obviously, our review of this volume can only provide some brief highlights of the developing trends, but these should give the reader a sense of the direction in which our distinguished authors see the field moving and also the ideas behind this direction. The area of language and communication training promises to continue as a basic area of research and intervention into the challenging problems of autism. We feel the chapters that follow provide important and exciting new directions in the study and remediation of communication problems in autism.

# REFERENCES

Bartak, L., & Rutter, M. (1974). The use of personal pronouns by autistic children. *Journal of Autism and Child Schizophrenia, 4*, 217–222.

Bettelheim, B. (1967). *The empty fortress: Infantile autism and the birth of the self.* New York: The Free Press.

Cunningham, M. A., & Dixon, C. A. (1961). A study of the language of an autistic child. *Journal of Child Psychology and Psychiatry, 2*, 193–202.

DeMyer, M. K., Barton, S., DeMeyer, W. E., Norton, J. A., Allen, J., & Steel, R. (1973). Prognosis in autism: A follow-up study. *Journal of Autism and Childhood Schizophrenia, 3*, 199–246.

Despert, J. L. (1951). Some considerations relating to the genesis of autistic behavior in children. *American Journal of Orthopsychiatry, 21*, 335–350.

Eisenberg, L., & Kanner, L. (1956). Early infantile autism 1943–55. *American Journal of Orthopsychiatry, 26*, 556–566.

Hermelin, B., & O'Connor, N. (1970). *Psychological experiments with autistic children.* London: Pergamon Press.

Kanner, L. (1943). Autistic disturbances of affective contact. *Nervous Child, 2*, 217–250.

Kanner, L. (1946). Irrelevant and metaphorical language in early infantile autism. *American Journal of Psychiatry, 103*, 242–246.

Kanner, L. (1971). Follow-up study of eleven autistic children originally reported in 1943. *Journal of Autism and Childhood Schizophrenia, 1*, 119–145.

Lane, H. (1976). *The Wild Boy of Aveyron.* Cambridge, MA: Harvard University Press.

Lockyer, L., & Rutter, M. (1970). A five to fifteen year follow-up study of infantile psychosis. IV. Patterns of cognitive ability. *British Journal of Sociology and Clinical Psychology, 9*, 152–163.

Lovaas, I. (1977). *The autistic child: Language development through behavior modification.* New York: Irvington.

Rimland, B. (1964). *Infantile Autism.* New York: Appleton-Century-Crofts.

Rutter, M. (1983). Cognitive deficits in the pathogenesis of autism. *Journal of Child Psychology and Psychiatry, 24*, 513–531.

Rutter, M., & Schopler, E. (Eds.). (1978). *Autism: A reappraisal of concepts and treatment.* New York: Plenum Press.

Rutter, M., Greenfeld, D., & Lockyer, L. (1967). A five to fifteen year follow-up study of infantile psychosis. II. Social and Behavioural Outcome. *British Journal of Psychiatry, 113*, 1183–1199.

Schopler, E. (1971). Parents of psychotic children as scapegoats. *Journal of Contemporary Psychotherapy, 4*, 17–22.

Schopler, E. (1983). New developments in the definition and diagnosis of autism. In B. B. Lahey & A. E. Kazdin (Eds.), *Advances in Clinical Psychology, Vol. 6* (pp. 93–127). New York: Plenum Press.

Schopler, E., & Reichler, R. J. (1971). Parents as cotherapists in the treatment of psychotic children. *Journal of Autism and Childhood Schizophrenia, 1*, 87–102.

Tinbergen, N., & Tinbergen, E. A. (1983). *Autistic children: New hope for a cure.* Winchester, MA: Allen & Unwin.

Wing, L. (Ed.) (1976). *Early childhood autism: Clinical, educational and social aspects* (2nd ed.). Oxford: Pergamon Press.

Wolff, S., & Chess, S. (1965). An analysis of the language of fourteen schizophrenic children. *Journal of Child Psychology and Psychiatry, 6*, 29–41.

**II**

# Overview

# Models of Child Language Development

## LYNN S. SNYDER and D. ELISE LINDSTEDT

To those individuals interested in the nature of child language development, the major controversy of the twentieth century involved the class of two distinct schools of thought: behaviorism and nativism. The controversy came to the fore in 1957 with the publication of B. F. Skinner's *Verbal Behavior* and Noam Chomsky's *Syntactic Structures*. Emerging from different philosophical and scientific traditions, Skinner and Chomsky presented highly contrasting points of view. Skinner, on the one hand, came from the empiricist tradition. This tradition stressed the idea that theories could only be derived after documented observation of perceptible events. One did not begin an inquiry with a theory to test. Rather, one carefully observed repeated instances of events and from these data formulated a theory. Thus, knowledge was derived from the information that one could perceive and measure. Coming from this milieu, it is no surprise that Skinner (1957) viewed language as simple, one more form of human behavior, albeit verbal, that one could observe, count, and quantify.

On the other hand, Chomsky's views grew out of the rationalist tradition. This theoretical stance suggested that inquiries began first with a set of theoretical questions or rational analyses developed to test perceived information. Thus, knowledge was derived from a set of mental principles that one applied to information.

From the field of developmental psychology a middle ground arose that incorporated aspects of both theoretical biases. Constructivism was influenced by Piagetian notions of child development. Piagetian epistemology suggested that knowledge was derived and constructed from one's interactions with the environment and perceptible events. One applies a set of mental principles to the information one encounters in the world. The information may be known

LYNN S. SNYDER and D. ELISE LINDSTEDT • Department of Speech Pathology and Audiology, University of Denver, Denver, Colorado 80208.

through the mental structure or it may offer a new vantage point and change the mental structure itself. Thus, individuals construct new knowledge based upon the interaction between their mental structures and the world's information.

When professionals confront the question of how language should be taught to children, they must decide how language develops in children. This represents a theoretical and practical problem for the professional. Problems are often defined in terms of the problem space. Wickelgren (1979) suggested that the problem space can be viewed as containing three components: the givens, the operations, and the goal. In the case of the language development problem, the goal is fairly straightforward: the child's comprehension and/or use of a specified lanugage form(s). The givens or the knowledge that one uses to solve the problems lie in the professional's theory of how language develops. The operations or the procedures that one uses to solve the problem are those intervention strategies that implicitly "go with" or follow from one's theory of language development. Thus, the model of child language development is central to the professional's intervention.

Most models of child language development seem to reflect one of three major points of view: behaviorism, nativism, and constructivism. The chapter will review the basic stance taken by each school of thought, describe the givens—the most recent models of language development proposed by theorists working in each school—and discuss the operations—the language intervention strategies that follow from these models.

## BEHAVIORISM

Behaviorism, as a general movement introduced to psychology in the 1930s, insisted that psychologists study only that behavior that could be observed. Semi-mental states, introspection, and the unconscious were not observable, nor were they verifiable (Robinson, 1976). Behaviorists described observable events with respect to a stimulus and its response (Watson, 1930). The stimulus was anything in the environment or any physiological change occurring in the organism itself. The response was anything that the organism did (Watson, 1930).

Epitomizing this tradition, Skinner examined verbal behavior and its acquisition. He suggested that many behaviors, including verbal behaviors, operate on the environment; these are operant behaviors (1957). They are acquired and are maintained as part of the organism's repertoire due to the occurrence of environmental events that elicit and reinforce them. Thus, the environmental stimulus elicits the verbal behavior that is reinforced and strengthened by some environmental event. Language learning in children depends upon environmental events through the conditioning of their verbal operants with reinforcers.

The child's verbal responses can be elicited not only by the particular stimulus that originally elicited it, but also by stimuli with similar properties. This is called *stimulus generalization*. Skinner suggests that the child's early verbal responses are smaller units. As children get many vocabulary items under stimulus control, they will gradually be able to get phrases and sentence frames under control. The child is thought to proceed synthetically, putting together units into responses of increasingly larger size. Parental reinforcement is seen to play a critical role. Skinner suggested that when the child initially emits verbal responses, parents tend to reinforce or reward these responses, despite their crude form. However, when the child emits them more frequently, parents will tend to require a closer approximation to target before reinforcing the child. Thus, the child will be led to the target adult form through parental operant conditioning. This conditioning leads the child along a continuum of responses that are successive approximations to the norm. Sometimes, however, the child's verbal responses may be highly accurate imitations of the adult model and, therefore, will not need to be shaped into the adult target form.

In sum, the hallmarks of Skinner's (1957) behaviorist approach to child language development are that children's learning of language depends on the input available to them from the environment. The conditioning of their verbal operants with reinforcers or rewards is responsible for their learning the symbolic system. Thus, the child's role is somewhat passive in that learning is determined by the input and the reinforcement provided by the environment.

## Theoretical Model

The most comprehensive application of Skinner's notions of child language development is found in the work of Staats (Staats, 1971, 1974; Staats & Staats, 1964). Although his work hardly represents a "recent" formulation of the behaviorist view, it seems to be one of the few available. Neobehaviorist theories are notably absent from current developmental psycholinguistics. The behaviorist model was unable to predict the types of verbal responses produced by children, which in no way resembled verbal responses available to them in the environment. Further, it failed to explain how children discover the underlying implicit rule structure in their language (Slobin, 1978). This role structure is often opaque in the input available to the child. In addition, the model emphasizes the importance of parental reinforcement in the language learning process. Yet, parents rarely seem to attend to the grammatical form of their children's language (Slobin, 1975). Consequently, this model of child language acquisition was abandoned by most psycholinguists of the last decade. Despite its lack of popularity among researchers in child language development, this model has continued to be popular with some professionals providing language intervention to autistic children.

Staats' behavioral model proposes that language is a complex multiple repertoire system that the child learns. These repertoires function together to result in functional language. Among other things, they include a speech sound repertoire and an emotional response or meaning repertoire for words. Although the speech sound response repertoire is learned through an instrumental conditioning, the emotional response or meaning repertoire is learned through classical conditioning (Staats, 1971, 1974).

Initially, the child's internal state, for example, hunger, will elicit the production of social and speech-like sounds. These will be reinforced by their satisfaction, for example, being fed. From about five to seven months of age, the infant's sound repertoire or babbling contains syllable structures that are similar to the language of the adult community. Through the process of successive approximations, described earlier, the child's repertoire of speech sounds becomes differentiated to resemble sounds produced by adult users (Staats & Staats, 1964). In these initial stages, parental reinforcement seems to be the primary factor shaping the child's response repertoire. When the greater number of the child's speech responses are under stimulus control and the child's speech resembles the adult language community target more closely, he or she will begin to discriminate sounds more closely and match his or her productions to those heard. When a match occurs, the child will be reinforced (Staats & Staats, 1964). Through this process, the child will imitate a large repertoire of speech units in order to learn the phonology or sound system of the language (Staats, 1971, 1974). The process of speech sounds discrimination and matching will become reinforcing to the child.

The child not only learns the phonetic or sound shape of words, he or she also learns their meanings. Staats (Staats, 1971, 1974; Staats & Staats, 1964) suggests that this occurs through a classical conditioning process. Words occur repeatedly with other kinds of environmental stimuli that elicit responses until the words become conditioned to evoke those responses. Through the frequency of these pairings, an association is formed between the response typically elicited by the environmental object or event and the spoken word. For example, a spoon may usually elicit a sensorimotor action response, feeding schema, and a functional "eating tool" meaning response from a child. If it is frequently paired with the spoken word *spoon,* the word spoon can be conditioned to elicit those same sensorimotor and functional responses, even when the spoon is no longer present. This classical conditioning process gives the word its discriminative controlling value (Staats, 1971, 1974). It limits the field of responses, and thereby the meaning, that will come to be associated with or conditioned to the word. At the occurence of a particular word, a specific family of responses will be elicited.

A different process, stimulus generalization, was thought to be responsible for the child's production of novel sentences (Staats, 1971, 1974). Novel sentences are those not previously heard in the environment. Staats' model suggests that word classes can be elicited with similar stimuli. In this way novel utterances come about.

Staats' model, then, represents a traditional behaviorist point of view. Language learning is seen as the development of a response repertoire that depends upon conditioning. The environment elicits responses from the child and the satisfaction of that child's own internal physiological state and/or the environment reinforces those responses. Certainly, the environment shapes the form—sounds and structures—that the child learns as well as the meaning that is to become associated with it.

## Intervention

Behaviorist models of child language development have had a considerable impact on the nature of language intervention. Such models suggest that the input provided to the child is crucial. The language learning environment should provide stimuli that will elicit responses that can come under discriminative control and allow the learning of the specified domain of meaning associated with each word and, by their combination, phrases and sentences. Consequently, behavioral approaches to language intervention stress the presentation of those language stimuli that are at the child's ability level (Costello, 1982; Hart & Rogers-Warren, 1978; Spradlin & Siegel, 1982).

Although intervention has to provide for the development of discriminative control, it also has to provide for sufficient generalization of the stimulus. If a stimulus is not sufficiently generalized, the field of meaning associated with a word may be excessively narrow. The word "ball" could be associated with one particular ball in the child's home. Many behavioral researchers and clinicians feel that the verbal stimulus must not only be generalized across exemplars, but also be generalized across settings or the places in which those verbal stimuli can occur, across behaviors or social affects that can be associated with those verbal stimuli, and across time for maintenance of the behavior (Costello, 1982). Consequently, the behavioral model emphasizes that the professional provide the child with a sufficient number of exemplars (Carr, 1980; Costello, 1982; Siegel & Spradlin, 1978). These exemplars can be the objects or events themselves or even the locations or settings in which the verbal responses are emitted (Costello, 1982). Such models also stress generalization across settings by using more naturalistic stimuli in the intervention setting (Carr, 1980; Hart & Risley, 1980; Hart & Rogers-Warren, 1978). Stimulus generalization across behaviors is thought to be facilitated by selecting responses that will be functional for the child to allow the achievement of a social goal (Costello, 1982; Hart & Roger-Warren, 1978). Thus, the role of input in language intervention must receive close attention from the behaviorist.

The behaviorist model also stresses the role of imitation in language learning. The child must be able to attempt to produce the adult target. Consequently, behaviorist approaches to language intervention put a great deal of energy into teaching children to become efficient imitators (Hart, 1981; Harris, 1975).

Lastly, the behaviorist model of child language development stresses the crucial role played by reinforcement. Stimulus generalization across settings is thought to be facilitated when the reinforcers themselves are selected from the natural environment (Hart, 1981; Spradlin & Siegel, 1982). Further, the generalization of responses across time is considered to be highly dependent upon reinforcement. Some behavioral theorists address this maintenance issue by suggesting that the relationship between the verbal response and its precise reinforcer be made opaque to the child (Stokes & Baer, 1977). This is usually done through the use of intermittent reinforcement (Costello, 1982).

The operations implied by the behaviorist model of child language development are direct consequences of its emphasis on input, imitation, and reinforcement. The most crucial of these processes, input and reinforcement, are determined by the environment. In language intervention, behaviorist models imply that the professional must accept responsibility for the careful selection and control of both the input and the reinforcers. In the behaviorist tradition, what children learn, how much they learn, how quickly they learn, and how long they will know it depend upon those variables. Although those variables are external to the child, they determine the course of that child's linguistic development.

## NATIVISM

The Chomsky–Skinner debate ignited the twentieth-century controversy about the nature of child language development. The vast differences between the points of view of these theorists threw their basic tenets into dramatic contrast. As noted, Skinner's views reflected the empiricist tradition, Chomsky's the rationalist tradition. The rationalist philosophy was based upon the idea that all knowledge was derived from the mind's analysis of perceived information. In fact, the mind's rational processes organize and direct incoming sensory information from the world. These processes consist of a set of innate organizing principles. Because these principles are subserved by similar innate brain structures in humans, their application results in a common body of knowledge called universals.

Although Chomsky's objective with *Syntactic Structures* (1957), and later, *Aspects of a Theory of Syntax* (1965), was to introduce a grammar that would account for all the grammatical utterances produced by language, he ventured some ideas about the nature of language development. Chomsky (1965) suggested that the child is born with an innate set of language-specific organizing principles that predisposes the child to learn language. As the child receives linguistic information from the environment, some of these organizing principles are activated. Once activated, they analyze the information and construct a set of hypotheses or guesses about the underlying rules or structure of the language. As the children produce language, they test their guesses. By comparing productions against the increasing instances of language structures that are encountered, they confirm or alter their hypotheses.

Chomsky (1968) argues strongly for the innate source of the child's ability to learn language. He does this by appealing to the existence of linguistic universals. He believes that these common denominators, which can be found in all languages, demonstrate that they must be produced by linguistic organizing principles that exist across the species, regardless of language community. These universals include the observation that all languages seem to possess a deep and a surface level of structure. The *deep structure* level refers to the abstract underlying structure of a sentence. The *surface structure* level refers to the surface arrangements of words. When one surface arrangement is difficult to understand, or seems ambiguous, it may be the result of two underlying deep structures. For example, "we gave her dog biscuits to eat" is ambiguous because one does not know which deep structure underlies it. Further, every language forms sentences with certain sets of grammatical relations. Another universal is that speakers are able to make judgments about the grammaticality of an utterance. There are other universals, all of which, the nativist argues, are evidence for a language-specific set of innate organizing principles.

Unlike Skinner, Chomsky has continued to develop his thinking about child language development. In recent responses to cognitively-oriented constructivist concepts, Chomsky (1975, 1980) has emphasized different aspects of his position. He has suggested that language is a unique faculty of a person's mind. It is so dissimilar from other cognitive organizing principles that these other principles could never account for the complex rules specific to language. Yet, children can discover these rules because their innate language principles predispose them to do so. Children can do this despite the relatively incomplete information available to them: fragmented conversations, incomplete sentences, etc. To Chomsky, this argues even more strongly for the presence of an innate, genetically determined rule discovery mechanism specific to language.

Although few behaviorist models of child language development have emerged since 1971, the explanatory power of the nativist theory spawned by

Chomsky led to a number of nativist models of child language development. Because Chomsky (1957, 1965, 1980) places syntax at the center of linguistic activity and assigns it the dominant and autonomous role in language, most nativist models concern themselves with the child's development of syntactic structures. In particular, these models are designed to specify what the child's innate principles allow him or her to discover and how they do this. These current models will be described and the implications that they contain for language intervention will be discussed.

## Theoretical Models

The Little Linguist Model. One recent version of the nativist hypothesis follows Chomsky's thinking quite closely. Studying the development of syntactic structures in children, Valian (Valian, Winzimer, & Errich, 1981; Valian & Caplan, 1979) has proposed that children learn a grammar similar to that described by Chomsky. A child's innate "syntactic acquisition device" thus allows him or her to learn a transformational grammar that contains phrase structure rules and transformational rules. The organizing principles that comprise the child's syntactic acqusition device are linguistic universals. As the child needs them, they make formal elements and operations available to him or her that can be used to formulate hypotheses about the structure of language.

Valian proposes that the child's hypotheses consist of phrase structure and transformational rules. The child then tests these candidate rules against the linguistic input available and uses the regularities in the distribution of forms in the language input that is heard. This information, however, is used only to test his or her language hypotheses. The child is thought to examine the match between his or her hypothesis rule and the incoming linguistic information. Depending upon how closely the candidate rule and the incoming data match, the child will then keep, discard, or revise the rule. In a sense, then, the child is a little linguist who uses inductive reasoning to formulate the rules for grammar, testing them against the data provided by informants—the fluent native speakers of the language community. The linguistic training provides a set of strategies about how to induce linguistic rules from the regularities and other characteristics of language structure. The child's innate rule discovery system, the "syntactic acqusition device," gives him or her a set of strategies to induce grammatical rules from the linguistic information presented.

The Lexical Model. Roeper and his colleagues suggest that children may gain access to the linguistic code through a strategy not couched in the early construction of candidate rules (Roeper, Lapointe, Bing, & Tavakolian, 1981). Rather, they suggest that the lexical items themselves, the words, may provide the child with a key to figuring out the grammar of the language. Observing the children learn words before they learn the rules that manipulate them, Roeper *et al.* suggest that children learn something about grammatical rules in learning about words. Specifically, the lexical model postulates that as the child learns words, a set of subcategorization frames that are associated with the lexical items are also learned. These subcategorization frames tell the child (or any speaker of the language) what parts of the sentence the item can enter into, what parts it cannot, and the combinations that are and are not permissible. For example, the child learns when and where the word *push* can be used, as opposed to *pushable,* and with which words each can occur. Thus, the lexicon is the way in which the child learns about syntactic categories and frames. Once the child figures out these categories and relations, he or she becomes alert to those syntactic rules that change those relations in some way.

Roeper and his colleagues suggest that once the child formulates a hypothesis about the syntactic relations into which words enter, a hypothesis formation process is triggered in the child. He or she will quickly be led to the formulation of a series of successive hypotheses until a rule that handles the incoming linguistic information is formulated, a rule that works. It is almost as if Roeper *et al.* see the hypothesis-formation process as some type of self-actualizing mechanism within the organism: Once begun, it continues with increasing momentum until a coherent explanation has evolved.

The Learnability Model. Wexler and Culicover (1980) have focused their efforts on describing those principles of mind that seem to make learning language an attainable objective for the child. They suggest that these principles are used by the child to discover the grammar of the language and they, hence, make language "learnable."

Wexler and Culicover describe a lengthy set of specific linguistic constraints, the majority of which are syntactic principles, and subject them to a series of tests of linguistic logic. They concede that it is possible that these linguistic constraints may reflect more general constraints on learning. However, since such cognitive constraints have yet to be well described and supported by data, they propose to remain with their well-specified nativist set of linguistic principles.

## Summary

Recent nativist models, then, continue to argue that the child possesses an innate language-specific set of organizing principles that allows the child to discover how language works. The thrust of their efforts has been to describe the contents of these innate organizing principles and how the child learns the system. Valian *et al.* (1981) suggest that they are linguistic universals. Roeper *et al.* (1981) feel that sensitivity to the subcategorization rules affecting lexical items gives the child the first clues. Wexler and Culicover (1980) describe an extremely detailed set of syntactic principles that operate on incoming information.

## Implementation

Nativist models of child language propose that each child has an inherent set of language-specific rule discovery principles. Consequently, reinforcement is not a concern. Over the years, nativist studies of child language development have attended to parental reinforcement only in terms of the linguistic information that their *verbal* reinforcement provides the child. Their interest in this linguistic information lies in the opportunities that it provides the child to test his or her hypotheses about language.

Language intervention approaches influenced by nativist models, then, look at the way in which the professional provides feedback to the child. One technique incorporated by these approaches involves the process of *expansion*. Expansion is a phenomenon observed in the speech of mothers to their young children (Brown & Bellugi, 1964). It involves the mother taking the child's utterance, such as "kitty sleep," and adding some elements to it to make it a syntactically complete sentence, for example "the kitty is sleeping." This type of parental feedback would seem to provide the child with a well-defined syntactic instance against which he or she can match his or her own production and rule. This technique is used by such approaches as reactive language therapy (Weiss, Hansen, & Hubelein, 1979; Miller & Yoder, 1972, 1974).

Another technique that has emerged is that of modeling (Leonard, 1981). This technique has the child observe someone produce the linguistic form that is the intervention target. The child is told that the clinician will be speaking in a "special way." The child will then be given a turn to speak. Although this could be interpreted as a type of imitation, this technique actually forces the child to analyze the clinician's production and to discern the linguistic rule being presented. In a sense, this technique seems to prod the child into the hypothesis formation that nativists believe is the very process of language development. This technique has been successfully used by Leonard (1975) and Wilcox and Leonard (1978).

The focused stimulation (Leonard, 1981) offered by Lee, Koenigsknecht, and Mulhern's (1975) intensive language teaching approach is another recent technique. It seems to be nativist in that the child is presented with a number of well-formed instances of a rule embedded in a story or an activity narrative. Subsequently, the child is asked questions that are designed to elicit the target rule. Thus, the child is provided with information that can be used for rule formation and then he or she is given the opportunity to try out his or her guesses.

Another instance in which language intervention might be influenced by nativist models may lie in those approaches that strive to keep a highly naturalistic context and simply provide general unfocused stimulation, for example, those of Whitehurst, Novak, and Zorn (1972). If each child has an innate language-specific rule discovery mechanism that operates with input encountered, more information of the same type might be helpful. Such reasoning would lead one to adopt an approach of providing general language stimulation much like that observed in the parent–child interactions of normally developing children. This approach is one in which the professional interacts with the child in a naturalistic play setting that provides additional opportunities for linguistic interchange.

As our earlier discussion emphasized, recent nativist models have tried to describe how the child discovers the rules of the language system. Language intervention programs influenced by such models would present and sequence language content to reflect these concerns. For example, language intervention influenced by Valian's little linguist model (Valian *et al.*, 1981) would be first concerned that the child gain mastery of simple phrase structure and later acquire sentence transformations. The professional would try to provide contexts that would elicit the child's production of a targeted rule and then try to provide the child with a variety of instances of the rule in its adult form. The instances provided to the child could be used to make a decision about the hypothesis or guess that was made about the rule.

By contrast, language intervention influenced by the lexical model would focus on one lexical item or word and use it in many different sentences to illustrate or present the child with information about its subcategorization. The lexical item might also be contrasted with a family member of a somewhat different morphological form, for example, *wash* with *washable,* so that the different subcategorization rules affecting the two words might become more salient for the child.

If the professional, however, were influenced by the learnability model, the language intervention program would have to be structured and sequenced to reflect Wexler and Culicover's (1980) syntactic principles, one at a time. The sentences presented would have to be restricted to those syntactic forms to which each principle applied. In this case, the goal of intervention would be to get the child to try to guess the underlying principle and then try to apply it in appropriate instances.

## CONSTRUCTIVISM

The third major theoretical point to be discussed is constructivism. First applied by Jean Piaget (1962, 1963), it did not gain status as a formal psycholinguistic theoretical orientation until recently. Its status was achieved not by Piaget himself, but rather by developmental psycholinguists looking for an alternate explanation for their observations of child language.

Piaget (1963) has argued that children come to know the world through their interactions with it. They apply their mental or—at the earliest stages of development—their sensorimotor schema to the world and incorporate its information. Or, the world may provide information that leads children to change their schemas. The reciprocity of this interaction—the assimilation of information and the accomodation of schemas—is the way in which the child develops cognitively. Among the cognitive attainments of the child is the ability to represent entities, conditions, and events even when they are no longer perceptually present. Piaget (1962) has suggested that this representation is achieved with symbols. It may take place with the linguistic symbols of words or with the nonlinguistic symbols of pretend play. Both are simply reflections of the child's symbolic development and his or her common underlying cognitive attainment of symbolic representation.

Psycholinguists influenced by Piaget's thinking, then, feel that the child's language development is critically related to cognitive development—the way in which the child knows the world and interacts with it at any point in time. Constructivist models of language development differ in the way and the degree to which they see the relationship between language and cognitive development.

## Theoretical Models

The Strong Cognitive Model. Several theorists have argued for a strong cognitive mode. Such a model is based upon the idea that the development of specific cognitive structures is sufficient to account for the child's ability to learn language (Miller, Chapman, & Bedrosian, 1977). This model often implies that the acquistion of a nonverbal cognitive skill will precede the acquisition of the corresponding linguistic structure or form, (MacNamara 1972). Indeed, there is some consensus that specific cognitive attainments are critical to the development of language. Delineated by Bowerman (1974), these include the ability to engage in symbolic representation, to order, to classify, to embed and conserve, to understand basic invariance and object-action relations, and to be able to represent perceptual space. It is not clear, however, whether these attainments themselves are sufficient to explain language development.

Another form of this model is the operative model of Karmiloff-Smith (1979). Karmiloff-Smith's research on determiners suggests that language, as something to be learned by the child, can be seen as a problem space. She suggests that the child makes use of strategies, procedures, or operations as one does in all types of problem-solving. She feels that the child's general cognitive development only partially explains language development. Rather, language-specific operations—phonological, syntactic, semantic, and pragmatic—facilitate the child's language development. Which particular procedure is acquired by a child at any one time is determined by the nature of the input. If the input tends to provide better phonological cues to a form, and the syntactic cues are more subtle, then the phonological procedure tends to be learned first. For example, in Italian it is easier to acquire the gender distinction by attending to differences in the phonology than it is in German, in which the same part of the word provides a different type of information.

Karmiloff-Smith suggests that once the child acquires the strategy or procedure and gets it under automatic control, he or she can analyze the procedure itself. The organism's drive toward an organized equilibrium and cognitive economy leads the child to reorganize his or her strategies until they can work in a coherent and balanced way. As the child's interactions with the world act to construct changes in his or her view of the world, these changes will also be reflected in language development, so that the organism's system will continue to seek an organized equilibrium. This reasoning, then, seems to represent a strong form of the cognitive model (Chapman, 1982). Further, Karmiloff-Smith (1979) proposes that the language-specific procedures acquired by the child are ultimately based on the child's cognitive development and ability to organize and make sense of all types of incoming information. This also argues for a strong cognitive model, despite her concern about the child's development of language-specific procedures.

The Weak Cognitive Model. The weak form of the cognitive model (Cromer, 1974, 1976) suggests that cognitive development is necessary and important for language to develop. However, it is not sufficient in itself to account for the development of language. The weak cognitive model can be discerned in Cromer's analysis, in which cognitive development provides the child with the meaning or concepts that language maps. Other, highly specific skills are needed, however, for the child to be able to learn the language system, and cognitive development does not seem to provide any significant input into these. Thus, cognitive development allows the child to develop the concepts that words will encode or represent, but nothing more.

The Correlational Model. The last constructivist model is one that seems to be gaining increased favor with researchers and theorists. Its popularity lies in the fact that it seems to have good explanatory power, that is, it seems to offer a coherent explanation of the events that occur in child language development. It takes a slightly different form with each theorist; the underlying theme, however, is the same for each. Essentially, this point of view suggests that cognitive and linguistic development are strongly related because they are subserved by common underlying structures or mechanisms. When a developmental change occurs in one of the underlying structures, it may be reflected in either the linguistic *or* the nonlinguistic cognitive domains or in both. However, there often may be a time lag between expression in one content domain and expression in the other. There are now three current interpretations of this viewpoint: those of Bates (Bates, Benigni, Bretherton, Camaioni, & Voltera, 1977, 1979; Bates & Snyder, 1982), Johnston (1982), and Schlesinger (1982).

Bates and her colleagues have put forward a *local homology* model. They argue that cognition and language development are linked by a common set of underlying cognitive structures or mechanisms. The development of a specific skill in one domain may be observed before development in the other domain. However, this is similar to the Piagetian notion of horizontal decalage: a time gap between the expression of a skill in one content area and expression in another. The two developments or attainments are not related because they are analogous or similar in structure; rather, they may share the input of the same underlying structure. For example, if the attainment of specific cognitive skill required the child to develop "software" programs A and C, and the attainment of a specific language skill required that the child develop programs B and C, the cognitive skill and the language skill may look correlated developmentally. If programs A and B have already developed, the emergence of program C in the child's software library will allow the child to attain both the cognitive and the linguistic milestones.

Specific milestones of cognitive and language development typically require the input of more than one underlying program. Thus, the relationship between cognitive and linguistic development is multidimensional. Further, the relationship between specific skills is not constant. As the child's way of viewing the world and language change developmentally, the types of software subserving his or her further development change. More of a particular underlying operation will not result in increased development. Rather, one more or many more different programs will be needed to facilitate further linguistic and cognitive development.

Although Bates' viewpoint stresses the role that operations or strategies play in the relationship between language and cognitive development, Johnston (1982) stresses the way in which conceptual and organizational knowledge affect the acquisition of language. Looking at a series of diverse achievements in child language, Johnston demonstrates a number of ways in which conceptual development constrains the development of some linguistic forms. This relationship extends beyond the mere notion of acquiring the concept to be mapped by the word. Other linguistic forms, such as the auxiliary system, do not seem to be related to cognitive development. Thus, the relationship between linguistic and cognitive achievements appears to be correlated for Johnston in some but not all areas.

Schlesinger (1982) proposes that underlying or deep structures of the child's language reflect the relationship between the child's cognitive development or his or her way of knowing the world and the way that language maps those relationships. The child's understanding is not simply a conceptual one; it is also relational, that is, there are relationships between concepts. The latter aspect is most often represented by word order and inflections. Schlesinger proposes that the child learns language by hearing utterances used in meaningful contexts. The child processes the context or situation in terms of an *I-marker* (input marker) or I-markers, concepts and the relations between them, and associates those elements with structures and forms in the utterance he or she hears. In this respect, his viewpoint is similar to that expressed by Slobin (1978).

Schlesinger also suggests that concepts may develop in the process of linguistic development. He further suggests that language concepts involve linguistic categorization. As the child learns a word, then, he or she also forms the linguistic categories underlying it. In a sense, language makes a contribution to the categorization processes for the child. It seems to add another set of cues that can be used to organize the world.

### Summary

Constructivist theories of child language development propose that the child is an active participant in the language learning process. The child's active interface with the world and the knowledge that results from that interaction provides a source for his or her hypotheses or guesses about language. Those proponents of the strong cognitive models see that this knowledge, the child's cognitive development, as a necessary and sufficient prerequisite to language development. Those who adhere to the weak cognitive model believe that it is necessary, but only for the acquisition of meaning. By contrast, the correlational model suggests that there is a series of highly specific links between cognitive and linguistic development that are more akin to shared underlying operations.

## Implementation

The constructivist view on language intervention has significantly changed the manner and the setting for intervention. Regardless of the particular model involved, they all share a common thread: the role of cognition in language development. The consequence of this point of view is that language should always be presented to the child in a meaningful situation. These models also perceive the child developing cognitively and, to some degree, linguistically from his or her interaction with the world. Consequently, constructively influenced language intervention programs tend to involve the child in activities in which he or she is engaged in manipulating the environment. Another consequence is that the setting for language intervention has changed from the therapy room to that place in the environment in which the child happens to be learning. Thus, professionals involved in the child's language development have gone into the classroom, as seen in reactive language therapy (Weiss *et al.*, 1979). Others also are encouraged to go out into the playground, the cafeteria, or wherever the child is involved, as in the transactional language approach (McLean & Snyder-McLean, 1978). Even highly behaviorist models have begun to acknowledge the effectiveness of this thinking, for example, milieu therapy of Hart and Rogers-Warren (1978).

The content and strategies of language intervention have also been heavily influenced by constructivist models. Those that are guided by the strong cognitive models will devote a great deal of effort to facilitating the child's cognitive development. The professional may focus on providing materials, activities, and discussions that are designed to facilitate specific cognitive developments, for example, classification, and not attend to the form and level of the linguistic stimuli being presented. The expectation is that the facilitation of cognitive development will have a positive effect on the child's language development. Usually, the activities presented to the child are Piagetian in nature. Or, if one adopted Karmiloff-Smith's (1979) point of view, one would work first on prerequisite general cognitive developments and then attempt to teach the linguistic procedures that are founded on these general principles.

If, however, professionals are guided by the weak cognitive model, they would first teach the conceptual bases for linguistic meaning that the child is to encounter. Subsequently, they would have to teach each of the specific linguistic rules and forms, apart from and in addition to the cognitive-oriented activities. This is the implication of this model that suggests that language requires processes and input that are beyond the scope of cognition.

Last, language intervention that is influenced by correlational models will take on a somewhat different appearance. Such intervention approaches will take care to work on *specific* cognitive attainments, for example, tool use or embedding, and carefully pair them with the linguistic forms that map these ideas. If the homology model is used, the intervention program may work on the achievement of more than one attainment within a given time period. This is related to the Batesian notion that specific linguistic and cognitive developments may be subserved by more than one underlying program. The influence of this thinking can be seen in the transactional approach to language training (McLean & Snyder-McLean, 1978) and reactive language therapy (Weiss *et al.*, 1979), among others. The transactional approach reflects even more closely the types of cues provided by Schlesigner's (1982) I-markers. The transactional approach makes heavy use of carefully defined conceptual referencing strategies and the semantic relations expressed by the grammar of the language.

Thus, constructivist theories of language can also influence language intervention in systematic ways. They offer an impressive alternative to the nativist and behaviorist models.

## THE PROBLEM SPACE REVISITED

At the outset of this chapter, we likened the task of developing language in the autistic child to a problem that must be solved. It can be solved in a number of ways. In order to solve problems, one must identify the "given" information in order to know what type of operation to apply. This chapter focused on one type of given or available information: models of child language development. In order to facilitate language development, one must have some idea of how it is that language develops. Our discussion has highlighted some prominent options and their implications for language development.

Unfortunately, there is another piece of "given" information that one must use in conjunction with those described in this chapter. This piece of information is what we know about the nature of autism and why and how it interferes with or delays a child's language development. As professionals we need to deal not only with this new piece of information, but also with how it interfaces or interacts with what we know of child language development. Thus, the problem space is far larger than we had imagined. There seem to be many more places where we can make erroneous decisions. This problem space, however, presents us with many more opportunities to make correct choices. And, there may be more than one operation or set of operations that will allow us to solve the problem.

## REFERENCES

Bates, E., & Snyder, L. (1982). The cognitive hypothesis in language development. In I. Uzgiris & J. M. Hunt (Eds.), *Research with the scales of psychological development in infancy.* Champaign–Urbana: University of Illinois Press.

Bates, E., Benigni, L., Bretherton, I., Camaioni, L., & Volterra, V. (1977). From the gesture to the first word: On cognition and social prerequisites. In M. Lewis & L. Rosenblum (Eds.), *Interaction, conversation and the development of language* (pp. 247–308). New York: Wiley.

Bates, E., Benigni, L., Bretherton, I., Camaioni, L., & Volterra, V. (1979). *The emergence of symbols: Cognition and communication in infancy.* New York: Academic Press.

Bowerman, M., (1974). Discussion summary—development of concepts underlying language. In R. Schiefelbusch & L. Lloyd (Eds.), *Language perspectives: Acquisition, retardation and intervention* (pp. 191–210). Baltimore; MD: University Park Press.

Brown, R., & Bellugi, V. (1964). Three processes in the child's acquisition of syntax. *Harvard*

*Educational Review, 34,* 133-151. (Reprinted in E. H. Lenneberg (Ed.), *New directions in the study of language,* 1964, Cambridge, MA: M.I.T. Press, pp. 131-162 (Reprinted in R. Brown, *Psycholinguistics,* 1970, New York: The Free Press)

Carr, M., (1980). Conversational therapy for adolescents with marginal to severe language disorders. In M. Burns & J. Andrews (Eds.), *Current trends in the treatment of language disorders.* Evanston, IL: Institute for Continuing Professional Education.

Chapman, R., (1982). Issues in child language acquisition. In N. Lass, J. Northern, D. Yoder, & L. McReynolds (Eds.), *Speech, language and hearing* (pp. 377-472). Philadelphia: W. B. Saunders.

Chomsky, N. (1957). *Syntactic structures.* The Hague, The Netherlands: Moulton Press.

Chomsky, N. (1965). *Aspects of a theory of syntax.* Cambridge, MA: M.I.T. Press.

Chomsky, N. (1968). *Language and mind.* New York: Harcourt Brace Jovanovich.

Chomsky, N. (1975). *Reflections on language.* New York: Pantheon Books.

Chomsky, N. (1980). On cognitive structures and their development: A reply to Piaget. In M. Piatelli-Palmerin (Ed.), *Language and learning: The debate between Jean Piaget and Noam Chomsky* (pp. 35-56). Cambridge, MA: Harvard University Press.

Costello, J. M. (1982). Generalization across settings: Language intervention with children. In J. Miller, D. E. Yoder, & R. Schiefelbusch (Eds.), *Contemporary issues in language intervention* (pp. 275-297). Rockville, IL: The American Speech-Language-Hearing Association.

Cromer, R. (1974). The development of language and cognition: The cognition hypothesis. In D. Foss (Ed.), *New perspectives in child development* (pp. 184-252). Baltimore, MD: Penguin.

Cromer, R. (1976). The cognitive hypothesis of language acquisition for child language deficiency. In D. Morehead & A. Morehead (Eds.), *Normal and deficient child language* (pp. 283-334). Baltimore, MD: University Park Press.

Harris, S. L. (1975). Teaching language to nonverbal children—with emphasis on problems of generalization. *Psychological Bulletin, 82,* 562-580.

Hart, B. (1981). Pragmatics: How language is used. *Analysis and Intervention of Developmental Disorders, 1,* 299-313.

Hart, B., & Risley, T. (1980). *In vivo* language intervention: Unanticipated general effects. *Journal of Applied Behavioral Analysis, 13,* 407-432.

Hart, B., & Rogers-Warren, A. (1978). A milieu approach to language teaching. In R. Schiefelbusch (Ed.), *Language intervention strategies* (pp. 193-238). Baltimore, MD: University Park Press.

Johnston, J. (1982). Cognitive prerequisites: Some evidence from children learning English. In D. Slobin (Ed.), *Proceedings of the Conference on Cross-Linguistic Studies in Language Acquisition.* Berkeley: University of California at Berkeley Press.

Karmiloff-Smith, A. (1979). *A functional approach to child language: A study of determiners and reference.* London: Cambridge University Press.

Lee, L., Koenigsknecht, R., & Mulhern, S. (1975). *Interactive language development teaching.* Evanston, IL: Northwestern University Press.

Leonard, L. (1975). Modeling as a clinical procedure in language. *Speech and Hearing Services in the Schools, 6,* 72-85.

Leonard, L. (1981). Facilitating linguistic skills in children with specific language impairment. *Applied Psycholinguistics, 2,* 89-118.

MacNamara, J. (1972). The cognitive basis of language learning in infants. *Psychological Review, 79,* 1-13.

McLean, J., & Snyder-McLean, L. (1978). *A transactional approach to language training.* Columbus, OH: Charles D. Merrill.

Miller, J., & Yoder, D. (1972). A syntax teaching program. In J. McLean, D. Yoder, & R. L. Schiefelbusch (Eds.), *Language intervention with the retarded.* Baltimore, MD: University Park Press.

Miller, J., & Yoder, D. (1974). An ontogenetic language teaching strategy for retarded children. In R. L. Schiefelbusch & L. Lloyd (Eds.), *Language perspectives: Acquisition retardation and intervention* (pp. 505–528). Baltimore, MD: University Park Press.

Miller, J., Chapman, R., & Bedrosian, J. (1977). *Defining developmentally disabled subjects for research: The relationship between etiology, cognitive development, language and communicative performance.* Paper presented at the Second Annual Boston University Conference on Language Development, Boston, MA.

Piaget, J. (1962). *Play, dreams and imitation in childhood.* New York: Norton.

Piaget, J. (1963). *The origins of intelligence in children.* New York: Norton.

Robinson, D. N. (1976). *An intellectual history of psychology.* New York: Macmillan.

Roeper, T., LaPointe, S., Bing, J., & Tavakolian, S. L. (1981). A lexical approach to language acquisition. In S. Tavakolian (Ed.), *Language acquisition and linguistic theory* (pp. 35–58). Cambridge, MA: M.I.T. Press.

Schlesinger, I. M. (1982). *Steps to language: Toward a theory of native language acquisition.* Hillsdale, NJ: Lawrence Erlbaum Associates.

Siegel, G. M., & Spradlin, J. E. (1978). Programming for language and communication therapy. In R. L. Schiefelbusch (Ed.), *Language intervention strategies* (pp. 352–398). Baltimore, MD: University Park Press.

Skinner, B. F. (1957). *Verbal behavior.* New York: Appleton-Century-Crofts.

Slobin, D. (1975). On the nature of talk to children. In E. H. Lenneberg & E. Lenneberg (Eds.), *Foundations of language development: A multi-disciplinary approach* (Vol. 1) (pp. 283–298). New York: Academic Press.

Slobin, D. (1978). *Psycholinguistics* (2nd ed.). Glenview, IL: Scott, Foresman.

Spradlin, J. E., & Siegel, G. M. (1982). Language training in natural and clinical environments. *Journal of Speech and Hearing Disorders, 47,* 2–6.

Staats, A. (1971). Linguistic–mentalistic theory versus an explanatory S–R learning theory of language development. In D. Slobin (Ed.), *The ontogenesis of grammar* (pp. 103–150). New York: Academic Press.

Staats, A. (1974). Behaviorism and cognitive theory in the study of language: A neopsycholinguistics. In R. Schiefelbusch & L. Lloyd (Eds.), *Perspectives in language—acquisition, intervention, retardation* (pp. 615–646). Baltimore, MD: University Park Press.

Staats, A. W., & Staats, C. K. (1964). *Complex human behavior.* New York: Holt, Rinehart & Winston.

Stokes, T. F., & Baer, D. M. (1977). An implicit technology of generalization. *Journal of Applied Behavioral Analysis, 10,* 349–367.

Valian, V., & Caplan, J. (1979). What children say when asked "What?": A study of the use of syntactic knowledge. *Journal of Experimental Child Psychology, 28,* 424–444.

Valian, V., Winzimer, J., & Errich, A. (1981). A "little linguist" model of syntax learning. In S. L. Tavakolian (Ed.), *Language acquisition and linguistic theory* (pp. 188–209). Cambridge, MA: M.I.T. Press.

Watson, J. B. (1930). *Behaviorism.* New York: Norton.

Weiss, R., Hansen, K., & Hubelein, T. (1979). *Pragmatic psycholinguistic therapy for language disorders in early childhood.* Short course presented at the meeting of the American Speech and Hearing Association, Atlanta, GA.

Wexler, K., & Culicover, P. (1980). *Formal Principles of language acquisition.* Cambridge, MA: M.I.T. Press.

Whitehurst, G., Novak, G., & Zorn, G. (1972). Delayed speech studied in the home. *Developmental Psychology, 7,* 169–177.

Wickelgren, W. W. (1979). *Cognitive Psychology.* Englewood Cliffs: Prentice-Hall.

Wilcox, M. & Leonard, L. (1978). Experimental acquisition of *wh*-questions in language disordered children. *Journal of Speech and Hearing Research, 21,* 220–239.

# Behavioral Approaches to Language and Communication

## EDWARD G. CARR

In the 1950s, there was a spirited and sometimes acrimonious debate between psycholinguists and behaviorists concerning the proper way of conceptualizing language (Chomsky, 1959; Skinner, 1957). It appears, in retrospect, that much of the controversy stemmed from the fact that proponents of the two viewpoints had legitimate but orthogonal goals. Thus, psycholinguists were most interested in being able to construct a grammar, that is, a system of rules capable of accounting for all possible language outputs, outputs that were of interest only as a reflection of underlying linguistic competence. Since competence is determined by the interaction of a number of cognitive processes, an individual's performance, that is, his or her verbal behavior, is peripheral to this approach. Behaviorists, in contrast, had little interest in understanding the formal properties of language or its underlying cognitive determinants, but they had a great deal of interest in understanding how language could be used by one individual to influence the behavior of another. Thus, for the behaviorist, systematic manipulation of verbal behavior became of paramount importance and educational intervention quickly assumed a central place in the research literature of the field. Today, much of the *Stürm und Dräng* that characterized the early period of behaviorism has increasingly given way to a sense of curiosity about nonbehavioral approaches to understanding language. There are two reasons for the calm that now follows the storm. First, it has become obvious to many behaviorally oriented researchers that language intervention efforts are constantly stymied by unanswered questions pertaining to subject

EDWARD G. CARR • Department of Psychology and Suffolk Child Development Center, State University of New York at Stony Brook, Stony Brook, New York 11794-2500.

differences, choice of curriculum items, problems in generalization, and the lack of communicative use of language by children involved in training. These difficulties have spurred behavior therapists into examining data and concepts derived from nonbehavioral viewpoints. A second important development has been the emergence of pragmatics within the field of psycholinguistics. Pragmatics focuses on the communicative functions that language may have. It is the study of language as it exists within the social context. This focus of interest interdigitates well with the traditional functionalist emphasis of behaviorism, an emphasis very much concerned with the effects of language as a social tool (Skinner, 1957). The result has been that there is now a convergence of interests in the field of language intervention with the developmentally disabled. In what follows, I would like to document this convergence, as well as address some of the problems that behaviorists will need to deal with in order to better help those children who have severe language handicaps. First, however, it is necessary to outline the studies from which current behavioral approaches and issues have evolved.

## THE TRADITIONAL BEHAVIORAL EMPHASIS ON FORM

The majority of studies carried out in the 1960s and 1970s were concerned with teaching specific linguistic forms to developmentally disabled children (Lovaas & Newsom, 1976; Sloane & MacAuley, 1968) or eliminating forms that were viewed as undesirable (Carr, Schreibman, & Lovaas, 1975; Lovaas, 1977; Schreibman & Carr, 1978). It can be argued that these approaches represented a breakthrough in the field of special education, especially when viewed against the prevailing pessimism that characterized the attitude of professionals toward instruction of the handicapped in the 1950s and early 1960s. However, critics of these approaches, both inside and outside behavioral circles, soon began to describe a number of problems that persisted in spite of intervention efforts. As noted above, these problems centered on four areas:

1. There were dramatic subject differences following treatment; that is, some children made considerable progress whereas, for others, progress was minimal.
2. The behavioral approach typically failed to provide educators with detailed guidelines for choosing curricular items.
3. Treatment gains often failed to generalize beyond the original training situation.
4. Teaching the child particular language forms was no guarantee that the child would use these forms in order to communicate with others in the day-to-day social context of home and school.

It is important to realize that, by and large, these problems are not unique to behavioral intervention, since no current approach can claim to have resolved these issues. The state of knowledge in the field calls for much humility and open-mindedness with respect to the philosophy of intervention and the conceptualization of the language learning process. This statement applies to non-behaviorists and behaviorists alike. The strength and promise of behaviorism lies in its commitment to empiricism and not on its reliance on any specific set of treatment procedures. This generic notion of behaviorism paves the way for a consideration of concepts and data derived from a variety of sources and informs much of the discussion that follows.

## INDIVIDUAL DIFFERENCES AMONG CHILDREN

Outcome data suggest that the highest levels of language performance are attained by children who already have good language skills at the start of treatment and/or were very young when treatment began (Howlin, 1981; Lovaas, Koegel, Simmons, & Long, 1973; Lovaas, 1982). The fact that subject variables appear to make a difference in spite of behavioral intervention suggests that it is incumbent upon investigators conducting outcome studies to report data on these variables so that clinicians and educators will be able to assess the extent to which gains are a function of treatment intervention rather than judicious subject selection.

From a behavioral perspective, the specification of such subject variables as initial language ability or age at onset of treatment is only a beginning. What is ultimately needed is an approach that attempts to identify variables that are not only related to performance differences, but that can also be potentially *manipulated* in order to eliminate or minimize these differences. To date, there has been relatively little research emphasis on the resolution of subject differences using this strategy. Therefore, in what follows, I can offer only a modest example of how one might proceed.

One difference that is often observed between children is in the very basic area of receptive language acquisiton. Even on an elementary task, such as receptive speech labeling, some children do well, while others make no progress. In this case, the basic question is whether we can identify a variable that discriminates among those children who succeed on the receptive task and those who fail. Then, we must manipulate the identified variable in order to improve the performance of those who fail. Our own research suggests that verbal imitative ability predicts differential outcome with respect to receptive labeling. Specifically, it appears that children who are poor at imitating simple sounds fail to acquire receptive speech labels in spite of hundreds of training trials. In contrast, children who are good verbal imitators quickly acquire receptive speech labels (Carr, 1982a,b; Carr, Pridal, & Dores, 1984). This finding has recently been replicated (Remington & Clark, 1983). Perhaps, then, verbal imitative skill is an important prerequisite for receptive speech as was implied in earlier research (Lovaas, 1966). Since this skill is manipulable, it might be possible to facilitate the acquisition of receptive speech by means of verbal imitation training. Interestingly, preliminary data suggest that children who exhibit poor verbal imitative skill may acquire receptive speech labels following a program that includes training in verbal imitation (Schaeffer, Kollinzas, Musil, & McDowell, 1977). These data are promising and bear out the potential utility of the strategy proposed above for dealing with individual differences. However, one must say that, in the field as a whole, the approach we have been describing is currently the exception rather than the rule.

## CHOOSING CURRICULAR ITEMS

### Functionality

Within behavioral circles, the major criterion for selection of curricular items has been that of functionality (Brown, Nietupski, & Hamre-Nietupski, 1976; Goetz, Schuler, & Sailor, 1981; Guess, Sailor, & Baer, 1978). That is, with respect to the question "How shall we choose which items to include in language training?" the behaviorist answer has been "choose those items that produce an immediate reinforcing consequence for the child such that the consequence that occurs is meaningfully related to the child's verbal behavior and is readily available to the child in his or her everyday environment." Thus, one might train the child to answer "I want juice" in response to the question "What do you want?" This interaction meets the functionality criterion just defined because (a) the child's response is likely to produce a glass of juice either immediately or after a short delay; (b) juice is a reinforcer for most children; (c) the consequence, namely, receiving juice, is directly related to the request for juice, a point that is not trivial and will be explained further below; and (d) juice is a reinforcing event that is commonly available in the child's day-to-day environment.

One could, however, train a child to answer "Monday" in response to the question "What day is it today?" Further, one might reinforce correct responding in this instance by allowing the child 5 seconds of access to a toy kaleidoscope. This sequence does not meet the functionality criterion because (a) there is only a very small probability that most adults will give a child toy kaleidoscopes for correctly identifying the day of the week; (b) the consequence, namely receiving the kaleidoscope, is not related in any meaningful way to saying "Monday," and this stands in sharp contrast to the meaningful relationship that exists between saying "I want juice" and receiving juice; and

(c) toy kaleidoscopes are typically not as available as juice is in the child's day-to-day living situation. It is true that the kaleidoscope may function as a reinforcer, a property that it shares in common with juice, but, with respect to the issue of functionality, all similarity ends there, as is evident from the three nonfunctional aspects of the interaction just listed.

Apart from the functionality criterion, behaviorists have developed relatively few guidelines as to how to select curriculum items. In light of this, I think there is perhaps some truth to the statement that behaviorism is a method in search of content, whereas psycholinguistics is content in search of a method. That is, over the years, behaviorists have evolved a number of highly effective teaching procedures (i.e., methods), but they have been rather reticent about suggesting systematic decision criteria concerning what tasks these procedures should be applied to (i.e., content). In contrast, psycholinguists have developed a detailed data base describing the developmental language characteristics of children (i.e., potential curriculum content). However, they have not provided very much in terms of elucidating specific teaching procedures for facilitating the acquisition of developmentally desirable language skills. At present, the two fields seem to have converged to the point at which it might be possible to combine behavioral methods with psycholinguistically derived curricular suggestions in order to benefit autistic children and others with severe developmental handicaps. In what follows, I would like to illustrate the potential benefits of this convergence by means of an example drawn from the recent research literature.

## Concept Acquisition

To begin, we may note that one important, yet difficult to achieve language goal for autistic children concerns concept formation (Hermelin & O'Connor, 1970). That is, a child must not only acquire labels for discrete parts of his or her environment, but must also be able to group aspects of the environment into broader classes in which all the members of a given class share some attributes. As an example of the problem that needs to be confronted, let us consider an everyday concept that normal children readily acquire quite early in life, namely an animal concept such as "bird." In a typical park, a child might encounter robins, sparrows, crows, pigeons, swans, ducks, and geese, as well as a variety of other birds. The question arises as to how best to teach an autistic child that all these different animals are members of the concept class "bird."

A common behavioral procedure that could be used is the method of training multiple exemplars (Stokes & Baer, 1977). Using this method, an adult would teach the child to label several different types of animals as "bird." For example, one might teach the child to label a swan, a crow, and a pigeon as "bird." Sometimes, following this mode of training, a child is more likely to label other types of animals, such as ducks and sparrows, as birds, too. At this point, the child is described as having mastered the concept. Although the method described is undoubtedly useful, no guidelines are provided concerning how one should choose particular training items. Should one train robin and pigeon as the exemplars, or turkey and chicken, or does item choice not matter?

Basic research in psycholinguistics provides some guidelines. Specifically, investigators in this area have discovered that some examples of a given concept class are better representatives of that class than are others. The good examples are referred to as prototypes and the other examples are referred to as nonprototypes. Thus, robins, sparrows, and finches are considered better examples of birds than are swans, chickens, and hawks.

This best-example theory of categorization (Rosch, 1973, 1975; Rosch & Mervis, 1975) has some important clinical implications. Specifically, it suggests that if one wishes to facilitate concept formation, it would be wise to select prototypes as training items rather than nonprototypes. Interestingly, recent research carried out with developmentally handicapped children demonstrates the superiority of prototype training over nonprototype training in concept acquisition (Hupp & Mervis, 1981, 1982). Let us consider what this means from the standpoint of training the concept "bird." The best procedure would be to select such prototypes as robin, sparrow, and finch as the training items. This should produce a good generalization of the concept label to other types of birds, such as ducks, geese, and crows. A less desirable procedure would be to select such nonprototypes as swans, chickens, and hawks as the training items. This should produce poorer generalization of the concept label to other types of birds, such as ducks, geese, and crows.

In essence, what we have been describing is the combination of a behavioral method (i.e., multiple exemplar training) with a psycholinguistically derived curriculum (i.e., selection of training items on the basis of whether or not they are prototypes). The combination helps us to attain a major language instruction goal, namely concept formation. This model has great potential as an aid to fostering language development. Just as importantly, it raises the general possibility that when behaviorism and psycholinguistics are combined, they may be able to address problems together that they are unable to address alone.

## THE ISSUE OF STIMULUS GENERALIZATION

Stimulus generalization involves the transfer of language skills from the original training situation to a variety of other situations that have not been involved in training. This phenomenon may be observed across adults, across settings, and across instructional tasks.

A number of review papers have documented some of the difficulties involved in producing generalized treatment gains (Garcia & DeHaven, 1974; Harris, 1975). The fact that such difficulties exist and are honestly acknowledged has created a misconception in the field, namely that failures in generalization are a unique characteristic of the behavioral approach. In fact, no approach has yet presented a coherent body of evidence demonstrating that its own particular assumptions and methods routinely lead to a complete resolution of the issue. It is worth emphasizing that the issue of generalization comes up only when treatment effects can be demonstrated; in the absence of treatment effects, there is nothing to be generalized. Given the ineffectiveness of many teaching procedures in traditional special education, it is perhaps not suprising that the problem of generalization did not become salient until the last decade. It was only then that data that systematically documented treatment effects were obtained.

## Tactics for Promoting Generalization

An important contribution of behavior modification has been the identification of tactics for promoting generalization. These tactics have been summarized in several sources (e.g., Baer, 1981; Carr, 1980; Stokes & Baer, 1977). A recurring theme has been the notion that many generalization problems stem from the practice of using restricted training environments (Baer, 1981). That is, training is undertaken by one adult, in one setting, using a limited set of instructional tasks. In what follows, I will describe one way that behavioral clinicians have attempted to overcome some of these difficulties.

In the section dealing with choice of curricular items, I briefly alluded to the method of multiple exemplar training as a means for helping to produce generalization across instructional tasks involving language concepts. In fact, multiple exemplar training is the most commonly employed procedure for enhancing generalization effects. There are data demonstrating its successful use in producing generalization across language instruction tasks (Carr, 1982c; Frisch & Schumaker, 1974; Lutzker & Sherman, 1974; Schumaker & Sherman, 1970; Stevens-Long & Rasmussen, 1974), across adults (Carr & Kologinsky, 1983; Garcia, 1974; Stokes, Baer, & Jackson, 1974), and across settings (Carr & Kologinsky, 1983; Griffiths & Craighead, 1972; Handleman, 1979). The basic strategy is the same irrespective of the type of generalization desired. Consider, for example, a situation in which one desires to produce generalization across adults. Rather than having a single adult provide all the training, one arranges for several adults to provide training. When this strategy is employed, one typically finds that new adults who have not been involved in training are able to evoke the desired response from the child.

## Implications for Educational Programs

The data on generalization cited above have broad implications for the design or redesign of educational programs as a whole. To begin, we may note that the current educational model used in most schools calls for each adult trainer (e.g., speech pathologist, art therapist, gym instructor, and regular classroom teacher) to tutor the child in a separate setting, and on completely different tasks. According to the analysis outlined above, this approach to educational programming is almost ideal for preventing generalization. A much better strategy would be to have various professionals decide on *common* language goals and then to implement these goals in a consistent and coherent fashion. To understand this point more clearly, one can consider the difference between the traditional approach versus the approach being proposed here vis-à-vis teaching an important concept such as *yes/no*. The traditional way to teach this concept would be to have the speech pathologist show the child several Peabody cards and ask the child to indicate agreement or disagreement with the question "Is this a ____?" As each card is presented, the relevant response is trained. But this normally involves a single adult working in a single setting using restricted instructional materials. Under these circumstances, generalization would be improbable. In contrast, a multiple exemplar strategy might have the speech pathologist carry out the above procedure until the child was proficient at the task and then, most importantly, a number of other adults would become involved as well. Thus, the art therapist might ask "Is this a____?" with respect to various materials related to drawing, painting, and papier-mâché while the child was in the art room. The gym teacher might ask the child the same question with respect to different items of playground equipment while the child was outside. Finally, the regular classroom teacher could ask the child the question as it pertained to materials involved in self-help training, lunch and snacks, and desk work items. In short, a particular skill would be trained using multiple exemplars of the same task, multiple trainers, and multiple settings. The data suggest that this should be a most effective intervention. Unfortunately, territoriality persists in most schools today. Each trainer is "responsible" for his or her own "area" and an eclectic, multidisciplinary approach is extolled as the treatment of choice. Yet, when eclecticism leads to educational mediocrity and the multidisciplinary approach quickly deteriorates into an amorphous curriculum that prevents generalization, who is the beneficiary? Certainly not the child. Perhaps the lesson here is for educators to be guided more by data and less by a territorial imperative. If so, then the generalization problem may be resolved.

## USING LANGUAGE TO COMMUNICATE

No language program can be considered complete until the issue of language use (i.e., communication) is addressed. The problem of restricted communication is a significant one for autistic children and has been documented repeatedly in the published literature (Lovaas *et al.*, 1973; Rutter, 1978a). Interestingly, the behaviorist position articulated by Skinner (1957) and the pragmatic orientation that is current within the field of psycholinguistics (Bates, 1976; Halliday, 1975; Searle, 1976) both seem relevant to the solution of this problem. Recent reviews (e.g., Hart, 1980) have stressed that many similarities exist between behaviorism and pragmatics, at least at the level of taxonomy. Given these similarities, it is reasonable for the behaviorist to ask what implications pragmatics might have for the design of treatment interventions.

## Implications of Pragmatics for Treatment Intervention

To answer the above question, I would like to contrast two methods of behavioral intervention, namely discrete-trial teaching (Koegel, Russo, & Rincover, 1977; Lovaas, 1981) and incidental teaching (Hart & Risley, 1982). Discrete-trial teaching is the major method used for facilitating the acquistion of language *forms*. It is the traditional method of language instruction through drill. Incidental teaching is a newer method, one that concentrates on facilitating language *use*, that is, communication. It is the method employed for teaching language within the everyday context of conversational exchange. Table 1 outlines the major differences that exist between these two procedures. I will elaborate upon these differences below.

First, however, it is necessary to place the procedures in perspective. As I have argued elsewhere (Carr & Kologinsky, 1983), the two methods are best viewed as complementary rather than antagonistic. The discrete-trial procedure is a powerful one for helping children acquire forms, but there are no data suggesting that it helps children to learn to communicate with others. The incidental teaching procedure has shown great promise in facilitating children's language use, but there are no data demonstrating that it can be employed alone; apparently, the forms that are to be used later in communication must typically be taught first through a discrete-trial procedure. In what follows, I will outline the major characteristics of the discrete-trial method and then contrast this procedure with incidental teaching, a method consistent with and partially derived from the literature on pragmatics.

## Discrete-Trial Teaching: The Traditional Method

In the following vignette, a child is taught to label "shoe" versus "sock," using a variant of the discrete-trial procedure. For clarity of exposition, several features of the procedure have been accentuated in order to highlight a number of language-training issues. These issues will later serve as a counterpoint when incidental teaching is discussed.

Table 1.   Some Differences between the Discrete-Trial and the
Incidental Teaching Method of Language Instruction

| Discrete-trial teaching | Incidental teaching |
|---|---|
| 1. Teaching episodes are initiated by the adult. | 1. Teaching episodes are initiated by the child. |
| 2. The adult chooses the location in which the teaching episode will take place. The location is often isolated from the natural context for language use. | 2. The child chooses the location in which the teaching episode will take place. The location is part of the natural context for language use. |
| 3. The adult chooses the entire content of the teaching episode. | 3. The child chooses all or part of the content of the teaching episode. |
| 4. A teaching episode typically consists of many (i.e, massed) training trials. | 4. A teaching episode consists of only a few training trials. |
| 5. Correct responding is often followed by arbitrary reinforcers. | 5. Correct responding is followed by natural reinforcers; that is, reinforcers that are meaningfully related to the child's communicative response. |
| 6. The method is typically employed to help the child acquire new language forms. | 6. The method is typically employed to help the child *use* language forms to influence others or to help children *elaborate* upon acquired forms in order to communicate better. |

The typical session takes place in a one-to-one therapy room located in a school building but isolated from the regular classrooms. The therapy room has been designed to be free of distractions on the assumption that an environment that is devoid of toys, sound, and other children will be most conducive to learning. All sessions are carried out by a specialist, in this case, a speech pathologist (S.P.).

S.P.: O.K., it's time for our lesson. (*Holds up a shoe.*) What's this?
CHILD: (*No response.*)
S.P.: Say "shoe."
CHILD: Shoe.
S.P.: Good talking. (*Puts away shoe. Gives the child a candy. Pauses. Then holds up the sock.*) What's this?
CHILD: Shoe.
S.P.: No! (*Puts away sock. Pauses. Holds up sock again.*) What's this? Say "sock."
CHILD: Sock.
S.P.: Good talking. (*Puts away sock. Gives child a candy.*)

The sequence just described may be repeated 50 times or more in a single session. Over trials, the adult will slowly fade out the imitative prompts; that is, by the end of training, the adult no longer provides the child with the correct answer.

There are several features of this procedure that are worth noting. First, the session was initiated by the adult (i.e., the speech pathologist) and not by the child. Second, the adult chose the location in which instruction was to take place, in this case, a one-to-one therapy room. The therapy room was isolated from the natural context in which language use would normally be expected to occur, namely the regular classroom, home, playground, restaurant, etc. Further, the teaching environment, given its distraction-free quality, did not resemble the kinds of settings that the child would typically confront on a day-to-day basis. Third, the adult chose the content of the language session, namely, labeling items of clothing. Fourth, the teaching episode was carried out in drill format; large numbers of trials were run in which the same two labels were practiced over and over. Fifth, when a correct response occurred, the child received an arbitrary reinforcer; that is, a reinforcer that was not meaningfully related to the response. Thus, if the child were to use the label "shoe" in the everyday community environment, it is very unlikely that he or she would be rewarded with a candy for doing so. Sixth and finally, the focus of the training sessions was on teaching new forms, rather than on teaching the child to *use* the forms that had been mastered.

If the only intervention that is employed is the one just described, there will typically be problems in getting the child to exhibit improved communication skills. It is at this point that a pragmatic orientation to language instruction is most helpful. The analysis and suggestions that follow have been drawn from several sources (Carr, 1982c; Hart, 1980; Hart & Risley, 1982; Seibert & Oller, 1981; Rogers-Warren & Warren, 1981; Yoder & Calculator, 1981), all of which address the potential problems, vis-à-vis communication, of the discrete-trial training method outlined above.

## Incidental Teaching: A Pragmatic Orientation

In order to promote the communicative *use* of language, clinicians and educators must adopt a different focus than that associated with discrete-trial teaching. As mentioned, this new focus finds its clearest expression in the procedure known as incidental teaching (Hart & Risley, 1982). To begin, a pragmatic analysis suggests that teaching episodes should be initiated by children rather than adults. To do otherwise would merely strengthen the child's tendency to wait for the adult to ask a question or deliver a prompt before using a particular language form communicatively. Since the language of autistic children already shows a strong tendency to be prompt-reliant, it is important to avoid intensifying this pattern.

Second, the practice of having a single professional (such as a speech pathologist) train the child in an isolated environment (such as a one-to-one therapy room) is likely to inhibit communicative development. It may be necessary to begin training by having one professional responsible for all intervention so as to ensure maximum consistency and control over what is being taught. However, it is important to realize that a specialist is not a person whom the child is likely to encounter with any frequency in the day-to-day living environment. The individuals with whom the child will communicate are most often parents, classroom teachers, and peers (including siblings). Therefore, it is these people who must quickly be incorporated into the fabric of instruction. Further, since these individuals are rarely found in isolated therapy rooms, a pragmatic model suggests that the notion of "therapy room" be expanded to include *any* setting in which an autistic child spends significant portions of his or her time. As implied above, this means that the instructional environment will not be distraction-free but, rather, will include many settings that contain a great diversity of stimuli. These settings may include the home, the neighborhood playground, shopping malls, and restaurants. Indeed, it is the use of these natural contexts for instruction that is one of the hallmarks of the pragmatic approach to language intervention embodied in incidental teaching.

Third, with the discrete-trial procedure, the adult completely determines the content of the session. This feature seems to be necessary in order to teach the child a variety of language forms pertaining to items that he or she may initially display no interest toward (e.g., clothing). However, once these forms have been taught, steps must be taken to encourage their use. One means for achieving this goal is to have the adult incorporate the newly acquired labels into the flow of a conversation, as in the following example of incidental teaching:

CHILD: Play on the swings?
PARENT: O.K., but first you have to put on your shoes and socks. Say, "Where are my shoes and socks?"
CHILD: Where are my shoes and socks?
PARENT: They're in the closet. Go get them. (*Child complies and is allowed to play on the swings.*)
CHILD: (*After several weeks of incidental teaching in a variety of situations related to the above example.*) Go to swimming pool?
PARENT: O.K., but first you have to put on your bathing suit.
CHILD: Where is my bathing suit?
PARENT: It's in the bottom drawer of your bedroom chest. Go get it. (*Child complies and is allowed to swim.*)

After incidental teaching has been in effect for a period of time, it is clear, based on the example just given, that the adult is no longer in total control of the content of a conversational exchange. Rather, the determination of content is a responsibility shared by both child and adult. The child determines, on a moment-to-moment basis, what topics will be the focus of instruction. The adult, in turn, attempts to take advantage of the topic at hand to get the child to display a greater variety of language use.

The above example relates to a fourth point, namely, the use of natural rather than arbitrary reinforcers in incidental teaching. When the child said "bathing suit," the adult did not respond by giving the child a candy and saying "good talking." That would have constituted arbitrary reinforcement, since the reinforcer would have had no meaningful connection with the child's communicative phrase. Instead, the adult permitted the child to have access to the reinforcer ultimately requested (i.e., first the bathing suit then the swimming pool). This is what is meant by the term *natural reinforcement*. It should be clear that the concept of natural reinforcement is related to the notion of functionality, discussed at length in the section on choosing curricular items. A functional response, it will be recalled, is one that regularly produces a reinforcing consequence that is meaningfully related to the child's verbal behavior. From the standpoint of facilitating communication, natural reinforcement is desirable because it strengthens the connection between a particular language form and a linguistically relevant reinforcer. In contrast, if we choose to train an autistic boy to expect candy whenever he says "bathing suit," we will, in a sense, be preparing him for a world that does not exist, since virtually no adult will recognize that the phrase "bathing suit" is functionally a request for candy. If on the other hand, we train the child to say the words "bathing suit" whenever he wants that item preparatory to going swimming, we will, in effect, ensure that his request will be honored by adults, at least some of the time, since most adults will recognize that the words do indeed represent a request for that particular item.

Perhaps the greatest value of using natural reinforcement in incidental teaching is that it may facilitate the *maintenance* of language gains. A frequently encountered problem in educating autistic children concerns the lack of durability of treatment effects (Carr, 1980; Lovaas *et al.,* 1973). By helping the child to develop a language repertoire that regularly and predictably produces a variety of desired reinforcers, we ensure that the child will continue to use language over a long period of time. This result will occur simply because language has become functional or, more colloquially, because it pays off.

In connection with the functionality issue, one can raise a fifth point, namely, whether a natural reinforcement approach could ever involve massed training trials. Within the domain of discrete-trial training, repeated practice may be seen as beneficial, since the goal is to strengthen the child's mastery of a particular form. Once that form has been acquired, however, pragmatic considerations suggest that language use will be facilitated by interventions that involve relatively few trials per training episode. The reason for this statement is that, in the natural context, a child's interests typically fluctuate from moment to moment. Therefore, it is improbable, if only for reasons of satiation, that the child would spontaneously ask for the same item 50 or 100 times in a row. This would suggest that any attempt to force the child to use the same language form repeatedly would violate the child-initiation aspect of incidental teaching and merely extinguish or perhaps punish spontaneous communication.

Finally, we may consider a point that has been implicit in much of the above discussion on the issue of encouraging language use and elaboration. Specifically, allowing a child an opportunity to choose the location of training or to help determine the content of a teaching episode will mean nothing unless the child is in an environment that contains a variety of stimuli capable of evoking communicative attempts and unless there are individuals present who are prepared to respond to those attempts. In this regard, although a barren environment may initially be helpful in developing a repertoire of language forms, it would ultimately inhibit the communicative use of those forms.

In a related vein, it is unfortunate that so many autistic children are forced to live in environments that are either stripped down for reasons of "safety" or contain a variety of communicatively irrelevant stimuli, such as puzzles, pegboards, and posters of cartoon characters. None of these stimuli are likely to function as reinforcers for a child, and therefore, they do not provide the kind of environment that is conducive to facilitating attempts at communication.

A pragmatic perspective suggests that some element of environmental reorganization will almost certainly be necessary in order to increase a child's motivation to communicate. One basic strategy is to create opportunities for communication by making a child's access to reinforcers depend upon adult assistance. Thus, the first step would be to alter the environment so that it includes a diverse array of reinforcing toys, foods, and activities. Importantly, the child should not be provided with free access to these reinforcers (as is commonly done), since to do so would deprive the child of valuable opportunities to request adult aid. Instead, access to snacks and extra treats, for example, should depend on the child's making specific requests of adults in an incidental learning paradigm. Further, attractive toys should be placed in a location that is visible, but out of reach, thereby again compelling the child to seek adult assistance.

One may also take steps that encourage communication related to self-care. For example, a teacher may provide an autistic girl with many glasses of juice and other fluids so as to heighten the probability that she will have to toilet herself. This provides an opportunity to teach the child a phrase, such as "potty" or "I have to go to the bathroom please."

Finally, once we have identified a situation in which the child desires something, we can build upon any simple acts of communication that occur (e.g., "Want cookie") by requiring that the child elaborate upon the language form initially used. This can be seen in the following example:

CHILD: Want cookie.
ADULT: (*Shows child several cookies varying in size and color.*) What color cookie?
CHILD: Brown cookie.
ADULT: (*Shows child several brown cookies varying in size.*) There are big cookies and little cookies. Which cookie do you want?
CHILD: Big cookie.
ADULT: (*Holds out two big brown cookies.*) How many?
CHILD: Two cookies.
ADULT: Oh, I see. You want two big brown cookies. (*Gives the child the cookies.*)

Clearly, such elaboration must be developed slowly over many incidental teaching episodes, but it can be done and the result is that the child's use of language has a more natural, conversational quality than is the case when the command "want cookie" is repeated over and over again.

## Incidental Teaching and Nonverbal Behavior

The above discussion assumes that the adults who are present in the child's environment will be responsive to the child's attempts to communicate. This assumption is a reasonable one, given that the adults have been trained to respond to the child's verbal requests and are knowledgeable in the use of incidental teaching techniques. However, there are many situations in which a child's language repertoire is so rudimentary that communicative attempts will not occur in the speech modality. Instead, the child will exhibit a variety of primitive and sometimes subtle *nonverbal* behaviors that may serve a communicative function. If the adult is not alert to this possibility, many important opportunities for incidental teaching will be lost and the child will be less likely to acquire a functional communicative repertoire. For example, an autistic boy who wants to have a piece of cake may grasp the hand of a nearby adult and place it on a fork positioned next to the cake. The adult should not view this behavior simply as a primitive autistic gesture nor should the adult immediately give the child the cake. Instead, the child's nonverbal behavior should be viewed as an attempt to communicate and the adult should try to teach the child, via incidental methods, to say the word "cake," thereby transforming a nonverbal request into a verbal one. Often, the child's behavior will be more subtle than in the example described. Thus, a child may merely glance at the desired object from time to time or make indecipherable grunts. At this level of interaction, incidental teaching will require that adults have the motivation and the sensitivity to recognize and act upon the subtle protocommunicative attempts that these children periodically display.

Another important insight provided by a pragmatic orientation is that *behavior problems* may constitute a primitive form of communication. It has been traditional to view behaviors such as self-injury, tantrums, or aggression simply as dangerous aberrations that must be eliminated as quickly as possible. However, there is an alternative, pragmatic viewpoint, namely, that behavior problems can provide helpful clues for communication training efforts. The literature on normal child development indicates that infant cries can serve a variety of simple communicative functions pertaining to attention-seeking and avoidance (Bruner, 1979; Wolff, 1969). Interestingly, data on developmentally disabled children suggest that behavior problems may have the same functions (Carr, 1977; Carr, Newsom, & Binkoff, 1976, 1980; Lovaas, Freitag, Gold, & Kassorla, 1965; Wolf, Risley, Johnston, Harris, & Allen, 1967).

In view of these data, we have recently suggested that it may sometimes be useful to assume that a given behavior problem represents a form of communication. Therefore, it may be worthwhile to attempt to remediate the problem by teaching the child an alternative, socially appropriate form of communication (Carr, 1982d; Carr & Lovaas, 1982). For instance, once it is determined that a child becomes aggressive or has tantrums when presented with a difficult classroom task (i.e., an avoidance response), one may choose to teach the child a phrase, such as "help me," in order to express frustration more appropriately. Likewise, once one discovers that a child has tantrums or engages in self-injury to get the teacher's attention, one may consider teaching the child an alternative means of getting attention, such as the phrase "Am I doing good work?" Our initial research in this area demonstrates that this type of communication training can be an effective means of replacing behavior problems with more socially desirable interactions (Carr & Durand, 1983; Durand & Carr, 1982).

## Incidental Teaching and Social Motivation

Although some autistic children may communicate in order to receive attention from adults, the majority either do not or do so rarely. This fact is not surprising when one considers that severe social isolation is typically cited as one of the hallmark characteristics of autism (Rutter, 1978b). Generally, one is able to teach autistic children to use adults in order to obtain tangible reinforcers; that is, one can help the children to make requests. The problem that has not yet been resolved in the field pertains to our inability to get autistic children to communicate in order to receive social attention. Thus, we are generally not able to help the child to make descriptive statements spontaneously. Few autistic individuals are likely to approach an adult and emit a phrase such as "it's my birthday today." In simple terms, they do not seem to care whether the adult attends to them.

Until we are able to deal with this lack of social motivation, it is likely that communication by autistic children will retain a stilted and artificial quality. There is, of course, a literature on social bonding and attachment that may be helpful in trying to address this problem (e.g., Ainsworth, 1973; Cairns, 1979). However, to date, there have been no programmatic attempts to translate this information into a form that is useful for intervention. Apart from a handful of studies conducted more than 15 years ago (Lovaas, Schaeffer, & Simmons, 1965; Lovaas, Freitag, Kinder, Rubenstein, Schaeffer, & Simmons, 1966), there has been virtually no research focusing on the remediation of social reinforcement deficits. Only recently have behavioral researchers begun to look again at the issue of social reinforcement and its effects on interaction between autistic children and other people (Nordquist, Twardosz, & McEvoy, 1982). If we can make the children more social, then there is the possibility of broadening their communicative repertoire beyond the narrow focus imposed by the use of requests alone. Applied researchers would do well to make the attainment of this goal their highest priority.

## Incidental Teaching and the Autistic Client

Finally, it is worth noting that although the pragmatic orientation and its associated method of incidental teaching offer much promise in enhancing the development of communication in autistic children, most treatment research using this approach has been conducted with mildly handicapped children (Hart & Risley, 1976, 1978, 1980). Until recently, there has been relatively little downward extension of these techniques to children with autism and other developmental disabilities (Carr & Kologinsky, 1983). Fortunately, however, the situation now appears to be changing (Hart, 1981; Rogers-Warren & Warren, 1981). It is likely that behaviorists will focus more heavily on pragmatic considerations in the years to come, with the result that the nature of behavioral language intervention will be dramatically altered. However, it is worth emphasizing again that incidental teaching does not invalidate the discrete-trial method. Rather, it should be viewed as an extension of behavioral language intervention to the domain of teaching children to use previously acquired forms communicatively.

## CONCLUDING STATEMENT

I have refrained from writing a lengthy exposition on the many successes that behaviorists have had in teaching specific language forms. Instead, I have focused on four problem areas in which the road has been rockier: individual differences, choosing curricular items, generalization, and language use (i.e., communication). Further, I have tried to outline strategies for dealing with each of these problems within a modified behavioral paradigm, a paradigm that is open to a variety of concepts and that uses data generated by nonbehaviorists. We are making headway in the four problem areas discussed, and we now have more to offer children and their families than we did 10 years ago. However, the resolution of these problems will ultimately require a substantial research effort that is characterized by curiosity and tolerance of many points of view among all who work in this field. If this occurs, and I think it will, then the future of the behavioral paradigm will be as vibrant as its past.

ACKNOWLEDGMENTS

I would like to thank June Lindquist for her helpful comments on earlier drafts of this manuscript.

## REFERENCES

Ainsworth, M. D. S. (1973). The development of infant–mother attachment. In B. M. Caldwell & H. N. Ricciuti (Eds.), *Review of child development* (Vol. 3). Chicago: University of Chicago Press.

Baer, D. M. (1981). *How to plan for generalization.* Lawrence, KS: H & H Enterprises.

Bates, E. (1976). *Language and context: The acquisition of pragmatics.* New York: Academic Press.

Brown, L., Nietupski, J., & Hamre-Nietupski, S. (1976). The criterion of ultimate functioning. In M. A. Thomas (Eds.), *Hey don't forget about me!* (pp. 2–15). Reston, VA: Council for Exceptional Children.

Bruner, J. (1979). Learning how to do things with words. In D. Aaronson & R. W. Rieber (Eds.), *Psycholinguistic research.* (pp. 265–284). Hillsdale, NJ: Lawrence Erlbaum Associates.

Cairns, R. B. (1979). *Social development: The origins and plasticity of interchanges.* San Francisco: W. H. Freeman.

Carr, E. G. (1977). The motivation of self-injurious behavior: A review of some hypotheses. *Psychological Bulletin, 84,* 800–816.

Carr, E. G. (1980). Generalization of treatment effects following educational intervention with autistic children and youth. In B. Wilcox & A. Thompson (Eds.), *Critical issues in educating autistic children and youth.* (pp. 118–134). Washington, DC: U.S. Department of Education, Office of Special Education.

Carr, E. G. (1982a). Some relationships between sign language acquisition and perceptual dysfunction in autistic children. In R. N. Malatesha & L. C. Hartlage (Eds.), *Neuropsychology and cognition: Vol. 2* (pp. 364-371). The Hague, The Netherlands: Martinus Nijhoff Publishers.

Carr, E. G. (1982b). Sign language acquisition: Clinical and theoretical aspects. In R. L. Koegel, A. Rincover, & A. L. Egel (Eds.), *Educating and understanding autistic children.* (pp. 142-157). San Diego: College-Hill Press.

Carr, E. G. (1982c). *How to teach sign language to developmentally disabled children.* Lawrence, KS: H & H Enterprises.

Carr, E. G. (1982d). Analysis and remediation of severe behavior problems. In D. Park (Ed.), *Proceedings of the 1981 International Conference on Autism* (pp. 313-317). Washington, DC: The National Society for Children and Adults with Autism.

Carr, E. G., & Durand, V. M. (1983, August). *The application of pragmatics to conceptualization and treatment of severe behavior problems in children.* Invited address presented at the meeting of the American Psychological Association, Anaheim, CA.

Carr, E. G., & Kologinsky, E. (1983). Acquisition of sign language by autistic children. II. Spontaneity and generalization effects. *Journal of Applied Behavior Analysis, 16,* 297-314.

Carr, E. G., & Lovaas, O. I. (1982). Contingent electric shock as a treatment for severe behavior problems. In S. Axelrod & J. Apsche (Eds.), *Punishment: Its effects on human behavior* (pp. 221-245). New York: Academic Press.

Carr, E. G., Schreibman, L., & Lovaas, O. I. (1975). Control of echolalic speech in psychotic children. *Journal of Abnormal Child Psychology, 3,* 331-351.

Carr, E. G., Newsom, C. D., & Binkoff, J. A. (1976). Stimulus control of self-destructive behavior in a psychotic child. *Journal of Abnormal Child Psychology, 4,* 139-153.

Carr, E. G., Newsom, C. D., & Binkoff, J. A. (1980). Escape as a factor in the aggressive behavior of two retarded children. *Journal of Applied Behavior Analysis, 13,* 101-117.

Carr, E. G., Pridal, C., & Dores, P. A. (1984). Speech versus sign comprehension in autistic children: Analysis and prediction. *Journal of Experimental Child Psychology, 37,* 587-597.

Chomsky, N. (1959). Verbal behavior by B. F. Skinner. *Language, 35,* 26-58.

Durand, V. M., & Carr, E. G. (1982, August). Differential reinforcement of communicative behavior. In R. L. Koegel (Chair), *Research on clinical intervention with autistic and psychotic children.* Symposium presented at the meeting of the American Psychological Association, Washington, DC.

Frisch, S. A., & Schumaker, J. B. (1974). Teaching generalized receptive prepositions in retarded children. *Journal of Applied Behavior Analysis, 7,* 611-621.

Garcia, E. (1974). The training and generalization of a conversational speech form in nonverbal retardates. *Journal of Applied Behavior Analysis, 7,* 137-149.

Garcia, E. E., & DeHaven, E. D. (1974). Use of operant techniques in the establishment and generalization of language: A review and analysis. *American Journal of Mental Deficiency, 79,* 169-178.

Goetz, L., Schuler, A. L., & Sailor, W. (1981). Functional competence as a factor in communication instruction. *Exceptional Education Quarterly, 2,* 51-60.

Griffiths, H., & Craighead, W. E. (1972). Generalization in operant speech therapy for misarticulation. *Journal of Speech and Hearing Disorders, 37,* 485-494.

Guess, D., Sailor, W., & Baer, D. M. (1978). Children with limited language. In R. L. Schiefelbusch (Ed.), *Language intervention strategies* (pp. 101-143). Baltimore, MD: University Park Press.

Halliday, M. A. K. (1975). *Learning how to mean: Explorations in the development of language.* London: Edward Arnold.

Handleman, J. S. (1979). Generalization by autistic-type children of verbal responses across settings. *Journal of Applied Behavior Analysis, 21,* 273-282.

Harris, S. L. (1975). Teaching language to nonverbal children—with emphasis on problems of generalization. *Psychological Bulletin, 82,* 565-580.

Hart, B. (1980). Pragmatics and language development. In B. B. Lahey & A. E. Kazdin (Eds.), *Advances in clinical-child psychology* (pp. 383–427). New York: Plenum Press.

Hart, B. (1981). Pragmatics: How language is used. *Analysis and Intervention in Developmental Disabilities, 1,* 299–313.

Hart, B., & Risley, T. R. (1976). Community-based language training. In T. D. Tjossem (Ed.), *Intervention strategies for high risk infants and young children* (pp. 187–198). Baltimore, MD: University Park Press.

Hart, B., & Risley, T. R. (1978). Promoting productive language through incidental teaching. *Education and Urban Society, 10,* 207–229.

Hart, B., & Risley, T. R. (1980). *In vivo* language intervention: Unanticipated general effects. *Journal of Applied Behavior Analysis, 13,* 407–432.

Hart, B. M., & Risley, T. R. (1982). *How to use incidental teaching for elaborating language.* Lawrence, KS: H & H Enterprises.

Hermelin, B., & O'Connor, N. (1970). *Psychological experiments with autistic children.* London: Pergamon Press.

Howlin, P. A. (1981). The effectiveness of operant language training with autistic children. *Journal of Autism and Developmental Disorders, 11,* 89–105.

Hupp, S. C., & Mervis, C. B. (1981). Development of generalized concepts by severely handicapped students. *The Association for Severely Handicapped Journal, 6,* 14–21.

Hupp, S. C., & Mervis, C. B. (1982). Acquisition of basic object categories by severely handicapped children. *Child Development, 53,* 760–767.

Koegel, R. L., Russo, D. C., & Rincover, A. (1977). Assessing and training teachers in the generalized use of behavior modification with autistic children. *Journal of Applied Behavior Analysis, 10,* 197–205.

Lovaas, O. I. (1966). A program for the establishment of speech in psychotic children. In J. K. Wing (Ed.), *Early childhood autism.* (pp. 115–144.) Oxford: Pergamon Press.

Lovaas, O. I. (1977). *The autistic child.* New York: Irvington.

Lovaas, O. I. (1981). *Teaching developmentally disabled children.* Baltimore, MD: University Park Press.

Lovaas, O. I. (1982, August). An overview of the young autism project. In O. I. Lovaas (Chair), *Critical factors in successful treatment of young autistic children.* Symposium presented at the meeting of the American Psychological Association, Washington, DC.

Lovaas, O. I., & Newsom, C. D. (1976). Behavior modification with psychotic children. In H. Leitenberg (Ed.), *Handbook of behavior modification and behavior therapy* (pp. 303–360). Englewood Cliffs, NJ: Prentice-Hall.

Lovaas, O. I., Freitag, G., Gold, V. J., & Kassorla, I. C. (1965). Experimental studies in childhood schizophrenia: Analysis of self-destructive behavior. *Journal of Experimental Child Psychology, 2,* 67–84.

Lovaas, O. I., Freitag, G., Kinder, M. I., Rubenstein, B. D., Schaeffer, B., & Simmons, J. Q. (1966). Establishment of social reinforcers in two schizophrenic children on the basis of food. *Journal of Experimental Child Psychology, 4,* 109–125.

Lovaas, O. I., Koegel, R., Simmons, J. Q., & Long, J. S. (1973). Some generalization and follow-up measures on autistic children in behavior therapy. *Journal of Applied Behavior Analysis, 6,* 131–166.

Lovaas, O. I., Schaeffer, B., & Simmons, J. Q. (1965). Experimental studies in childhood schizophrenia: Building social behavior in autistic children by use of electric shock. *Journal of Experimental Research in Personality, 1,* 99–109.

Lutzker, J. R., & Sherman, J. A. (1974). Producing generative sentence usage by imitation and reinforcement procedures. *Journal of Applied Behavior Analysis, 7,* 447–460.

Nordquist, V. M., Twardosz, S., & McEvoy, M. A. (1982, November). *A naturalistic approach to the problem of establishing social reinforcers in autistic children.* Paper presented at the meeting of the Association for Advancement of Behavior Therapy, Los Angeles.

Remington, B., & Clarke, S. (1983). The acquisition of expressive signing by autistic children: An evaluation of the relative effects of simultaneous communication and sign-alone training. *Journal of Applied Behavior Analysis, 16,* 315–328.

Rogers-Warren, A., & Warren, S. F. (1981). Form and function in language learning and generalization. *Analysis and Intervention in Developmental Disabilities, 1,* 389–404.

Rosch, E. (1973). On the internal structure of perceptual and semantic categories. In T. E. Moore (Ed.), *Cognitive development and the acquisition of language* (pp. 111–144). New York: Academic Press.

Rosch, E. (1975). Universals and cultural specifics in human categorization. In R. Brislin, S. Bochner, & W. Lonner (Eds.), *Cross-cultural perspectives on learning* (pp. 177–206). New York: Halsted Press.

Rosch, E., & Mervis, C. B. (1975). Family resemblances: Studies in the internal structure of categories. *Cognitive Psychology, 7,* 573–605.

Rutter, M. (1978a). Language disorder and infantile autism. In M. Rutter & E. Schopler (Eds.), *Autism: A reappraisal of concepts and treatment* (pp. 85–104). New York: Plenum Press.

Rutter, M. (1978b). Diagnosis and definition. In M. Rutter & E. Schopler (Eds.), *Autism: A reappraisal of concepts and treatment* (pp. 1–25). New York: Plenum Press.

Schaeffer, B., Kollinzas, G., Musil, A., & McDowell, P. (1977). Spontaneous verbal language for autistic children through signed speech. *Sign Language Studies, 17,* 287–328.

Schreibman, L., & Carr, E. G. (1978). Elimination of echolalic responding to questions through the training of a generalized verbal response. *Journal of Applied Behavior Analysis, 11,* 453–463.

Schumaker, J., & Sherman, J. A. (1970). Training generative verb usage by imitation and reinforcement procedures. *Journal of Applied Behavior Analysis, 3,* 273–287.

Searle, J. R. (1976). A classification of illocutionary acts. *Language in Society, 5,* 1–23.

Seibert, J. M., & Oller, D. K. (1981). Linguistic pragmatics and language intervention strategies. *Journal of Autism and Developmental Disorders, 11,* 75–88.

Skinner, B. F. (1957). *Verbal behavior.* New York: Appleton-Century-Crofts.

Sloane, H. N., & MacAuley, B. (Eds.). (1968). *Operant procedures in remedial speech and language training.* Boston: Houghton Mifflin.

Stevens-Long, J., & Rasmussen, M. (1974). The acquisition of simple and compound sentence structure in an autistic child. *Journal of Applied Behavior Analysis, 7,* 473–479.

Stokes, T. F., & Baer, D. M. (1977). An implicit technology of generalization. *Journal of Applied Behavior Analysis, 10,* 349–367.

Stokes, T. F., Baer, D. M., & Jackson, R. L. (1974). Programming the generalization of a greeting response in four retarded children. *Journal of Applied Behavior Analysis, 7,* 599–610.

Wolf, M. M., Risley, T., Johnston, M., Harris, F., & Allen, E. (1967). Application of operant conditioning procedures to the behavior problems of an autistic child: A follow-up and extension. *Behaviour Research and Therapy, 5,* 103–112.

Wolff, P. H. (1969). The natural history of crying and other vocalizations in early infancy. In B. M. Foss (Ed.), *Determinants of infant behavior* (Vol. IV, pp. 81–109). London: Methuen.

Yoder, D. E., & Calculator, S. (1981). Some perspectives on intervention strategies for persons with developmental disorders. *Journal of Autism and Developmental Disorders, 11,* 107–123.

# Contribution of Behavioral Approaches to the Language and Communication of Persons with Autism

## CATHERINE LORD

One way of evaluating the contribution of a specific theoretical approach to language and communication in the field of autism is to ask what it is that we want from a theory. As Carr has pointed out, the two major approaches to communication, behavioral and psycholinguistic perspectives, have typically had quite different goals. This seems an appropriate place to discuss the goals in communication and language most important to those of us who work with people with autism and then to ask how behaviorism, in theory and practice, has helped or failed to help us obtain those goals.

While establishing goals for research or intervention is an individual matter in the end, two major objectives would appear to be relatively free from controversy. A first goal is practical and straightforward: to increase the ability of persons with autism to communicate in everyday settings. Although we may differ in how communication is best defined, the goal of facilitating functional communication is usually foremost for the clinician, educator, or family of a person with autism.

Second, a longer-term objective is to increase our understanding of the nature of autism. A primary aspect of this goal would be to use our knowledge of the communication skills and deficits associated with autism as clues to etiologies and risk factors. The eventual aim would be to prevent or to treat basic biological causes of autism. In the meantime, a better understanding of

CATHERINE LORD • Department of Pediatrics, University of Alberta, Glenrose Hospital, Edmonton, Alberta T5G 0B7, Canada.

communication abilities and disabilities of autistic persons should allow us to individualize education and treatment of specific deficits and, perhaps, to prevent secondary problems (e.g., social isolation, inappropriate behavior, cognitive delays) that are compounded by difficulties in language. Furthermore, a better understanding of language in autism should allow us to predict responses to various treatments more accurately. Finally, from the broadest perspective, a better understanding of language in autism should add to our knowledge about communication and language development, in general.

This chapter will discuss how recent trends in behaviorism, many identified by Carr (Chapter 3), have contributed to these goals. Suggestions are made about possible modifications in this approach that might help us better meet the two major objectives of facilitating communication in everyday settings and of increasing our understanding of the nature of autism.

## BEHAVIORAL APPROACHES TO MODIFYING FUNCTIONAL COMMUNICATION

Behavioral methods, more than any other treatment approach, have focused on the first goal, increasing the ability of autistic persons to communicate. Most documented changes related to specific treatments have used such behavioral methods as prompting and differential reinforcement. Operant procedures have become a standard part of the repertoires of most clinicians and educators working with autistic people, regardless of the declared orientation of the professional (Howlin, 1981). As Carr delineated, behavioral methods have been used to teach productive and receptive labels, grammatical morphemes (e.g., such word endings as -ed and -s, such functors as the and is), and sentence structures. Operant procedures have also resulted in decreased inappropriate language, such as some forms of echolalia or idiosyncratic use of words (see Chapter 3).

Although clear changes in children's language have been observed, the extent to which behavioral methods have met the primary goal of increased communication in daily living has recently been questioned (Lord & O'Neill, 1983; McLean & Snyder-McLean, 1978; Seibert & Oller, 1981). Carr described four concerns about the efficacy of behavioral interventions in producing meaningful changes: individual differences, problems in selecting curricula, generalization of observed changes, and actual use by children of the language they have been taught. As Carr mentioned, these problems do not necessarily belong to behaviorism alone, but may well hold true for any intervention for which treatment effects are evaluated. Two of the above problems, difficulties in generalization and limitations in the extent to which children use in everyday life the aspects of language they were taught during specific behavioral interventions, have significantly limited the ultimate impact of even well-documented changes. Although behaviorists have been able to show increases within teaching contexts in the production of specific terms or grammatical structures, typically it has been much more difficult to show that children generalize these new situations or that these changes can be maintained even in the same situation without excessive environmental manipulation (Seibert & Oller, 1981).

Furthermore, individual differences before and after intervention have often been found to be far better predictors of eventual outcome than differences attributed to treatment. Independent of treatment, echolalic children who have some receptive vocabulary, produce a few words spontaneously, and do well on nonverbal intelligence tests have a much better prognosis for communicative language than do children without these characteristics (Howlin, 1981). This finding has held true across treatment programs from a variety of orientations, not just behavioral approaches (Menyuk & Wilbur, 1981). However, the lack of control groups and the use of individual data reported primarily for successful subjects (Lord, 1978) have made the results of some behaviorists more obviously misleading than others.

A final difficulty in evaluating language treatment programs is that response to treatment is typically nonspecific. There are seldom clear relations between what is actually taught children and what children learn, when learning is measured in contexts outside the teaching situation (e.g., informal home observations, standardized tests). Improvements in most aspects of communication appear to be much the same, regardless of the nature of the program (Bartak & Rutter, 1973). Thus, Howlin (1979) found similar changes occurring for children in a home-based behavioral program and a clinic-based program and for children with no treatment at all. Bartak and Rutter (1973) and Howlin (1979) both found complexity of language to be one of the least responsive treatment measures in the classroom, clinic, or home-based treatment programs, although the programs emphasized grammatical skills. Lovaas (1977) observed remarkable changes in the connected discourse and narratives of a few autistic children who were being taught very rote passages or such simpler structures as grammatical morphemes. He attributed these changes to generalization of general language ability. However, the link between the linguistic structures these children were taught and the changes in the language they produced is very tenuous. Clearly some children make remarkable gains in the complexity of their language, but in many cases, these gains seem to occur regardless of the specific content of their language treatment.

As Carr pointed out, the difficulties of choosing a curriculum using only a behavioral paradigm may account for some of the nonspecificity of treatment effects. If what is being taught in a curriculum has little relationship to the ideas and needs children want to communicate, it is not surprising that children do not use what they have learned or that changes in what they *do* use show little relation to the curriculum. In addition, if *how* the child is taught to communicate is not applicable to situations that arise in his or her daily life, then it is not surprising that greater changes are observed in response to environmental demands than to artificial treatment situations.

What then is the contribution of behavioral approaches to increasing the communicative ability of people with autism? We are left with the encouraging finding that behavioral treatments *do* seem to produce reliable, measurable gains in the frequency, appropriateness, and communicativeness of children with autism (Howlin, 1981). Although other methods of intervention might do as well (Seibert & Oller, 1981), to date, it is primarily behaviorists who have consistently provided evidence of improvement. On the other hand, it is less apparent that the most useful aspects of communication that change in response to behavioral interventions are the aspects of language that are taught in behavioral programs. Curtiss (1981) distinguished between acquiring linguistic skills (e.g., sounds that form words that form rule-based sentences) and acquiring communication skills (e.g., effective ways of conveying socially directed messages). It is ironic that, although behavioral programs in the past generally focused on teaching linguistic forms, the greatest changes observed were in communication (Menyuk & Wilbur, 1981).

Real benefits do seem to be reliably associated with behavioral treatment. What is still unclear is how these changes come about: Are improvements in frequency of communicativeness due to direct effects of increased experience communicating or to indirect effects of changes in parental language or expectations for comprehension? Or are these improvements direct or indirect effects of even more general changes such as bringing behavior under control or structuring the environment so that it makes sense to the child? What are the specific relationships and factors that mediate between treatment and behavior change? In order to differentiate between these relationships, the results of different treatments must be compared. More specific information is needed, with controls for the content of the interventions, behavioral and otherwise, and the content of the expected improvements. Then, specific relationships between treatments and changes could be better understood. In a way, it is precisely because behaviorists have provided us with an effective treatment that we can now move beyond asking if the treatment works to asking when and why.

## A BEHAVIORAL PERSPECTIVE ON
## LANGUAGE DISORDER AND DEVELOPMENT

Earlier, I identified a second goal for communication research in autism—the contribution of behaviorism to our understanding of the language skills and deficits associated with autism. Simple behavioral attempts to account for the deficits associated with autism (Ferster, 1961) or language acquisition in general (see Brown & Hanlon, 1970, or deVilliers & deVilliers, 1978) have received very little empirical support and will not be discussed here (see Chapter 3 and 4, this volume). Yet language itself has proved to be a powerful predictor of long-term educational and residential outcome for people with autism. On the basis of epidemiological studies, functional language by early school age has been shown to be as powerful an indicator of later skills as intelligence (Rutter, 1978a). Carr suggested another predictive relationship between vocal imitation and receptive language that might also prove to be important. The potential complexities of the association between imitation and comprehension provide a useful illustration of the conceptual difficulties in adapting a primarily behavioral approach to understanding the language deficits of autistic persons.

One problem is the propensity of many behaviorists to focus on a specific behavior in isolation, without placing it in a broader framework of other behaviors or development. Complex behaviors and relationships may come to seem deceptively simple. At the same time, this approach may eventually interfere with our understanding of the nature of autism, an unarguably complex disorder. For example, Carr, Pridal, and Dores (1984) and others (e.g., Howlin, 1981) found that children who can imitate sounds or words are more likely to acquire receptive labels during behavioral treatment than are children who do not imitate. Carr therefore suggested that verbal imitation may be an important prerequisite for receptive language. Yet why or how imitation might serve as a prerequisite for comprehension is not clear. The finding that imitation typically predicts comprehension does not necessarily imply that one process is a prerequisite for the other (Flavell, 1982). Although knowing that a child can use a spoon allows the prediction that he or she may soon use a fork, a child does not have to use a spoon in order to use a fork, nor does the acquisition of one skill ensure the other.

Several investigators have found that spontaneous imitation in young, normally developing children occurs with wide variations in frequency. Although some children imitate very frequently, others imitate rarely, if ever (Bloom, Hood, & Lightbown, 1974). Thus, spontaneous imitation cannot be viewed as a prerequisite for normal language acquisition. In addition, some parents appear to engage frequently in routines designed to elicit verbal or vocal imitation from their infants and toddlers. Others do not. There is little evidence from normal developmental research that elicited imitation is either a necessary or an important process in language acquisition (Bloom & Lahey, 1978; Snow, 1977). To reach the conclusion that imitation is a prerequisite for language acquisition by children with autism, one would have to hypothesize that the mechanisms underlying language development are quite different for the autistic child than they are for other children. Since there are many similarities to the course of normal language development for those children with autism who learn language (Rutter 1978b), this position seems unnecessary and extreme. Imitation skills may certainly be useful to the child with autism, but that is not to say that they are prerequisite.

Since children with autism show such a vast range of abilities, from severe retardation to superior skills in some areas, another problem is the familiar one of nonspecificity. Is learning to imitate of particular value for acquiring receptive labels or is there just a general relationship between performing well on two language-related tasks? Children who imitate may not only learn receptive labels faster than children who do not, they may also have better articulation and more sophisticated syntax. In fact, they may be taller, complete puzzles more rapidly, have better social skills, and be more likely to be toilet trained. Certainly, the importance of measuring the degree of general intellectual retardation associated with autism has been one of the major contributions of epidemiological research in the last 15 years (Rutter, 1978a). It would appear more parsimonious to conclude that autistic symptoms and general delay are negatively related to task performance in many areas than it would be to identify each possible relationship between specific skills.

I do not mean to discourage innovative ideas such as facilitating language comprehension through imitation training, but rather to say that previous experience with research in which causal inferences have been made on the basis of correlative data between isolated behaviors suggests that a measure of caution is warranted (Flavell, 1982). This skepticism, however, could be counteracted in several ways. First, the behaviorist could use the research in normal development to derive some reason, besides proximity in the steps of an intervention program, as to why verbal imitation training should enhance the acquisition of receptive labels more than other kinds of training. We need to know why this particular relationship is seen to be potentially more important than others. We then would have an hypothesis that should be testable on multiple levels.

Second, the behaviorist could provide some methodological controls to show not only that children who were taught to imitate understood more words faster than other children, but also that these results were not due to pretreatment differences among subjects. For example, we need to know that (a) "imitative" children (meaning children who were successfully taught to imitate) could not imitate before the intervention began; (b) imitative children did not understand more words than nonimitative children before treatment; (c) imitative children were equivalent to nonimitative children on nonverbal, social, and other sensorimotor skills from the start as well; and (d) those children who failed to learn to imitate were similar on most measures to children who had never been taught to imitate, except on acquisition of receptive vocabulary (e.g., they were not more generally delayed). With such information, we could appropriately conclude that there was a specific treatment effect of learning to imitate that was not due to subject selection or abilities already possessed by the children before the treatment program began.

Third, one would also want to control for the specificity of the treatment program by showing that teaching children behaviors other than verbal imitation (e.g., motor imitation, block-building, sorting, doll play) did not result in the same gains.

Beyond the difficulties that arise out of the failure to place communicative behaviors in some theoretical framework, the contribution of behaviorism to our understanding of autism has also been limited by the failure of many researchers (noted by Carr to be not just behaviorists) to apply information concerning language acquisition in normally developing young children to children with disorders. For example, the notion of bringing a child's receptive language under the "stimulus control" of a word or words is almost directly antithetical to recent evidence indicating that normally developing, language-learning children typically determine what someone is saying by attending to many nonlinguistic sources of information, apart from the specific words they hear (Chapman, 1978). Attempts to make children rely only on words for understanding may make initial comprehension unnecessarily difficult. In the long run, an approach that emphasizes well-defined stimulus control may be counterproductive for comprehension (although it may be important for other reasons), since these methods discourage children from using valuable sources of information available in their everyday environments.

Even the innovative methods, such as incidental teaching, that Carr describes as attempting to be more ecologically valid by "spacing trials" (i.e., because young children do not spontaneously request the same item 50 times in a row) seem to have been designed without reference to common sense or to an extensive literature on mother–child interaction. This literature has shown very high levels of repetitions (although perhaps not 50 repetitions, certainly 10 or 20 repetitions of the same term in the same context are not rare) and cognitive constraints in communicative sequences for young, language-learning children (Snow, 1977). This is not to advocate massed trials to the exclusion of more communication-oriented, child-initiated teaching sequences. However, research in normal development would sugguest that critical differences between discrete-trial formats presented *en masse* and more normally occurring contexts for communicative development do not lie in the spaced versus massed trial distinction, but rather relate to the meaningfulness of the topics, the underlying social behaviors, and the continual, predictable changes in form (e.g., word order, word ending, intonation) made by most parents when speaking to very young children (Seibert & Oller, 1981). Isolating specific behaviors to be changed, without attending to how these behaviors fit into more complex aspects of social and language development, may amount to not seeing the forest for the trees.

A similar point could be made concerning the failure of children and adults with autism to respond to social reinforcement. Carr stated that the majority of autistic children rarely communicate in order to receive attention. Yet, in several independent studies in which the spontaneous language of school-age children with autism was observed and recorded utterance by utterance, the authors included "comment" or "tacts" (that is, utterances with no apparent objective except to maintain social contact) as one of the two or three most frequent pragmatic categories used by autistic children in everyday situations (O'Neill & Lord, 1982; Watson, Chapter 9, this volume). Although the overall amount of spontaneous language for most of the children with autism was much smaller than expected for normally developing children, the pattern of functions was not radically different from that of younger, preschool-age, normally developing children. It has been argued that defining these utterances as socially directed requires making unfounded inferences about the child's motivations. However, behaviorally, the inferences required for autistic children need be no greater than those made during "rich interpretations" of normally developing children's language (Brown, 1973).

If we use as a criterion whether or not the child would have produced the same utterance if there was a different listener or no listener at all, an autistic child who says "flower" under his breath as he is handed a flower by his teacher may be commenting in the same way pragmatically as a normally developing child who says "pretty flower, mommy" as she smiles and takes a flower from her mother's hand. Again, if we look carefully, the difference in the quality of the two children's behavior may be better accounted for by their ability to use gaze, facial expression, gesture, intonation, delayed imitation, and social initiative (i.e., taking the flower themselves) and by specific aspects of language (i.e., vocabulary, syntax) than by their intentions or social motivation. Carr suggests drawing upon developmental theories related to attachment and bonding to explain what he perceives as lack of motivation. An alternative way of using normal developmental research might be to observe communicative behaviors in normally developing children in similar contexts (rather than leaping back to infancy and attachment paradigms) and then determine when and where these positive social behaviors occur for children with autism.

The example of the "flower" statements is also related to an earlier point. When complex behaviors are oversimplified or treated in isolation, the possibility of identifying individual patterns of communicative abilities is greatly lessened. The opportunity to use these patterns both to design individualized interventions and to better understand the complex nature of autism is forfeited. It is in this sense that behavioral approaches to language and autism have been particularly uninformative. Many behaviorists may respond that they chose to focus on the first goal, that of increasing communication, to the exclusion of the second, that of enhancing our understanding of language and communicative deficits. However, it now seems that this choice is no longer necessary or justifiable.

Carr suggested several instances in which behavioral and psycholinguistic approaches could be used together. Similar statements could be made about the potential for reconciling practical and conceptual goals in the area of communication and autism. For behaviorists, success should now motivate reconceptualization and expansion. The short-term positive results of behavioral intervention are well established. Thus, it is no longer sufficient to show that autistic children *can* learn certain aspects of language if we do not know why or how or what, exactly, they have learned or if their new skill will have any practical benefit. On the other hand, emphasizing one goal (e.g., functionalism) and ignoring the other (e.g., the question of the specific nature of autism) is also not sufficient, for the answer to what constitutes useful communication for a person with autism is not a simple one either. Given the wide acceptance of behavioral methods and the general rejection of behavioral conceptualizations of both autism and language development, the question of who is or is not a behaviorist becomes moot. It may be more useful to ask what our goals in the area of communication skills for people with autism are and how we expect to obtain them?

# REFERENCES

Bartak, L., & Rutter, M. (1973). Special educational treatment of autistic children: A comparative study I. Design of study and characteristics of units. *Journal of Child Psychology and Psychiatry, 14,* 161–179.

Bloom, L. & Lahey, M. (1978). *Language development and language disorders.* New York: Wiley.

Bloom, L., Hood, L., & Lightbown, P. (1974). Imitation in language development; if, when and why. *Cognitive Psychology, 6,* 380–420.

Brown, R. *A first language.* (1973). Cambridge, MA: Harvard University Press.

Brown, R., & Hanlon, C. (1970). Derivational complexity and order of acquisition in child speech. In J. R. Hayes (Ed), *Cognition and the development of language* (pp. 11–54). New York: Wiley.

Carr, E. G., Pridal, C., & Dores. P. A. (1984). Speech versus sign comprehension in autistic children: analysis and prediction. *Journal of Experimental Child Psychology, 37,* 587–597.

Chapman, R. S. (1978). Comprehension strategies in children. In J. F. Kavanagh and W. Strange (Eds), *Speech and language in the laboratory, school and clinic* (pp. 308–327). Cambridge, MA: M.I.T. Press.

Curtiss, S. (1981). Dissociations between language and cognition: cases and implications. *Journal of Autism and Developmental Disorders, 11,* 15–30.

deVilliers, J. G., & deVilliers, P. A. (1978). *Language acquisition.* Cambridge, MA: Harvard University Press.

Ferster, C. B. (1961). Positive reinforcement in behavioural deficits of autistic children. *Child Development, 32,* 437–447.

Flavell, J. H. (1982). Structures, stages and sequences in cognitive development. In W. A. Collins, (Ed.), *The concept of development: The Minnesota symposium on child psychology, Vol. 15* (pp. 1-28). Hillsdale, NJ: Lawrence Erlbaum Associates.

Howlin, P. (1979). *Training parents to modify the language of their autistic children, a home-based approach.* Unpublished doctoral dissertation, London University, London.

Howlin, P. (1981). Effectiveness of operant language training with autistic children. *Journal of Autism and Developmental Disorders, 11,* 89-106.

Lord, C. (1978). Review of O. Ivar Lovaas' *The autistic child. Journal of Autism and Childhood Schizophrenia, 8,* 123-128.

Lord, C., & O'Neill, P. J. (1983). Language and communication needs of adolescents with autism. In E. Schopler & G. Mesibov (Eds.), *Autism in adolescents and adults* (pp. 57-77). New York: Plenum Press.

Lovaas, O. I. (1977). *The autistic child.* New York: Irvington.

McLean, J., & Snyder-McLean, L. (1978). *A transactional approach to early language training.* Columbus, OH: Merrill.

Menyuk, P., & Wilbur, R. (1981). Preface to special issue on language disorders. *Journal of Autism and Developmental Disorders, 11,* 1-14.

O'Neill, P. J., & Lord, C. (1982). Functional and semantic characteristics of child-directed speech of autistic children. In D. Park (Ed.), *Proceedings from the International Meetings for the National Society for Autistic Children* (pp. 47-48). Washington, DC: National Society for Autistic Children.

Rutter, M. (1978a). Developmental issues and prognosis. In M. Rutter & E. Schopler (Eds.), *Autism: A reappraisal of concepts and treatment* (pp. 497-505). New York: Plenum Press.

Rutter, M. (1978b). Language disorder and infantile autism. In M. Rutter & E. Schopler (Ed.), *Autism: A reappraisal of concepts & treatment* (pp. 85-104). New York: Plenum Press.

Seibert, J. M., & Oller, D. K. (1981). Linguistic pragmatics and language intervention strategies. *Journal of Autism and Developmental Disorders, 11,* 75-88.

Snow, C. (1977). Mother's speech research: From input to interaction. In C. Snow & C. Ferguson (Eds.), *Talking to Children* (pp. 1-10). New York: Cambridge University Press.

# 4

# Psycholinguistic Approaches to Language and Communication in Autism

## HELEN TAGER-FLUSBERG

## INTRODUCTION

During the past decade, there has been a concerted effort to begin applying some of the basic concepts of developmental psycholinguistics to our understanding of the primary language and communication problems of autistic children. Most of these efforts have addressed two fundamental issues. First, In what ways are autistic children who acquire some functional language similar to, or different from, normal children acquiring language? And second, How can we apply psycholinguistic principles to the treatment of mute or minimally verbal autistic children? In this chapter, I will briefly review the research directed at both these issues and will then present an alternative approach to these issues demonstrating how I believe developmental psycholinguistics can make its greatest impact in furthering our understanding of the autistic child's language and communication deficits.

## RESEARCH COMPARING AUTISTIC AND NORMAL CHILDREN

Research that has addressed the central question of how the language acquired by autistic children compares to the language acquired by normal children has generally followed the path taken by child language researchers.

HELEN TAGER-FLUSBERG • Department of Psychology, University of Massachusetts, Boston, Massachusetts 02125. Preparation of this chapter was supported by a grant from the National Institute of Mental Health (MH-37074).

Early work, conducted during the mid-seventies, was directed toward the acquisition of structural properties of language, primarily phonology and syntax. More recently, interest has shifted to pragmatic functioning and communicative competence in autistic children. This line of comparative research has relied on the approaches and methodology developed within normal language acquisition research, but like other applied research, it has tended to lag behind basic developmental work by a number of years.

Studies conducted within this developmental psycholinguistic framework have typically examined one particular aspect of language, such as phoneme production, the use of certain grammatical constructions, or a specific pragmatic ability, in a cross-sectional sample of autistic children matched to one or more control groups. There are thorny methodological questions concerning the appropriate control groups to be used and the kinds of measures on which subjects should be matched. Studies typically use normal children as one control group and may add mentally retarded or developmental aphasic children as additional controls. Matching is usually accomplished on the basis of mental-age level, either verbal or nonverbal, and, in some cases, both. We have learned a good deal about how autistic children function with language, although, by definition perhaps, this research has focused exclusively on verbal autistic children.

The major findings from this body of work have led to the proposal that autistic children who develop at least some functional language show no significant deviations from the normal developmental path in their acquisition of phonology and syntax (Tager-Flusberg, 1981a). The seminal studies conducted by Bartolucci and his colleagues have provided much of the data leading to these conclusions, many of which have been supported by more recent research.

In one study, Bartolucci, Pierce, Streiner, and Eppel (1976) elicited phonemes from autistic, mentally retarded, and normal children matched on nonverbal mental age in a picture-naming task. They found the same frequency distribution of various phonemes across the subject groups, as well as the same distribution of error patterns. These findings were replicated by Boucher (1976a) in England. In a later study, Bartolucci and Pierce (1977) looked at how well autistic children could discriminate differences in speech sounds and found that their performance was comparable to that of retarded and normal children. Overall, then, there are no significant phonological deficits in autistic children.

Similar findings have been reported, with respect to syntactic development, in those children who develop productive language. For example, Pierce and Bartolucci (1977) analyzed 50 utterances from matched autistic, retarded, and normal children. They found that all the children were developing a rule-governed grammatical system that was similar across the subject groups. The autistic children, however, were less advanced in the kinds of rules that they employed compared to the control groups, a finding that has not been explained in the literature. We will return to this issue later in the chapter. The general finding that autistic children use appropriate syntax has been confirmed by Cantwell and his colleagues (Cantwell, Baker, & Rutter, 1978; Cantwell, Howlin, & Rutter, 1977), and it is true both for spontaneous speech and echolalic speech (Howlin, 1982). In addition to using syntactic rules in production, I found that autistic children were comparable to matched normal control children in their use of syntactic rules and strategies in sentence comprehension (Tager-Flusberg, 1981b).

Although there are general similarities in the way phonology and syntax develop in autistic and normal children, there are some differences that have been reported in other aspects of language development. Bartolucci, Pierce, and Streiner (1980) examined the use of grammatical morphology in the spontaneous speech of autistic, retarded, and normal children. Overall, children in all the groups demonstrated proficient use of the morphemes examined; however, the autistic children tended to omit certain ones to a greater extent than the control subjects. Specifically, they had some difficulty with verb endings (e.g., past tense -ed) and articles (e.g., a, the). Bartolucci and his colleagues explain these findings in terms of a problem that autistic children have in encoding the meanings encompassed by these morphemes, rather than a grammatical deficit.

More profound deficits have been identified in the way autistic children make use of language as a system of communication in social contexts. It is now generally accepted that autism involves a primary deficit in pragmatics (e.g., Baltaxe & Simmons, 1981; Fay & Schuler, 1980; Tager-Flusberg, 1981a), which may also be linked to their deficits in nonverbal communication. Of course, Kanner himself identified the communication problems of autistic children in his original definition of the syndrome (Kanner, 1943), and they remain one of the cardinal features at the intersection of language and social dysfunction.

Recent psycholinguistic research has led to a more precise definition of the nature of the pragmatic and communicative deficits and to the development of a methodology with which to measure and compare autistic and normal pragmatic functioning. Although no control subjects were employed, the work of Shapiro and his colleagues, in the early seventies, was important for first demonstrating, empirically rather than clinically, the severe communicative deficits in a group of profoundly disturbed psychotic children, which included some children fitting the diagnostic characteristics of autism (Shapiro & Fish, 1969; Shapiro, Chiarandini, & Fish, 1974; Shapiro, Fish, & Ginsberg, 1972; Shapiro, Huebner, & Campbell, 1974).

More recently, Ball (1978) compared a small number of autistic, developmental aphasic, and normal children matched on verbal mental age. Using transcripts of spontaneous speech, she found that the autistic children were more significantly delayed and limited in their development of speech acts than either control group. Baltaxe (1977) identified a number of pragmatic impairments in the dialogues of high-functioning autistic children, which persisted into adolescence. In general, autistic children have the most severe difficulties in conducting a dialogue (Baltaxe, 1977), maintaining a topic (Tager-Flusberg, 1981c), and monitoring their listeners' needs (Langdell, 1981).

Other research has illustrated that some aspects of communicative functioning may not be affected by autism. For example, Prizant and Duchan (1981) demonstrated that highly echolalic autistic children may use echolalia for a variety of communicative purposes (see also Fay, 1969; Schuler, 1979). Hurtig and his colleagues (Hurtig, Ensrud, & Tomblin, 1980) showed that repetitive questioning in verbal autistic children also served important communicative functions. And Paccia-Cooper, Curcio, and Sacharko (1981) and Tager-Flusberg (1981c) reported a fairly high degree of appropriate responding in verbal autistic children, although these children differed from normal children in their lack of initiating conversation. Echolalia and stereotyped language are now seen as primitive strategies for communicating, especially in the context of poor comprehension. The current picture of autistic children is that they do attempt to communicate, albeit using primitive and idiosyncratic means, and that they can at times, in some contexts, but never under all circumstances, use language appropriately. Nevertheless, pragmatic deficits are a significant feature of the syndrome.

Despite the recent proliferation of psycholinguistic studies, there remain serious gaps in our knowledge of language acquisition in autism. For example, because there have been no longitudinal studies since Cunningham's in 1966 (which predated the current era in language acquisition research), we know very little about the sequence in which phonemes, grammatical constructions, and vocabulary develop or the processes by which they are acquired. Thus, we do not know whether the same developmental processes are involved in acquiring language by autistic and normal children. The lack of detailed work in this area severely limits any conclusions about such issues that can be drawn from the meager data scattered in the literature. Even more surprising is the virtual absence of any empirical research on semantic development in autism. Although numerous researchers have postulated that autism involves a primary semantic and related conceptual deficit (e.g., Bartolucci *et al.*, 1980; Caparulo & Cohen, 1977; Fay & Schuler, 1980; Menyuk, 1978; Ricks & Wing, 1976; Schwartz, 1981; Tager-Flusberg, 1981a), there are no studies that directly test the hypothesis. Finally, very little has been done on the interrelationships in development of the various aspects of language in autistic children and the relationships among language acquisition, cognitive development, and social development. These are just a few areas in which new research is sorely needed. Clearly, there is still a great deal of work to be done in this vein before we have a complete answer to the question of how autistic children compare with normal children or with other language-disordered and -delayed children in their acquisition of language.

## PSYCHOLINGUISTIC APPLICATIONS
## TO TREATMENT PROGRAMS

The psycholinguistic approach not only provides a framework for investigating language acquisition in verbal autistic children, it can also contribute to the treatment of autistic children who are more limited in their language skills. Far fewer studies have focused on this applied issue, perhaps because most psycholinguists see themselves as primarily concerned with basic research questions. One exception is the work of Blank and Milewski (1981) on a training program, designed according to current psycholinguistic principles, that was used successfully with one autistic child. Their subject was 4 years old, high functioning, and hyperlexic, but minimally verbal. The researchers were concerned with teaching this child to use grammatical morphemes productively. The ways in which the morphemes combined with nouns and verbs were taught through imitation (taking advantage of the child's echolalia), and their semantic properties, or meaning, were taught using a question–answer format. The child had to use complete sentences to answer questions about situations, pictures, and events that were posed by the therapist. Unlike other remediation programs, these researchers included many different sentence types and taught many new grammatical forms simultaneously in order to maximize generalization [an approach based on a proposal by Maratsos and Chalkley (1980), on how syntactic categories are acquired in normal children]. The results of the training, which was continued by the parents, were dramatic: The child showed significant improvement in his language and related nonlinguistic skills. He spontaneously began learning new constructions, and also mastered the morphemes that were explicitly trained. He began playing symbolically and markedly reduced his stereotyped activities. Interestingly, Blank and Milewski (1981) report that he still showed some pragmatic deficits, especially when he could not understand language addressed to him.

The main contribution that psycholinguistics can make to intervention programs is to provide guidance on the content of such programs. For example, the therapist can use psycholinguistic principles in deciding answers to such questions as What features of language should the child be taught? In what order should they be presented? How should the content of the intervention program be organized? Psycholinguistic principles can be applied to deal with these issues in a variety of programs: in training sign language, speech, or other communication modes and in using a variety of training methods and even behavior modification techniques. The role of psycholinguistics in language therapy for the autistic child has been discussed recently by Fay and Schuler (1980) and Prizant (1982a), although not much has been published on the topic. Still, many training programs, and speech-language pathologists and educators have, during the past few years, made implicit, if not explicit, use of psycholinguistic concepts in grappling with these issues.

Thus far, I have reviewed two important approaches through which psycholinguistics has contributed to our understanding of the language and communication deficits of the autistic child. There is a third approach through which I believe developmental psycholinguistics can add to the eventual solution of these problems in a potentially significant way, an approach that has been relatively neglected until now, but that I hope will characterize much of the research of the next decade.

## RESEARCH ROOTED IN THEORIES OF LANGUAGE ACQUISITION

Most of the past research on the basic and applied issues of language in autistic children, summarized above, was not rooted in the theoretical foundation that has been rapidly developing within the field of developmental psycholinguistics. Instead, what it has taken from normal language acquisition research has been limited to methodological innovations and a way of analyzing the linguistic system. I would like to propose that research questions that are based on theories of language acquisition will ultimately prove to be the most fruitful.

Past psycholinguistic research on autism has clearly not been atheoretical; rather, it has been guided primarily by theories of autistic deficits and only minimally by general theories of the process of language acquisition. Probably 5 years ago, theories of language acquisition were not sufficiently developed to have been of use to those concerned with autistic language, so it is not surprising that they were essentially ignored. But that has changed recently, and in the rest of this chapter we will consider one domain of language, namely, syntax, in which there have been a number of significant theoretical advances that can be of potential importance in understanding language acquisition in autistic children. I will specifically address the kinds of predictions that emerge from theories of normal language development regarding the possible language deficits that one could uncover in autism, and discuss how such a theoretically based approach can integrate some of the research findings reviewed above. In essence, we can use theories of normal language acquisition to address the two issues (how autistic children's language compares to that of normal children;

the content of intervention programs) with which this chapter began. Such theories can provide more specific hypotheses and predictions around which future research on these issues can be designed. Ultimately, of course, language research on autism must consider both theories of language acquisition and theories of autistic deficits. By taking this route, psycholinguistic research on autistic language and communication will not only enrich our understanding of the nature of autism; it will also enrich our knowledge of the basic language acquisition process.

## Current Theories of Syntactic Development

The domain of syntax, which we will be exploring here, has received a good deal of attention from developmental psycholinguists in recent years. One of the primary lessons that has been learned from the field of linguistics is that syntax is a wondrously complex and abstract system. Indeed, it is quite remarkable that normal children, let alone autistic children, ever acquire the syntactic knowledge that they evidently possess about how morphemes and words combine to create sentences. That they do so in such a relatively short period of time is one of the key mysteries that child language researchers are trying to solve. In response to the obvious complexity of syntax, a number of major theorists propose that there is a language-specific system that governs certain aspects of syntactic processing that is independent of other aspects of language and other cognitive systems. For many, this autonomous component is innate; however, there is still a good deal of controversy about the precise nature of this putative innate component. Whereas the nature of the innate faculty is still being debated, the hypothesis that language, specifically syntax, has some independence from other cognitive systems has become generally (though not universally) accepted among child language researchers.

The history of this so-called "task-specificity" hypothesis in language acquisition has been far from straightforward. During the sixties, following the revolution in linguistics and psycholinguistics brought about by Chomsky (1957), the idea that language was innate and independent of other cognitive systems was quite readily accepted (e.g., McNeill, 1970). But child language research of the seventies began to focus on the role of the special properties of the linguistic input to which children are apparently exposed, as well as the possible cognitive and social bases of linguistic development. This led to new theories of language acquisition that denied the need for a language-specific component and, instead, proposed that language develops out of more primary social and cognitive accomplishments of the infancy period (e.g., Cromer, 1974; Snow, 1979). At the same time, the pendulum began to swing away from nativism. In the past few years, these newer developmental theories have been highly criticized for being simplistic and not having sufficient explanatory power (e.g., Bates, Bretherton, Beeghly-Smith, & McNew, 1982; Maratsos & Chalkley, 1980), primarily because many aspects of syntactic development are purely formal in nature and thus cannot be reduced to social interaction or general cognition. For example, in English the primary way meaning relations are expressed in a sentence is through the use of word order. Thus typically, sentence subjects (usually the semantic agent or initiator of action) come before the verb, and sentence objects (usually the semantic patient or thing acted upon) come after the verb. Other languages may express these same relations using different word order (e.g., Japanese), or they may rely on noun affixes rather than word order to indicate the basic relations in a sentence. Neither a particular word order nor a set of affixes could plausibly be derived from some non-verbal aspect of cognition or social interaction; instead, these are purely formal linguistic devices that children must learn for the particular language to which they are exposed. This realization has led to a return to a language-specific, partially nativist perspective among many child language researchers.

Although there is a consensus that syntax has some independence from other aspects of language and cognition, it is also generally recognized that syntactic development does not take place in a vacuum. There is an accumulating body of evidence that the course of syntactic development goes far beyond the autonomous, probably innate component. Syntactic development is also influenced (but not fully determined) by additional factors, including conceptual, semantic, contextual, and input factors. The work of Lois Bloom (e.g., Bloom, 1973; Bloom, Lahey, Hood, Lifter, & Fiess, 1980; Bloom, Lifter, & Hafitz, 1980), for example, has demonstrated the importance of semantics in the acquisition of a number of grammatical constructions, including verb inflectional morphology and sentence connectives. A recent review of research on the acquisition of English syntax by de Villiers and de Villiers (in press) illustrates the important role played by a variety of extra-syntactic factors in the development of grammatical rules.

One current viewpoint in developmental psycholinguistics is that not all syntactic rules are equal: They show different sensitivities to these extra-syntactic factors, and especially environmental factors. There are certain syntactic rules that are exceedingly robust and they develop under the most deprived conditions. These are rules that, for example, children acquiring language without the benefit of a rich and tailored input language (such as deaf children of hearing parents who were studied by Goldin-Meadow, 1977; or hearing children of deaf parents who were studied by Sachs, Bard, and Johnson, 1981) nevertheless make use of in their multi-word utterances. According to some theoretical accounts, these robust syntactic rules are likely candidates for the autonomous, innate language component; at least the child seems to be constrained to seek such rules for the grammars of language they construct.

One example of such a robust rule has been proposed by Gleitman and Wanner (1982), who argue that from the beginning children are highly sensitive to the order of words. They are likely to develop very early a rule that assigns the grammatical (subject, object) or semantic (agent, patient) roles of a sentence on the basis of word order. Not only do children extract word order information from the input, they also use strict sequences of words in their earliest multi-word utterances. Word order is typically the first syntactic rule that young children who are learning many different languages employ. It is a rule not readily influenced by extra-syntactic factors, and contrary to earlier accounts, it cannot be reduced to social interaction or general cognitive processing.

Other aspects of grammatical development in normal children are apparently more sensitive to external influences. For example, the acquisition of grammatical morphology and the auxiliary system of English has been shown to be influenced by the language input. In one study, Newport, Gleitman, and Gleitman (1977) showed that children who were extensively exposed to specific kinds of input, namely, many *yes/no* questions, learned auxiliaries at a faster rate than children whose mothers used fewer such questions. This result is interpreted as demonstrating the influence of input, as children who hear many *yes/no* questions hear auxiliaries in the highly salient initial position of the sentence. Gleitman and Wanner (1982) suggest that rules governing the use of closed class or function words, such as morphemes and auxiliaries, will be more susceptible, or sensitive, to environmental influence.

Thus far, we have considered a number of proposals about what the significant influences on syntactic development are. But we have not considered a crucial question: How does a child break into the grammatical system in the first place? The initial step requires breaking up the continuous stream of sound into words. This is an extremely complex task that the child faces; it has been likened to the problem of an adult listening to people speaking a foreign language. One hears what sounds like a continuous word composed of indistinct sounds that needs to be segmented into basic units. Beyond this phase, the child must then distinguish the major content words, primarily nouns and verbs, and perform some grammatical analyses in order to determine the basic form-meaning relations within a sentence; that is, who is doing what to whom, and so forth.

According to Gleitman and Wanner (1982), young normal children exploit their perception of stress to pick out the key content words of the language addressed to them. In this way, they selectively listen to content words (nouns and verbs) at the earliest stages, and they use only stressed content words in constructing their earliest two-word sentences. Thus Gleitman and Wanner hypothesize that normal children use stress as a "bootstrap" into the linguistic system, which nevertheless requires a high-level sophisticated analysis of input into its basic components. The initial rules the child develops are based solely on content words that are more salient and easily picked out by the child. These rules are word order rules, which, as we saw earlier, are considered to be fairly robust. Later, the child begins to develop grammatical rules that apply to closed class words, such as morphological rules, and auxiliary rules, which are more sensitive to extra-syntactic factors.

In this section I have provided a sketchy summary of the main proposals to have emerged from recent theorizing on constraints and processes in syntactic development in normal children. It is these proposals that can advance our understanding of how language might develop in the verbal autistic child and what impedes language acquisition in those autistic children who never develop productive language. In the next section we will consider some of the implications that emerge from this theoretical perspective and discuss the directions that future researach on autistic language might take.

## Implications for Syntactic Development in Autism

Let us examine how the theoretical proposals described above can shape our understanding of language acquisition in autism. We can begin with the currently accepted hypothesis that syntactic development involves language-specific, probably innate mechanisms and consider how this influences language development, specifically in those autistic children who do eventually acquire some functional language. We know that many of these children achieve this despite severe cognitive and communicative limitations, and some research supports this view. For example, I demonstrated in a group of verbal autistic children matched to a group of normal children on verbal mental age that for the autistic subjects, syntactic ability was independent of discourse ability (Tager-Flusberg, 1981c). In these autistic children, discourse ability, that is, knowledge about the rules governing conversations, including turn-taking and maintaining a topic, but not syntax, was closely related to social functioning. Similarly, there is some limited evidence that syntactic functioning is independent of semantic functioning in autistic children. In a study of sentence comprehension (Tager-Flusberg, 1981b), I found that the use of syntactic strategies (which was comparable to that of matched normal children) was unrelated to the use of semantic strategies in the autistic subjects. The use of a semantic strategy is closely tied to cognitive functioning and there is an apparent deficit in autism in making use of semantic knowledge (see also Hermelin & O'Connor, 1970; Menyuk, 1978; Schwartz, 1981). Clearly, then, autistic children are not using social interaction or general cognitive abilities on which to construct the grammar of their language. On the contrary, verbal autistic children can be taken as good evidence in support of the language-independence hypothesis, for in at least some of these children the syntactic system is not especially deficient (cf. Curtiss, 1982).

Because some proportion of the autistic population does develop some functional language, Boucher (1976b) and Fein and Waterhouse (1979) have argued that autism is not a disorder of language. At this time, there is too little data on the process of language acquisition in verbal autistic children to allow one to draw such dramatic conclusions. Nevertheless the fact that verbal autistic children show no specific deviances in phonology or syntax probably has some significant implications for models of neurological deficits in autism. Specifically, the hypothesis that the left hemisphere of autistic children is dysfunctional, which has been proposed by numerous researchers (e.g., Blackstock, 1978; Prior & Bradshaw, 1979; Ricks & Wing, 1976), is not supported by this pattern of language ability in autistic children (cf. Tager-Flusberg, 1981a). Our current knowledge of the developmental neurological underpinning of language and related functions is still in its infancy, and therefore, great caution is required in building neuropsychological theories of autism. Certainly, even a high-functioning autistic child does not resemble the children studied by Dennis and Whitaker (1976) whose left hemispheres were removed, and therefore a simple theory of left hemisphere deficit is *a priori* untenable. As we learn more about language ability and language deficit in the autistic child we can develop more sophisticated hypotheses about the neurological deficits associated with this syndrome.

Let us turn now to considering how syntax might indeed develop in these verbal autistic children. As was stated earlier, this crucial question has not been adequately studied, so little is actually known about the process of development. Nevertheless, based on what is currently known about normal syntactic development and the primary deficits in autism, one could predict that there will be some differences in the course of syntactic development in normal and autistic children.

Consider the proposal that there are two classes of syntactic rules: in one class, the rules are robust, develop early, even under quite deprived conditions, and are not easily influenced by extra-syntactic factors; in the second class, the rules are less robust, develop later, and are more susceptible to extra-syntactic influence. These distinctions in classes of syntactic rules can be used to construct hypotheses about syntactic development in autism. I would like to propose that the acquisition of those syntactic rules that are independent of other factors, for example, word order rules, will be similar in verbal autistic children and normal children (and indeed, other language-disordered children). However, linguistic rules that are sensitive in development to nonsyntactic factors, be they semantic, environmental, or conceptual, will not necessarily develop in exactly comparable ways in normal and autistic children. These grammatical rules may be more vulnerable; their acquisition may be more markedly delayed; and their order of emergence may vary from the normal order. As the nature of the cognitive–semantic and social deficits in autism is defined more clearly, it will be possible to predict exactly which of these sensitive apsects of syntax will be more affected in autistic children's language acquisition.

Much of the existing, but limited literature on syntactic development in autistic children fits this hypothesis. For example, I found no differences between autistic and normal children in their ability to use word order strategies in sentence comprehension (Tager-Flusberg, 1981b). Both groups of children showed that they used the sequence of words in sentences, or anomolous word strings, to infer the basic semantic relationships about agent and patient. Word order is a robust syntactic rule in both normal and autistic children. Similarly, in the study by Pierce and Bartolucci (1977) described earlier, it was shown that the grammatical system of autistic children was as rule-governed, with respect to rules of sequence, as matched mentally retarded and normal children.

Yet recall that the autistic children in this study were indeed more delayed, and used simpler rules, than the control subjects. We know from research on normal children learning English that many of the later developing syntactic constructions, such as questions, negatives, conjoined sentences, and passive sentences, are influenced in part by semantic and contextual factors (de Villiers & de Villiers, in press). If, as many researchers have proposed, autistic children suffer a primary semantic deficit, and are thus unable to use semantic information appropriately and are relatively unaware of their surroundings and therefore less efficient in using contextual information, then we could predict that those aspects of syntax that are differentially influenced by semantic and contextual factors will be adversely affected in autistic children. More research is clearly needed to test this hypothesis.

One study supports the hypothesis that at least some sensitive grammatical rules, as defined by Gleitman and Wanner (1982), are adversely affected in autistic children. In the study cited earlier by Bartolucci et al. (1980), which focused on the acquisition of 14 grammatical morphemes, there were differences between the autistic and control groups. Certain morphemes that are known to be influenced by linguistic input and that entail certain semantic properties were deviant in the autistic children. Thus it does appear that some grammatical rules are more adversely affected in autistic language development, as predicted by the hypothesis discussed here.

We cannot make extravagant claims about strong supporting evidence from these few existing studies, which were not designed to test the hypothesis under consideration. The purpose of presenting these studies again in this context is more to demonstrate the potential usefulness of this theoretical framework as a way of organizing investigations into syntactic development in autistic children. Even more important is the hope that future research can be based on more precise predictions in order to test the viability of the hypothesis that robust and sensitive syntactic rules will be differentially affected in autistic children.

Ultimately, training programs for autistic children will be of benefit, if indeed this hypothesis receives substantial empirical support. It makes strong claims about which areas of syntax should be given primary attention in therapy and which areas of syntax should not. Thus rules that are considered robust, like word order rules, need not be explicitly taught, whereas the vulnerable rules of morphology, auxiliary verbs, and complex syntax ought to become the focus of intervention programs. Before these suggestions are put into practice, though, more basic research on syntactic development in autistic children is needed to confirm or disconfirm this hypothesis.

Thus far, we have considered how theories of normal language acquisition can influence our understanding of syntactic development in verbal autistic children. But many, perhaps one-half of even the verbal autistic population do not acquire functional language; instead these children remain primarily echolalic, using little spontaneous speech. How can we begin to understand what distinguishes those children who develop functional language from those who are merely echolalic? There are a number of possible explanations, yet at this time they are tentative and none have sufficient support from the existing literature.

For example, one possibility is that echolalic children may suffer from organic impairments that damage the biological substrate of language, such as the left hemisphere. This is the least likely possibility: It makes assumptions about language localization that are still speculative. It also postulates qualitative differences in the neurological organization of verbal and echolalic autistic children, a proposal that some researchers would view with skepticism. Still, one could salvage this neurological explanation by suggesting that different syndromes might be associated with echolalic and verbal autistic children, although no one has yet offered this suggestion.

A different explanation might be that echolalic (as well as mute) autistic children lack the interest or ability to communicate and therefore have shunned spontaneous language, which is, after all, a system for communication. This proposal has the advantage over the neurological one in that it places echolalic autistic children more on a continuum with verbal autistic children, as they too show severe deficits in communicating effectively. This hypothesis essentially argues that mute and echolalic autistic children suffer primarily in their lack of social skill and motivation to communicate, both verbally and nonverbally. If one could increase their need and desire to communicate, functional language might at least begin to develop if the potential for language exists. The main problem with this hypothesis is that it is not consonant with some of the research cited earlier that demonstrates that even highly echolalic children attempt to use echolalia for a variety of communicative purposes (cf. Prizant & Duchan, 1981). Still, one could argue that since echolalic autistic children are so limited and ineffective in their communicative behavior, they have severe deficits in this domain. Some better theoretical understanding of communication and its relation to social interaction is needed to substantiate this hypothesis; even work on normal communication development has been primarily descriptive. Perhaps research on autistic children can inform basic theory building in this area of social and communicative development.

We can consider a third possible interpretation of why many autistic children fail to develop functional language, an interpretation that is more directly rooted in current theories of language development. Specifically, one might postulate that although echolalic autistic children do have the necessary biological substrate for language, and some minimal motivation to communicate, they may be incapable of entering the linguistic system. Recall the earlier discussion of Gleitman and Wanner's (1982) proposal that normal children rely on stress to segment incoming sounds into words and select key content words from which they begin to construct a basic grammar. One intriguing possibility is that echolalic and mute autistic children have specific difficulty in using this stress "bootstrap." From a quite different direction, Prizant (1982b) has also proposed that autistic children cannot analyze or segment an acoustic message into its discrete units—words. He suggests that their use of echolalia reflects an alternative, "gestalt" or wholistic method of language processing, which may be the only way that autistic children can ever break into the linguistic system. Austistic children cannot segment input into words; instead they treat sentences and phrases as unanalyzed chunks. We have here the beginnings of a convergence between theories of normal language acquisition and theories of autistic deficit, although there is obviously a great deal of research to be done to test these theories.

Why should autistic children not make use of stress to pick out key content words from input? There is contradictory evidence in the literature on the prosodic abilities and deficits of autistic children. In one of the few relevant and well-controlled studies, Frith (1969) showed that autistic children could, in fact, distinguish between stressed and unstressed words, especially if content words were stressed. This study grants autistic children precisely the requisite ability that Gleitman and Wanner (1982) suggest is needed to begin developing syntactic skills. In a different study, Cooper and Curcio (1979) found that autistic children who were echolalic mimicked the exact prosody of sentences that were presented to them, which they could not understand, thus showing that they must have been able to perceive the stress variations in the sentences in order to have reproduced them. But there are other researchers who claim that autistic children are deficient in their perception and production of prosody, for example, Baltaxe and Simmons (1981) and Simon (1975). Certainly many autistic children, both echolalic and highly verbal, have striking peculiarities in their intonation and voice quality, which points to some deficit in prosodic control. Thus there are conflicting views and seemingly contradictory evidence on the nature of prosodic functioning in autistic children.

The evidence itself is sparse and can be interpreted in a number of ways. Baltaxe and Simmons (1981) and Simon (1975) seem, in their arguments about prosodic deficits in autism, to equate production with perception, and not enough attention has been paid to distinct prosodic features (such as volume, pitch variation, voice quality, and timing). One way to resolve this conflict over hypothesized prosodic and stress deficits in autism is to consider that autistic children differ individually. Those who have less difficulty acquiring functional language and are not echolalic may not be impaired in their perception of stress. This would follow from Gleitman and Wanner's proposal, and there is some evidence of this in the literature. Frith's subjects appear to have been relatively highly verbal, although she does not report how much language they acquired, and so it is not surprising that they were able to perceive stress. Baltaxe and Simmons (1977) reported that among seven autistic subjects there were individual differences in prosodic functioning and that those children who showed more prosodic deficits were also less advanced in their syntactic development. Individual differences may hold the key to understanding the relationship between prosodic functioning and syntactic ability.

There are still large gaps in research on this topic that need to be filled. Only then will these issues be resolved and a number of important, yet unanswered questions will be addressed. There have been almost no systematic studies on stress and related prosodic features, either in normal or in autistic children. Some of the questions that need to be answered include: Do some autistic children have difficulty perceiving stress? If so, do they encounter problems in stress perception for nonverbal as well as verbal stimuli, or is their deficit restricted to verbal stimuli alone? Is their perception of other intonational features, such as pitch and timing, also impaired? Are their perceptual deficits linked to deficits in prosodic production? Can training help autistic children who show such deficits overcome their difficulties? And with respect to the hypothesis under consideration here, do those autistic children who are impaired in their perception of stress show related delays and abnormalities (such as excessive echolalia) in the early stages of syntactic development? From the theory that stress perception provides entry into the linguistic system, as proposed by Gleitman and Wanner (1982), we would predict such a relationship between deficits in stress perception and language development (except perhaps in those children who are hyperlexic, and latch onto reading as an alternative way of segmenting speech into words).

In this section I have tried to demonstrate how a hypothesis about the normal language acquisition process provides an underpinning for proposals from research in autism and, in turn, helps to frame critical research questions. The answers, which I hope will be forthcoming, will provide insight into autistic functioning and may suggest alternative intervention strategies for nonverbal autistic children. If these children cannot perceive stress and are hampered in the earliest stages of language development, alternative methods, such as using sign language or presenting modified input in the form of key content words only, might be helpful training techniques. In addition such research will provide a critical test of Gleitman and Wanner's important hypothesis.

## CONCLUSIONS

In the last part of this chapter, I have described a number of avenues by which current theories of syntactic development can increase our understanding of language development in highly verbal and nonverbal or echolalic autistic children. Theories from developmental psycholinguistics of phonological, semantic, and pragmatic development can also be exploited in a similar way. This approach of basing research on language in autism on theories of normal language acquisition can direct research comparing autistic and normal children toward the most promising areas for investigation and help formulate more precise questions and predictions. This will lead to an enriched understanding of language functioning in autistic children. This approach also has the potential for contributing to psycholinguistically oriented therapy by specifying more exactly which aspects of language should be targeted by the therapy.

## REFERENCES

Ball, J. (1978). *A pragmatic analysis of autistic children's language with respect to aphasic and normal language development.* Unpublished doctoral dissertation, Melbourne University, Melbourne, Australia.

Baltaxe, C. A. M. (1977). Pragmatic deficits in the language of adolescent autistics. *Journal of Pediatric Psychology, 2,* 176–180.

Baltaxe, C. A. M., & Simmons, J. Q. (1977). Bedtime soliloquies and linguistic competence in autism. *Journal of Speech and Hearing Disorders, 42,* 376–393.

Baltaxe, C. A. M., & Simmons, J. A. (1981). Disorders of language in childhood psychosis: Current concepts and approaches. In J. Darby (Ed.), *Speech evaluation in psychiatry* (pp. 285–328). New York: Grune & Stratton.

Bartolucci, G., & Pierce, S. J. (1977). A preliminary comparison of phonological development in autistic, normal, and mentally retarded subjects. *British Journal of Disorders of Communication, 12,* 137–147.

Bartolucci, G., Pierce, S. J., & Streiner, D. (1980). Cross-sectional studies of grammatical morphemes in autistic and mentally retarded children. *Journal of Autism and Developmental Disorders, 10,* 39–50.

Bartolucci, G., Pierce, S. J., Streiner, D., & Eppel, P. T. (1976). Phonological investigation of verbal autistic and mentally retarded subjects. *Journal of Autism and Childhood Schizophrenia, 6,* 303–316.

Bates, E., Bretherton, I., Beeghly-Smith, M., & McNew, S. (1982). Social bases of language development: A reassessment. In L. Lipsitt & H. Reese (Eds.), *Advances in child development and behavior, Vol. 16,* (pp. 7–75). New York: Academic Press.

Blackstock, E. G. (1978). Cerebral asymmetry and the development of early infantile autism. *Journal of Autism and Childhood Schizophrenia, 8,* 339-353.

Blank, M., & Milewski, J. (1981). Applying psycholinguistic concepts to the treatment of an autistic child. *Applied psycholinguistics, 2,* 65-84.

Bloom, L. (1973). *Language development: Form and function in emerging grammars.* Cambridge, MA: MIT Press.

Bloom, L., Lahey, M., Hood, L., Lifter, K., & Fiess, K. (1980). Complex sentences: Acquisition of syntactic connectives and the semantic relations they encode. *Journal of Child Language, 7,* 235-261.

Bloom, L., Lifter, K., & Hafitz, J. (1980). Sematic of verbs and the development of verb inflection in child language. *Language, 56,* 386-412.

Boucher, J. (1976a). Articulation in early childhood autism. *Journal of Autism and Childhood Schizophrenia, 6,* 297-302.

Boucher, J. (1976b). Is autism primarily a language disorder? *British Journal of Disorders of Communication, 11,* 135-143.

Cantwell, D., Howlin, P., & Rutter, M. (1977). The analysis of language level and language function: A methodological study. *British Journal of Disorders of Communication, 12,* 119-135.

Cantwell, D., Baker, L., & Rutter, M. (1978). A comparative study of infantile autism and specific developmental receptive language disorder: IV. Analysis of syntax and language function. *Journal of Child Psychology and Child Psychiatry, 19,* 351-362.

Caparulo, B. K., & Cohen, D. J. (1977). Cognitive structures, language, and emerging social competence in autistic and aphasic children. *Journal of the American Academy of Child Psychiatry, 16,* 620-645.

Chomsky, N. (1957). *Syntactic structures.* The Hague, The Netherlands: Mouton Press.

Cooper, J. P., & Curcio, F. (1979, September). *Language processing and forms of echolalia in severely disturbed children.* Paper presented at the Fourth Annual Boston University Conference on Language Development, Boston, MA.

Cromer, R. (1974). The development of language and cognition: The cognition hypothesis. In B. Foss (Ed.), *New perspectives in child development* (pp. 184-252). Baltimore, MD: Penguin.

Cunningham, M. A. (1966). A five-year study of the language of an autistic child. *Journal of Child Psychology and Psychiatry, 7,* 143-154.

Curtiss, S. (1982). Developmental dissociation of language and cognition. In L. K. Obler & L. Menn (Eds.), *Exceptional language and linguistics* (pp. 285-312). New York: Academic Press.

Dennis, M., & Whitaker, H. A. (1976). Language acquisition following hemidecortication: Linguistic superiority of the left over the right hemisphere. *Brain and Language, 3,* 404-433.

de Villiers, J. G., & de Villiers, P. A. (in press). The acquisition of English. In D. I. Slobin (Ed.), *The cross-linguistic study of language acquisition.* Hillsdale, NJ: Lawrence Erlbaum Associates.

Fay, W. (1969). On the basis of autistic echolalia. *Journal of Communication Disorders, 2,* 38-47.

Fay, W., & Schuler, A. (1980). *Emerging language in autistic children.* Baltimore, MD: University Park Press.

Fein, D., & Waterhouse, L. (1979, February). *Autism is not a disorder of language.* Paper presented at the New England Child Language Association, Boston, MA.

Frith, U. A. (1969). Emphasis and meaning in recall in normal and autistic children. *Language and Speech, 12,* 29-38.

Gleitman, L., & Wanner, E. (1982). Language acquisition: The state of the state of the art. In E. Wanner & L. Gleitman (Eds.), *Language acquisition: State of the art.* (pp. 3-48). New York: Cambridge University Press.

Goldin-Meadow, S. (1977). Structure in a manual communication system developed without a conventional language model: Language without a helping hand. In H. Whitaker & H. A.

Whitaker (Eds.), *Studies in neurolinguistics (vol. 4)* (pp. 125–209). New York: Academic Press.

Hermelin, B., & O'Connor, N. (1970). *Psychological experiments with autistic children.* Oxford: Pergamon Press.

Howlin, P. (1982). Echolalic and spontaneous phrase speech in autistic children. *Journal of Child Psychology and Psychiatry, 23,* 281–293.

Hurtig, R., Ensrud, S., & Tomblin, J. B. (1980, June). *Question production in autistic children: A linguistic pragmatic perspective.* Paper presented at the University of Wisconsin–Madison Symposium on Research in Child Language Disorders, Madison, WI.

Kanner, L. (1943). Autistic disturbances of affective contact. *Nervous Child, 2,* 217–250.

Langdell, T. R. (1981, July). *Pragmatic aspects of autism.* Paper presented at the National Society for Autistic Children International Symposium for Research on Autism, Boston, MA.

Maratsos, M.P., & Chalkley, M. A. (1980). The internal language of children's syntax: The ontognesis and representation of syntactic categories. In K. Nelson (Ed.), *Children's language* (Vol. 2) (pp. 127–214). New York: Gardner Press.

McNeill, D. (1970). *The acquisition of language: The study of developmental psycholinguistics.* New York: Harper & Row.

Menyuk, P. (1978). Language: What's wrong and why. In M. Eurrwe & E. Schopler (Eds.), *Autism: A reappraisal of concepts and treatment* (pp. 105–116). New York: Plenum Press.

Newport, E. L., Gleitman, H., & Gleitman, L. R. (1977). Mother I'd rather do it myself: Some effects and non-effects of maternal speech style. In C. E. Snow & C. A. Ferguson (Eds.), *Talking to children: Language input and acquisition* (pp. 109–149). Cambridge, England: Cambridge University Press.

Paccia-Cooper, J., Curcio, F., & Sacharko, G. (1981, October). *A comparison of discourse features in normal and autistic language.* Paper presented at the Sixth Annual Boston University Child Language Conference, Boston, MA.

Pierce, S. J., & Bartolucci, G. (1977). A syntactic investigation of verbal autistic, mentally retarded, and normal children. *Journal of Autism and Childhood Schizophrenia, 7,*121–134.

Prior, M., & Bradshaw, J. L. (1979). Hemispheric functioning in autistic children. *Cortex, 15,* 73–81.

Prizant, B. M. (1982a). Speech-language pathologists and autistic children: What is our role? *American Speech and Hearing Association, 24,* 463–468; 531–537.

Prizant, B. M. (1982b). Gestalt language and gestalt processing in autism. *Topics in Language Disorders, 3,* 16–23.

Prizant, B. M., & Duchan, J. F. (1981). The functions of immediate echolalia in autistic children. *Journal of Speech and Hearing Disorders, 46,* 241–249.

Ricks, D. M., & Wing, L. (1976). Language communication and the use of symbols. In L. Wing, (Ed.), *Early childhood autism: Clinical, educational and social aspects* (2nd ed., pp. 93–134). New York: Pergamon Press.

Sachs, J. S., Bard, B., & Johnson, M. L. (1981). Language learning with restricted input: Case studies of two hearing children of deaf parents. *Applied Psycholinguistics, 2,* 33–54.

Schuler, A. (1979). Echolalia: Issues and clinical applications. *Journal of Speech and Hearing Disorders, 44,* 411–434.

Schwartz, S. (1981). Language disabilities in infantile autism: A brief review and comment. *Applied Psycholinguistics, 2,* 25–31.

Shapiro, T., & Fish, B. (1969). A method to study language deviation as an aspect of ego organization in young schizophrenic children. *Journal of the American Academy of Child Psychiatry, 8,* 26–56.

Shapiro, T., Fish, B., & Ginsberg, G. L. (1972). The speech of a schizophrenic child from two to six. *American Journal of Psychiatry, 128,* 1408–1414.

Shapiro, T., Chiarandini, I., & Fish, B. (1974). Thirty severely disturbed children. *Archives of General Psychiatry, 30,* 819–825.

Shapiro, T., Huebner, H. F., & Campbell, M. (1974). Language behavior and hierarchic integration in a psychotic child. *Journal of Autism and Childhood Schizophrenia, 4,* 71–90.

Simon, N. (1975). Echolalic speech in childhood autism: Consideration of underlying loci of brain damage. *Archives of General Psychiatry, 32,* 1439–1446.

Snow, C. E. (1979). The role of social interaction in language acquisition. In W. A. Collins (Ed.), *Children's language and communication: The Minnesota symposia on child psychology* (Vol. 12, pp. 157–182). Hillsdale, NJ: Lawrence Erlbaum Associates.

Tager-Flusberg, H. (1981a). On the nature of linguistic functioning in early infantile autism. *Journal of Autism and Developmental Disorders, 11,* 45–56.

Tager-Flusberg, H. (1981b). Sentence comprehension in autistic children. *Applied Psycholinguistics, 2,* 5–24.

Tager-Flusberg, H. (1981c, July). *Pragmatic development and its implications for social functioning in autistic children.* Paper presented at the National Society for Autistic Children International Symposium for Research on Autism, Boston MA.

# 4A

# Converging Perspectives in Psycholinguistics and Behaviorism

## EDWARD G. CARR

It is comforting when two researchers who make widely differing assumptions regarding language and communication develop converging perspectives. Such convergence is enough to make one believe that there is an underlying order in nature. Dr. Helen Tager-Flusberg (Chapter 4) and I (Chapter 3) focus on a number of problems that each of us agrees are well worth addressing, regardless of theoretical orientation. That is not to say that we agree on everything. For instance, I suspect that she would attach much less importance to factors such as operant conditioning and modeling than would I. Nonetheless, there are several noteworthy commonalities that emerged from our respective chapters and it is on these commonalities that I would like to focus.

Tager-Flusberg notes that, traditionally, psycholinguists have been concerned primarily with developing general theories of language. Applied issues pertaining to intervention have therefore not been emphasized. The near-exclusive focus on basic questions has acted to drive a wedge between psycholinguists and behaviorists. The reason for this is that behaviorists have been most concerned with practical treatment issues, particularly those pertaining to children who have severe language disorders. I can remember reading many chapters dealing with psycholinguistic accounts of early language acquisition and coming away frustrated in that I saw no obvious way to apply the results to language-disordered children. Nor did I sense much enthusiasm on the part of psycholinguists to translate research findings so that they could be applied in an intervention format. This situation is now changing. The change is due to

EDWARD G. CARR • Department of Psychology and Suffolk Child Development Center, State University of New York at Stony Brook, Stony Brook, New York 11794.

the emergence of a field of applied psycholinguistics and the willingness of researchers like Tager-Flusberg to address applied issues without losing touch with the data core and methodology of basic language research.

An important point of contact between our respective positions concerns the communicative aspects of language, known technically, in psycholinguistic circles, as pragmatics. The fact that the jargon used by various professionals differs should not blind us to the fact that there are critical similarities at a functional level. Thus, when a behaviorist speaks of *mands* and a psycholinguist speaks of *directives* (or *imperatives*), they are both referring to the same language functions. All these terms refer to the communicative situation in which a child is attempting (e.g., "I want milk") to get an adult to provide a specific object. Similarly, the behavioral term *tact* and the psycholinguistic term *representative* (or *declarative*), are roughly synonymous. These terms pertain to the situation in which the child seeks to maintain a conversational exchange, presumably as a means of attracting social attention from adults (e.g., the child says "it's a doggie," and the adult replies "yes, it is a doggie. Do you know what kind of doggie?" and so on). As Tager-Flusberg points out, psycholinguists have been particularly interested in documenting how autistic and normal children differ in the way they communicate. Given the pervasiveness and seriousness of the pragmatic deficits in autism, it becomes important to isolate and identify the major features that distinguish autistic children from normal children. Knowing what these differences are makes it possible for a treatment agent to target certain skill areas for remediation.

This last point forces us to confront a very basic question, namely, *what should we remediate?* Implicit in my discussion thus far is a point that Tager-Flusberg makes quite explicitly in her chapter, namely, the major contribution that psycholinguistics can make to intervention efforts is in the area of choosing curricular *content*. Behaviorists are justifiably proud of the treatment methods they have developed. Techniques such as prompting, fading, differential reinforcement, and methods of generalization programming are basic to any intervention effort. However, having techniques is not the same as knowing to what areas of skill development these techniques should be applied. As Tager-Flusberg notes, psycholinguistic studies have begun to provide some guidelines concerning specific skill areas that are most in need of remediation. Information is beginning to be available concerning what skills should be taught and in what order they should be taught. Tager-Flusberg appropriately qualifies her enthusiasm for this potential contribution by noting that we do not as yet have enough psycholinguistic data to construct a complete curriculum with confidence. Nonetheless, any empirically minded individual will see the value of having on hand a body of data that would allow an intervention agent to select curriculum items systematically. The ultimate practical test of applied psycholinguistics would consist of a group comparison study in which the various currricula currently in use were pitted against a psycholinguistically derived curriculum. The time for this comparative evaluation is not far off.

In her chapter, Tager-Flusberg suggests that autistic children do not constitute a homogenous group, especially with respect to language. The possible existence of subgroups is a valuable notion clinically in that it suggests the need to identify variables that make distinctions among the subgroups so that appropriate remedial action can be taken. In other words, it is unlikely that we will be able to design a global treatment that works equally well for all children. The search for functional subgroups is one that is increasingly capturing the attention of behaviorists as well (cf. Lovaas, Koegel, Simmons, & Long, 1973).

In line with the notion of subgroups, Tager-Flusberg discusses a number of variables that may help explain why one-half the autistic population fails to acquire functional language. One variable of interest concerns the possible inability of some autistic children to break up the stream of sounds into words. Specifically, these children may not be able to use the stress cues that are present in speech to segment incoming speech into meaningful word units. Most clinicians will appreciate the face validity of this hypothesis, since it is common to find autistic children who use phrases such as "I want a cookie" as if the entire sentence were one word. The treatment implication here is that such children might profit from discrimination training conducted with respect to word stress features.

Continuing on the topic of communication, Tager-Flusberg mentions the possibility that some problems in this area might stem from low social motivation; that is, the children may have a "lack of interest" in interacting with others. In addition, she notes that perceptual dysfunctions, particularly those related to selective, or more precisely, overselective attention (cf. Carr, 1982; Carr & Dores, 1981; Lovaas, Koegel, & Schreibman, 1979) could effectively block the important modulating role that the external environment plays in syntactical development. Of course, insensitivity to external context would also be expected to disrupt conversational exchanges, and thereby inhibit normal communicative development. The important point that I would like to make is that the motivational and perceptual variables described by Tager-Flusberg are also those that concern behaviorists. Once again, then, we have an example of convergent interests among scientists who differ widely in theoretical orientation.

Continued convergence between psycholinguistics and behaviorism seems likely. Perhaps, in the manner of Hegelian dialectics, the disparate viewpoints represented by these two orientations will give rise to a new synthesis. This may cause sadness among some scientists and outright denial among others, but the fact is that evolution is an inevitable process in scientific inquiry, just as it is in nature. We should welcome the new synthesis as an important vehicle for providing better help to autistic children and their families.

# REFERENCES

Carr, E. G. (1982). Some relationships between sign language acquisition and perceptual dysfunction in autistic children. In R. N. Malatesha & L. C. Hartlage (Eds.), *Neuropsychology and cognition, Vol. 2* (pp. 364–371). The Hague, The Netherlands: Martinus Nijhoff Publishers.

Carr, E. G., & Dores, P. A. (1981). Patterns of language acquisition following simultaneous communication with autistic children. *Analysis and Intervention in Developmental Disabilities, 1,* 347–361.

Lovaas, O. I., Koegel, R. L., Simmons, J. Q., & Long, J. S. (1973). Some generalization and follow-up measures on autistic children in behavior therapy. *Journal of Applied Behavior Analysis, 6,* 131–166.

Lovaas, O. I., Koegel, R. L., & Schreibman, L. (1979). Stimulus overselectivity in autism: A review of research. *Psychological Bulletin, 86,* 1236–1254.

**III**

# Explanation of Language Problems

# 5

# Prosodic Development in Normal and Autistic Children

## CHRISTIANE A. M. BALTAXE and JAMES Q. SIMMONS III

### INTRODUCTION

Deficits in prosody have been consistently described as an integral part of the speech and language disorder in autistic children (Kanner, 1946; Ornitz & Ritvo, 1976). Such deficits still remain evident in the language characteristics of children whose speech showed considerable improvement over time (DeMyer, Barton, DeMyer, Norton, Allen, & Steele, 1973; Rutter & Lockyer, 1967; Baltaxe & Simmons, 1983). However, there is still a paucity of research investigating the deficits in this important aspect of speech and language. The present review is an effort to summarize prosodic studies in autism and to consider the findings to date in terms of what is known about prosody in normal language acquisition and in language pathology. Finally, we will present some speculation on how the prosodic deficits might fit into the general picture of the autistic language disturbance and brain dysfunction.

### PROSODY: ITS SCOPE AND DEFINITION

Prosody or the "melody of speech" is a complex and relatively unexplored area of linguistic function. Monrad-Krohn (1963) called it the "third element of speech," in addition to semantics and grammar. Cutler and Isard

---

CHRISTIANE A. M. BALTAXE and JAMES Q. SIMMONS III • Department of Psychiatry and Biobehavioral Sciences, University of California, School of Medicine, Los Angeles, California 90024.

(1980) colorfully characterized prosody as the "sauce of the sentence which subtly changes or enhances the favor of the original." Prosody is made up of intonation, stress (accent), and the rhythmic (timing) pattern of language. It also extends beyond the boundaries of the sentence and lends speech its emotional tone. Mood and other emotional aspects of a linguistic interchange are frequently solely expressed by changes in prosody. Acoustically, prosody is a composite of the parameters of pitch (fundamental frequency), intensity (amplitude), and duration and their co-variation.

Prosody is an important aspect of communicative behavior with regard to speech production and speech perception. From the perspective of speech production, prosody interacts significantly with other levels of language. Cutler and Isard (1980) indentified four sources of prosodic effect on speech production. These are lexical stress patterns for individual words, placement of sentence accent, syntactic structure, and a variety of semantic and/or pragmatic factors, including choice of speech act as well as attitudinal and mood indicators. All four of these sources influence the overall shape of the intonation contour of an individual utterance or of a sequence of utterances. The prosody of any stretch of speech thus is a blend of different ingredients and their effects are difficult to isolate and identify by the naive listener.

Prosody also plays a major role in the perception of speech, where it provides the listener with cues for the segmentation and interpretation of the linguistic signal and at the same time alerts the listener to the psychological state or mood of the interlocutor. For example, syntactically, prosodic cues help the listener reconstruct phrase and sentence boundaries (Darwin, 1975; Butterworth, 1980). Research has shown that major syntactic and phrase boundaries are typically signaled by a fall/rise pattern in fundamental frequency (Cooper & Sorenson, 1981). The prepausal lengthening of vocalic segments preceding phrase boundaries is another prosodic cue (LeHiste, 1972; Klatt, 1975, 1976). Similarly, differences in sentence types, such as declaratives and interrogatives, are signaled by differences in intonation contouring (Lieberman, 1968). Prosodic features also help the listener resolve linguistic surface structure ambiguities (LeHiste, 1973a; LeHiste, Olive, & Streeter, 1976; Nakatani & Schaffer, 1978). In addition, prosodic features provide semantic and pragmatic information to the listener (Klatt, 1976; Bates & MacWhinney, 1979). For example, differences in lexical categories, such as noun and verb, are frequently solely signaled by differences in stress placement. In a series of reaction time experiments, Cutler and Foss (1977) provided evidence that listeners use accentual cues in language processing and comprehension to locate points of information focus. Accented words have been shown to be carriers of information, whereas unaccented words have not. The above study shows that words with a greater degree of accent appear to be easier to process. Syllables in English are marked by a number of correlated acoustic phonetic cues for accent or stress, such as greater duration, greater intensity, and more precise vowel quality, along with pitch movement, and experimental studies for English have shown that there is an acoustic hierarchy of cues that assist the listener in identifying accent or stress in the speech signal (Fry, 1955, 1958). These are pitch modulation, duration, intensity, and segmental quality. Changing pitch, not necessarily higher pitch, has been shown to serve most effectively to signal accent or stress.

Accent or stress has also been shown to represent an important factor in the rhythmic structure of speech (Kozhevnikov & Chistovich, 1965; LeHiste, 1978). Little is currently known about the rhythmic structure of speech. However, based on available studies, English has been characterized as a stress timed language. Studies in speech production and perception have shown that, when sounds and words are produced in isolation, they have different, generally longer, durational values than when they are produced in connected speech and that sequences of sounds and words in connected speech seem to be synchronized toward a regular beat or rhythm, with stressed syllables occurring at equal intervals (Petersen & LeHiste, 1960; Kozhevnikov & Chistovich, 1965; LeHiste, 1970; Huggins, 1972; Martin, 1979). This means that when changes occur in the durational features of one segment or syllable, compensatory changes will take place in the remainder of the utterance, so that the overall durational characteristics remain unchanged. This tendency of stressed syllables to occur at equal time intervals has been called isochrony (LeHiste, 1973b, 1977). Listeners appear to make use of this principle perceptually in processing relevant information (Huggins, 1972; Martin, 1972, 1975; LeHiste, 1978). Cutler and Foss (1977) argue that by being able to predict the location of upcoming accents, the listener is greatly assisted in sentence comprehension, since the "language processing mechanism" can direct attention to the potentially most important element of an utterance.

Although the above prosodic cues relate more specifically to the processing of the communicative aspect of the speech signal, prosodic characteristics also play a role in signaling speaker attitude and mood. Although it is difficult to determine exactly how different acoustic cues and their combinations are utilized by the listener to infer a particular emotional state, such as discontent, sadness, anger, or happiness, changes in pitch, intensity, and the rate of speech all have been identified as prosodic carriers of affective information (Williams & Stevens, 1981; Scherer, 1979, 198la,b; Weitz, 1979).

An appraisal of the current state of studies in language leaves no doubt that an investigation of prosody represents a significant frontier in such studies and links the interests of speech scientists, applied and theoretical linguists, psycholinguists, psychoacousticians, clinicians, neuroscientists, and others. Hoever, it is a complex area of investigation, and current views still differ on a number of issues. These include which characteristics of prosodic structure are linguistically salient, the best methods for studying prosody, the relation-ship of prosody to other levels of language, and the status of prosody within a theory of grammar and language (Chomsky & Halle, 1968; Bolinger, 1964; Cutler & Isard, 1980; Cutler, 1983; LeHiste, 1982, 1983a,b; Fromkin, 1983; Martin, 1977, 1982, 1983; Garding, 1982, 1983).

Studies that have addressed the relationship between prosody and syntax range from theoretically supporting the complete or relative independence of prosody and syntax (Martin, 1983; Garding, 1983) to a complete dependence of prosody on syntax (Chomsky & Halle, 1968). Although the relationship be-tween prosody and syntax has received a great deal of attention over the past few years, that between prosody and semantics has not been studied to an equal degree (LeHiste, 1983b). Here again the views differ, ranging from assertions of the complete or relative independence of prosody and semantics (Martin, 1983), to those proclaiming a dependence of prosody and semantics (Bolinger, 1964; Butterworth, 1980; Cutler, 1983). In addition, prosody, which in the past has also been labeled the suprasegmental features of language, takes on a special status with respect to the phonological component of language (Ladd, 1983).

Liberman (1983) probably best summarizes the current state of prosodic studies in stating that

> there is no generally accepted practice for notating, naming, or even categorizing in-tonation. While a number of schools of description exist, their systems are usually difficult for outsiders to learn, the completeness of their coverage is often suspect, the intersubjective reliability of their descriptions is generally dubious, and the basic categories employed have (at least superficially) very little similarity from school to school.

In this regard, until quite recently, most prosodic studies have been based on listener judgment or native speaker intuition. Fortunately, in addition to careful and laborious studies using manual measurement of the acoustic speech signal, the advent of computer-assisted technology for speech analysis has recently ad-vanced the field, especially by providing the capacity for more precise specifi-cations of various production characteristics and for verification of perceptual parameters. This trend will also be seen in the following review of prosody in language development.

## STUDIES OF PROSODY IN NORMAL CHILDREN

Prosody appears to be an important variable from the perspective of child language acquisition. Although our current knowledge of prosodic develop-ment is limited, a review of studies carried out with normal children strongly supports the notion that early in language development prosody is more advanced than phonological, syntactic, and semantic development (Ervin, 1966; Lenneberg, 1967; Jakobson, 1968; Lieberman, 1968; Tonkava-Yampolskaya, 1969, 1973; Kaplan, 1970; Crystal, 1979). Early prosodic units seem to fulfill a facilitative function perceptually as well as productively.

Studies in speech perception during the first year of life have shown that very young infants already respond differentially to the various intensities, durations, and frequency ranges that make up the prosodic characteristics of the speech signal (Kaplan, 1970; Morse, 1972, 1974; Spring & Dale, 1977). Differential responses in these studies were defined using conditioning techniques, cardiac rate changes, and electroencephalogram (EEG) technology. For example, Morse (1972), using synthesized nonsense syllables, showed that infants as young as 1 and 2 months of age were able to differentiate between rising and falling intonation. With larger sequences, Kaplan (1970) found that 8-month-old infants were able to differentiate between rising and falling intonation contours of the same utterance. Spring and Dale (1976), using a high amplitude sucking paradigm, showed that 1-to 4-month-old infants were able to perceive location of stress on artifically synthesized, two-syllable sequences (bába–babá).

Moving from speech perception to language comprehension, it has also been suggested that the exaggerated intonation contours often used by mothers in their interaction with young children may enhance their children's language comprehension (Garnica, 1977). In addition, the slower rate adults use in speaking to young children may also enhance children's language comprehension (Broen, 1972). Bonvillian, Raeburn, and Horan (1979) also hypothesized that children may rely on intonation to increase comprehension when other (linguistic) abilities are stretched, for example, when they are processing a long sentence. Productively, Tonava-Yampolskaya (1969, 1973), Crystal (1979), and others have emphasized the importance of maternal and adult prosodic modeling in the acquisition of prosodic patterns by young children.

In studying prosodic production characteristics in young children, Crystal (1979) and Dore (1975) have proposed that prosodic development consists of a sequence of learned patterns that appear in the second half of the first year of life and that continue to unfold in a series of complex patterns after prosody is joined with the segmental aspects of speech. Early prosodic patterns seem to form templates for these segmental patterns. Bruner (1975) called these early primitive prosodic units "envelopes" or "matrices," while Dore (1975) labeled them "frames." Crystal (1979) claimed that such early prosodic units were more stable than the segmental dimensions accompanying the prosodic contour. Dore (1975) also remarked on the more stable prosodic shape of utterances in early language acquisition when compared to the segmental shape, and Menn (1976) referred to the distinctive prosodic shapes as "protowords" in the speech of a child she studied. Lenneberg (1967) pointed out that the linguistic development of an utterance did not seem to begin with the composition of individual independently moveable items, but rather as a "whole tonal pattern" and that this whole became differentiated into "further component parts."

The phonological and phonetic details of the development of these prosodic frames into determinate units with a definable internal structure are not clear at present; however, studies of the prosody of individual children have shown that there appears to be a developmental sequence with respect to the stabilization of the individual acoustic parameters of prosody. Kirk (1973) and Allen and Hawkins (1980) suggest that control of fundamental frequency appears to be acquired first, timing second, and segmental contrasts last. These authors relate such developmental differences to individual physiological and maturational processes involved in the various aspects of speech production and also to task complexity. Pitch contouring, largely signaled by changes in the larynx, is presumably easier to master than either timing, which requires cortical control, or segmental contrasts, which require a variety of articulatory processes in glottal and supraglottal control.

Control of fundamental frequency not only relates to its linguistic use, such as the signaling of word and sentence stress and different sentence types, but also to the fundamental frequency range in which such information is expressed. Although it is generally known that young children use higher pitched voices than older children and adults, only a limited number of studies have investigated the pitch ranges used by young children to produce speech. One such study, by Keating and Buhr (1978), examined the fundamental frequency contours of six infants and children, 33 to 169 weeks old, in non-cry utterances. The utterances consisted of babbling, words, and sentences. Analysis was carried out using sound spectrograms. Surprisingly, fundamental frequency values characterizing the Fo patterns of their subjects ranged from a low of 30 Hz to a high of 2500 Hz, with individual ranges as wide as 30 Hz to 1500 Hz. Based on the ages studied, Keating and Buhr concluded that very low as well as very high frequencies may be common at all stages of language acquisition. The findings of the above study appear to be at variance with those of earlier ones in which extremes of this magnitude were not reported. For example, Fairbanks (1942) showed a gradual rise of fundamental frequency of approximately 200 Hz between birth and 4 months (from 313 Hz at 1 month to 585 Hz at 4 and 9 months). Sheppard and Lane (1968), who investigated the vocalizations of two children from birth to 5 months, found the average fundamental frequency to be 438 Hz. Petersen and Barney (1952), in a study of older children (ages not specified) based on a citation paradigm, found that their subjects used fundamental frequencies between 250 and 275 Hz, and Lieberman (1975) noted that children use fundamental frequencies that range up to

500 Hz. Two other studies by Fairbanks, Wiley, and Lassman (1949) and Fairbanks, Herbert, and Hammond (1949) reported average fundamental frequencies in reading for 7-year-old boys (294 Hz), for 8-year-old boys (297 Hz), for
7-year-old girls (273.2 Hz), and for 8-year-old girls (286.5 Hz).

The above studies address the issue of the average fundamental frequency
(pitch) as well as the range of fundamental frequency infants and young children use in their vocalizations and verbalizations. These studies leave no doubt
that the controls and constraints on these two parameters seen in the adult are
either still absent or only partially present at the particular ages and language acquisition stages of the children studied. In addition to a high average fundamental frequency very early in development, which gradually decreases with
age, the above studies also show extreme ranges of fundamental frequency and
considerable variation. It is clear from a comparison with adult values for average fundamental frequency and range of fundamental frequency that physiological maturation, sex differences, and probably the acquisition of prosody itself
all play a role in development to achieve ultimate adult values. Further research is necessary to clarify the above findings and to trace more clearly the
longitudinal development of these two parameters. In addition, there are still
very few studies that have focused on the fundamental frequency characteristics of early prosodic production in terms of their linguistic salience. However,
studies by Kirk (1973) and Branigan (1979) have shown that a falling fundamental frequency contour seems to be one of the earliest prosodic devices
used linguistically to mark phrase boundaries and signal terminaltiy. A rising
fundamental intonation contour has been noted to develop in the second year of
life (Tonkava-Yampolskaya, 1973).

Available studies of the durational and timing characteristics in children's
speech productions have shown that, although such characteristics develop
early, children do not achieve adult durational values until mid-childhood and
some durational features may not be acquired until early puberty. Young children show longer segment, syllable, and phrase durations than do adults
(DiSimoni, 1974a, b, c; Smith, 1978; Kent & Forner, 1980). Smith (1978), in
a developmental study of the temporal parameters of the speech production of
a 2½- to 3- and 4- to 4½-year-old children, found, for example, that the younger group of children already differentiated vowel duration in stressed and unstressed syllables. Although this study showed greater variability in the youngest children's productions, by the age of 4, durational values were
comparable to those of adults. Smith also noted that, whereas the absolute duration increments due to language specific variables were greater for the children than for the adults, both groups of children behaved very much like their
adult control group when the durations between stressed and unstressed vowels
were considered proportionally. Based on these findings, Smith concluded that
children appear to possess timing control that is more sophisticated than had

been previously thought. Other studies (DiSimoni, 1974c; Tingley & Allen, 1975; Kent & Forner, 1980; Flege, 1982) have also provided evidence of greater temporal variability in early child speech productions, including a greater range of durations over repeated productions of a specific utterance. For example, in a study of the timing characteristics of 5, 7, 9, and 11 year olds, Tingley and Allen (1975), using the repeated productions of a nursery rhyme, found that timing control improved with age. A study by Kent and Forner (1980), using spectrographic analysis of sentence recitations by 4, 6, and 12 year olds, also showed longer segment durations and greater variability of such durations for the 4 year olds when compared to the older children. Kent and Forner (1980) suggest that the degree to which young children lengthen segments may depend on several unexplored segmental, suprasegmental, and linguistic factors. In a separate study, Kubaska and Keating (1981) examined word durations longitudinally in three children ranging in ages, by weeks, from 66 to 145, 69 to 128, and 121 to 153. They hypothesized that lexical familiarity may also affect greater durational constancy. However, results of their study, which was based on spectrographic analysis, only showed that variations in word duration were generally due to the effect of position in the utterance. Non-final words in two-word utterances were produced with a shorter duration than those in isolated or in final position. Although the results of the above studies varied somewhat, they do provide evidence that the temporal variability in children's speech productions tends to decline until as late as 11 or 12 years of age (Kent & Forner, 1980).

The current, most commonly proposed hypothesis to account for the greater durational values and variability is based on maturation. It proposes that children have less mature neuromotor systems than adults (Tingley & Allen, 1975; Allen & Hawkins, 1980; Smith, 1978). Kent and Forner (1980) had also suggested that individual timing characteristics may vary with unexplored factors that influence segment duration. Smith, Sugarman, and Long (1983), pursuing this line of reasoning, examined the effect of speaking rate on temporal variability in children's speech. Although their study partially confirmed the maturational hypothesis, it also suggested that artifacts of statistical analysis may contribute to the commonly observed variability in children's speech.

Studies on the linguistic use of prosody beyond the first year of life have focused heavily on the importance of stress in the acquisition process. Such studies have generally relied on perceptual listener judgement. Stress does appear to aid verbal memory function, and children exhibit sensitivity to stress perception in various ways. For example, stressed words (content words) seem to be retained more easily than unstressed words (function words) in imitation and in early telegraphic speech (Brown & Fraser, 1963; Brown & Bellugi, 1964; but see Eilers, 1975). These authors suggest that young children retain content words more readily in repetition paradigms precisely because they are stressed. Similarly, Blasdell and Jensen (1970) found word stress to be a significant factor in the recall of verbal material in children as young as 2½ years of age.

Individual observations and studies have generally shown that children appear to become sensitive to accentual or stress patterns of words and phrases by about the age of 2 and begin to signal accentual distinctions in their own speech soon after. For example, Weir (1962) noted that, at age 2½ years, her son already used stress appropriately and in consonance with the English adult system. Miller and Erwin (1964) found that 2½ year olds use contrastive stress patterns with which they marked possessives and locatives. Similarly, Wieman (1976) showed that children with a mean utterance length of only two words already demonstrated an established stress pattern. Wieman found that the children's sentence stress assignment also appeared highly correlated with the semantic content of the utterance, in particular with the introduction of new information. Adult syntactic categories appeared inconsequential in her subjects' stress assignment. From the child's point of view, it was unimportant, for example, whether the semantic notion of locative was expressed through a noun, preposition, or prolocative. Stress was assigned to each case, when the locative introduced new information. Hornby and Hass (1970) more specifically studied contrastive stress in the context of topic and comment. They found that children as young as 4 years of age already used contrastive stress as a primary device to mark topic–comment distinctions. Atkinson-King (1973) examined the acquisition of stress patterns in compound words and phrases in age groups ranging from 5 to 13 years. When she compared prosodic production to prosodic comprehension, she found that the production of prosodic patterns never exceeded their comprehension. Her findings also identified an age factor, which operated with regard to the various aspects of the use, perception, and comprehension of stress in the children she studied. An age factor was also identified by Cutler and Swinney (1980) in a reaction time experiment focusing on the perception of stressed versus unstressed words.

In summary, then, the currently available data on children's acquisition of prosody indicate that even though prosodic development initially appears to be in advance of other linguistic levels, children's knowledge of the full prosodic system remains inaccurate and does not reach adult refinement until about the age of 12 or onset of puberty (Atkinson-King, 1973; Allen & Hawkins, 1980; Cutler & Swinney, 1980). Empirical evidence supports the notion that the acquisition of prosody, despite its early lead in development, is complex and must be understood as a progression of steps interlocking the development of prosody with maturational, physiological, and cognitive factors, as well as with the developing syntactic, semantic, and pragmatic domains of language. In view of this complex interactional pattern, prosody must be considered an important variable in the acquisition process in children with developmental disorders of language as well.

## STUDIES OF PROSODY IN AUTISM

The speech of autistic children has been variously described as improperly modulated, dull, and wooden and as having a singsong quality. Distortions in rhythm, loudness, and pitch and overprecision in articulation have been noted (Goldfarb, Braunstein, & Lorge, 1956; Pronovost, Wakstein, & Wakstein, 1966; Goldfarb, Goldfarb, Braunstein, & Scholl, 1972). Also, autistic children have been reported to lack the prelinguistic intonation contouring commonly seen in normal children (Hicks, 1972). Even those children with high language function often continue to have demonstrable difficulties in the use and interpretation of the fine nuances of language. Such difficulties have led to their language being characterized as "extremely literal" and "concrete" (Rutter, 1966). The autistic child's failure to use and interpret prosodic features appropriately may be responsible, at least in part, for this "literalness," since fine nuances of meaning are most often signaled by changes in the prosodic patterns. The flat affect described in autistic children often relates to the fact that their speech sounds "atonal, arhythmic and hollow" (Ornitz & Ritvo, 1976). Goldfarb et al. (1972) observed that the description of the schizophrenic (autistic) child's speech patterns, in terms of flatness of affect, is the listener's reponse to the schizophrenic (autistic) child's broad range of errors in stress, pitch, phrasing, intonation, inflection, meaning, and mood expression.

Deficits in prosody have also been reported in the speech of non-English–speaking autistic children. For example, Sedlackova and Neshidalova (1975) found that Czech autistic children had abnormal prosody. Similarly, Baltaxe and Simmons (1977), in a comparison of English-and German-speaking autistic adolescents, found that abnormal prosody was also characteristic of their German subjects. Simon (1975) considered impairment in prosody as characteristic for autism in a differential diagnosis from aphasia. She maintained that aphasic children showed impairment in phonemic discrimination, but intactness of intonational features, whereas the reverse was true for the autistic children. However, more recent evidence fails to substantiate this differentiation (Baltaxe, 1981; Baltaxe, Simmons, & Zee, 1984).

Follow-up studies on the speech and language deficits of autistic subjects grown to adolescence still indicate residual difficulties in prosody despite the presence of much improved speech (Kanner & Eisenberg, 1956: Rutter, 1966; Rutter & Lockyer, 1967; DeMyer et al., 1973; Kanner, 1971). The prosodic deficits described in these follow-up studies refer to a lack of lability, or cadence, and difficulties with inflection and intonation. Simmons and Baltaxe (1975) and Baltaxe and Simmons (1977, 1983) also noted the persistence of intonational problems into adolescence, and Ornitz and Ritvo (1976) commented on their continued presence in adulthood.

To date, prosodic studies on autism have been limited primarily to the production of prosody and have consisted of those that have included the use of instrumentation in the analysis of speech. Despite some interesting findings, the characteristics of the prosodic deficits in autism still await complete exploration. The relationship of prosodic abnormalities to other aspects of the autistic dysfunction has also not been clarified. We will now review available prosodic studies in some detail and discuss some of their more relevant findings.

The earliest studies, which addressed themselves more specifically to prosodic abnormalities, were those by Goldfarb and his co-workers (Goldfarb *et al.*, 1956, 1972). Although these studies suffered from some limitations, they are noteworthy because they represent a pioneering effort in a difficult area. The 1956 Goldfarb study consisted of observations made by a trained speech pathologist on the prosodic patterns of spontaneous utterances in a group of 12 schizophrenic children and 6 children with reactive behavior disorders. Listener judgements were made regarding deviations from a hypothetical norm in the use of prosody. The results of this study showed that the schizophrenic children evidenced a greater number and a wider range of deviations in rhythm and intonation than did the control group. More specifically, the speech of the schizophrenic children was characterized by what these authors described as a kind of flatness not noted in the comparison group. The schizophrenic children were also more deviant in terms of voice volume, and their speech was characterized by insufficient change in volume. Even these limited changes in volume were usually unrelated to language content. Goldfarb and his colleagues further observed that the schizophrenic children sometimes had excessively high pitch, but most often showed insufficient pitch change and pitch change was frequently unrelated to meaning. A narrowed pitch range and a lack of pitch fall in utterance final position were more general observations. Insufficient, incorrect, or distorted intonation patterns were observed, and intonation insufficiency was sometimed linked to pitch insufficiency, Atypical durational characteristics, leading to the impression of chanting, were also noted. Some of the limitations of the first Goldfarb study included a lack of definitions, an unclear delineation of the prosodic categories to be rated, and an apparent limited understanding of the acoustic parameters of prosody. An assessment of reliability was not provided and the results were based on the listener impressions of a single rater. Nevertheless, some of these early observations have been subsequently verified through the use of instrumental acoustic measurements (Bagshaw, 1978; Baltaxe, 1981; Baltaxe, Simmons, & Zee, 1984).

In a 1966 study, Pronovost, Wakstein, and Wakstein examined the speech behavior of 14 children diagnosed as autistic or atypical and, based on listener judgement, found that the subjects exhibited wide variations in intensity, pitch, and extensive variation from normal voice quality, with hoarseness, harshness, and hypernasality occurring in addition to normal phonation. These authors also noted that the echoed speech did not imitate the rhythm or intonation of the adult stimuli, but rather tended to be monotonous in pitch, rhythm, and intensity.

In a 1972 study of the speech and language characteristics of 25 schizophrenic children matched with 25 normal children, Goldfarb and his coworkers again examined prosodic characteristics. Compared to their earlier study, a more complete prosodic rating scale had been developed and served as the basis for the observations. No specific clustering of linguistic deficits uniquely characteristic for childhood schizophrenia was noted in this study. However, the authors did report that their subjects exhibited a wide variation of deficits and that speech production was characterized by the "presence of antipodal phenomena fluctuating from one extreme to the other in many voices and speech elements" (p. 219). In other words, schizophrenic children showed either too much or too little of a given prosodic feature, or they exhibited both too much and too little. None of these studies interpreted these findings in more specifically linguistic terms.

Fletcher (1976), using sound spectrograms, compared the intonation patterns of six autistic and six normal subjects for fundamental frequency characteristics based on an imitation task. She found that the autistic children were not able to imitate the intonation contours as well as the normal subjects. However, the comparisons were based on the "visual" inspection of her spectrographic data, and actual measurements were not obtained. More recently, Bagshaw (1978) compared the frequency and durational characteristics of three autistic subjects, aged 5.9, 10.5, and 18 years, and one normal subject, aged 4.5 years. She used sound spectrographic analysis in two imitation tasks. Measurements of imitations of simple declarative utterances showed no significant differences between the autistic subjects and the normal subjects, except for a trend by the autistic subjects to show greater variability in total utterance duration. Bagshaw also examined the use of fundamental frequency and vowel lengthening in marking contrastive stress. Results showed that two of the three autistic subjects did not mark stress by either fundamental frequency modulation or vowel lengthening, whereas the normal child used both of these acoustic parameters appropriately. Bagshaw suggested the possibility of subgroups based on findings of her second experiment. Subgroups had also been suggested by Goldfarb et al. (1972), who divided the schizophrenic subjects into an organic and nonorganic group prior to examining their speech patterns. They were also able to link some of the deficits observed to that division.

The studies reviewed so far have focused exclusively on the characteristics of production deficits. A study of a somewhat different nature is that of Paccia and Curcio (1982), who used prosody as a tool to study the interaction of comprehension and echolalia. These authors hypothesized that, if echolalia reflected a comprehension deficit, then the incidence of echoing should vary depending on a given child's understanding of the words and/or the syntactic–semantic relations contained in a specific eliciting utterance. Echolalia, in their study, was also linked to replications of prosodic contours. They hypothesized that modification of the prosodic contours of the echoes also reflected some degree of comprehension. The intonation contours of echolalic responses were analyzed in the context of *yes/no* and *wh-* questions with respect to their fundamental frequency characteristics. The analysis was carried out with the use of a computer-aided program and by listener judgment. The contours were judged by two individual raters independently to determine whether they were imitative or contrastive with respect to the examiner's question. Judgement was made primarily in terms of the prosodic shape of the utterance final contours. Rising intonation was judged as being imitative and falling contour as contrastive.

Results showed that approximately 55% of echolalic utterances were prosodically imitative, whereas the remaining 45% were contrastive. However, their findings showed a wide range of individual variation. Contrastive prosody was also more likely to be used in response to questions requiring affirmation than when the identical question required negation. The authors concluded from these findings that pathological echolalia seemed not merely to present mimicry of what was heard, but actually consisted of prosodic restructuring, which they interpreted as evidence of some degree of comprehension. Prosodic restructuring also increased in the presence of mitigation of the echolalic responses. Crystal (1973) had proposed earlier that prosodic restructuring presented the earliest type of linguistic structuring. Paccio and Curcio suggest that echolalic autistic children who do not manipulate the prosodic features of their speech may also be more impaired linguistically than those who frequently restructure their echoes prosodically. The findings in the above study, which included the one that prosody was frequently replicated in echoic responses, can be considered at variance with the earlier observations by Pronovost et al. (1966) that echoed speech did not imitate the rhythm or intonation of the adult stimulus, but instead tended to be monotonous in pitch, rhythm, and intensity.

In a continuing series of studies at the University of California at Los Angeles, prosody in autism has received increasingly critical examination. The first study of prosody was linked to an investigation of the speech and language faults of autistic adolescents (Simmons & Baltaxe, 1975). These authors rated prosodic deficits using the scale established earlier by Goldfarb and his co-workers. They found that four of their seven subjects, between 14 and 21 years of age, still had prosodic deficits in speech production that included difficulties in pitch, volume, rhythmic elements, stress, and intonation as measured by that scale. These same subjects also had major difficulties in the semantic aspects of language despite an IQ on the WAIS that ranged between 86 to 120. Interestingly, the four subjects who did poorly in language and prosody also did poorly perceptually on the tone and rhythm subtests of the Seashore Test of Musical Talents (Seashore, Lewis & Saetit, 1956). No correlations based on age or IQ scores could be established to account for the differences between the autistic subjects showing these deficits and those who did not show them. One possible explanation of these results is that they are independent of each other and reflect a pervasive degree of impairment. Another possibility might be that, in these subjects such deficits are interrelated. Thus, the autistic subjects' deficits in perception of rhythm and tone on this test may be more specifically related to prosodic deficits that, in turn, may affect speech perception and/or comprehension. Although the subjects' division into two distinct groups based on these production and perception characteristics is not easily explainable, similar subgroupings are seen in some of the above studies and suggest heterogeneity within the diagnostic category.

In a later study, Baltaxe (1981), using an imitation task, studied the prosodic production characteristics of eight autistic children and eight normal controls matched by sex, social class, and psycholinguistic age. The task included declaratives, *yes/no* questions, *wh-* questions, and commands, all of which are noted to have distinctive intonation patterns in English. Acoustic tracings of fundamental frequency, intensity, and durational characteristics of each of the utterances were obtained under controlled conditions, using a pitch and intensity meter and an Oscillomink inkwriter. Manual measurements and statistical analysis then provided the basis for durational, fundamental frequency, and intensity findings regarding these utterances. Results showed that, as a group, the autistic subjects had greater durations and also showed greater variability in the production of each utterance type than did the normal subjects. In contrast, the normal children seemed to aim their utterances at a pretargeted time frame, regardless of whether an utterance was produced with omissions or misarticulations. In addition, when individual words, produced in isolation, were compared to the same words in the context of a sentence, the normal children showed durational differences. Such differences were smaller or absent for the autistic group. Based on these results, the author suggested that autistic children may differ from normal children in their temporal organization and rhythmic structure of speech. Whereas normal children may follow a rhythmic structure or relative timing model of speech production, the autistic subjects may follow a serial or chain model. As noted earlier, a relative timing model posits that any speech event is synchronized in connected speech toward a kind of regular rhythm or beat, with stressed syllables occuring at regular intervals (e.g., Kozhevnikov & Chistovich, 1965). In contrast, a serial or chain model posits that connected speech must be viewed linearly as a process of chaining or concatenation of individual elements, with no durational adjustments of individual segments, syllables, or words. Each utterance thus constitutes the sum of its individual elements (Lashley, 1951).

The 1981 study examined frequency and intensity configurations. Results showed that the normal group was characterized by greater frequency ranges, especially for *wh-* and *yes-no* questions. In contrast, the autistic group showed greater intensity ranges. Normal children used frequency characteristically to express differences in the sentence types examined, whereas autistic subjects used intensity, when such differences were expressed at all. In addition, the normal subjects also showed greater synchrony and covariation between frequency and intensity. The exceptions were *yes/no* questions when such synchrony is not expected (Lieberman, 1968; O'Hala, 1978). The author interpreted the autistic subjects' apparent predilection for intensity to convey linguistic prosodic information as a possible modality-specific overselectivity. Lovaas, Schreibman, Koegel, and Rehm (1971) have shown that autistic children overselect one modality when presented with competing stimuli in several modalities. This concept could be extended to events in which several stimuli (in this case, frequency, intensity, and duration) compete within the same modality.

In a recently completed study using different subject groups, but the same instrumental procedures, Baltaxe, Simmons, and Zee (1984) examined the intonation contours of a matched group of six normal, five autistic, and six aphasic children; the MLU was between 1.45 and 4.46 morphemes. The normal children ranged in age between 2.0 and 4.0 years, the autistic children between 4.6 and 12.2 years, and the aphasic children between 4.5 and 10.2 years. This study examined simple declarative utterances (subject–verb–object) produced spontaneously under controlled conditions. In addition to fundamental frequency range, a number of the other prosodic characteristics were examined. The first was terminal fall, which has been shown to develop early in child language (Branigan, 1979) and is generally associated with the declarative mode in English. Terminal fall begins with, and marks, the final stressed syllable in an utterance and seems to express terminality (O'Shaughnessey, 1979; Cooper & Sorenson, 1977). The second was the overall intonation contour of the utterance, as characterized by a series of pitch obtrusions expected on the stressed vowels of the utterance (Martin, 1982), and in this study predicted to occur for the first syllable of nouns and verbs in subject–verb–object positions. Another was the declination effect, which is the tendency of pitch to drift downward over a declarative intonation group (Pierrehumbert, 1979; Cooper & Sorenson, 1981). The last was covariation of frequency and intensity over the entire intonation contour (Lieberman, 1968; O'Hala, 1977; Cooper & Sorenson, 1981; Kutik, Cooper, & Boyce, 1983).

A comparison of the fundamental frequency ranges across the three groups showed that the normal group had the greatest range, followed by the autistic group; the aphasic group had the narrowest range. Significant differences occurred between normal and aphasic subjects and autistic and aphasic subjects. However, when the autistic subjects were considered individually, they showed either a highly exaggerated or a very narrow range. Narrow-range subjects were similar to the aphasic group. In an analysis of terminal fall, the normal subjects showed the highest percentage of occurrence, followed by the autistic group and then by the aphasic group. However, two of the autistic subjects and three of the aphasic subjects lacked terminal fall altogether. When the overall intonation contour was examined, results showed that stressed vowels could be marked by either pitch obtrusion, intensity obtrusion, or both, for all subject groups. None of the subject groups marked stress consistently by any one of these markers. However, greatest stability in marking stress was noted for subject position and normal subjects marked stressed syllables with the highest frequency. Declination again occurred with the highest percentage in the normal group, followed by the aphasic group and finally by the autistic group. In considering covariation of frequency and intensity over the entire contour, normal subjects showed the highest percentage in this case, followed by the autistic group and then the aphasic group. However, individual profiles also showed that some autistic subjects and some aphasic subjects lacked covariation altogether. The overall results of the above study again showed considerable between- and within-subject variability. They also point to the fact that some of the prosodic characteristics examined are more stable and consistent than others. Both language-deficient groups generally showed less stability and greater individual variation. Differential performance by the individual groups and individual subjects was also seen with respect to individual prosodic markers.

The results of this study support the notion that both frequency and intensity are important prosodic markers in the speech of young children and that the linguistic salience of these parameters may differ for individual children and individual groups. The study also provides evidence that covariation of frequency and intensity, expected in prosodic patterns of the type studied, may itself be the result of maturational factors and learned behavior. Although the frequency parameter was characterized as the most stable initially in prosodic development (Kirk, 1973; Allen & Hawkins, 1980), when considered from the perspective of its individual components, some components appear to be more stable than others. Results of this study suggest that some prosodic features relating to frequency, intensity, and their covariation may develop earlier, whereas others, less stable and consistent, may depend more on maturational factors, learned behaviors, and further linguistic development. For the language-impaired groups, such markers may then exhibit particular vulnerability.

A significant area in the review of studies on prosodic development was the role of the accentual system. One aspect of this system is that of contrastive stress, which is an important pragmatic device available to the speaker to mark topic–comment distinctions or to focus on a particular lexical element. Contrastively stressed elements present new information against a background of lesser stressed elements, which present old information. Other devices to mark the topic–comment distinction include word order, explicit lexicalization, the use of fully specific noun phrases, indefinite reference, and cleft constructions. According to Bates and MacWhinney (1979), contrastive stress is also the choice device when the point of an utterance is to contradict or replace some aspect of the listener's beliefs.

In a further study of prosody in autism, based on listener judgment, Baltaxe (1984) examined the use of contrastive stress in a group of seven autistic children matched with a normal and a language-delayed (aphasic) control group. Mean length of utterance for all subjects ranged between 1.5 and 4.0 morphemes. Contrastive stress in this study was again elicited for subject, verb, and object positions under controlled conditions. The task required that each subject deal with the presupposition of a *yes/no* question that was not supported by the accompanying extralinguistic situation. For example the question might be "Is the baby sleeping in the bed?" and the extralinguistic situation might show a dog sleeping in the bed. Results of this study, based on the judgment of two independent raters, showed that the response rate for all three subject groups was below criterion level in that responses were given only about 60% of the time. Significant between-group differences were seen in terms of correct responses, with normal subjects having the highest and the autistic subjects the lowest number of correct responses. Differences in error patterns for all three groups related to whether subject, verb, or object were to be contrasted as well as to the type of stress misassignment. Although errors for the normal and the aphasic groups consisted only of stress misassignment to stressable elements, the autistis subjects differed in that they also misassigned stress to function words that ordinarily do not bear stress. In addition, more than one-third of the incorrect responses by the autistic subjects could also be accounted for by the simultaneous assignment of stress to more than one element.

In placing these findings into perspective with regard to earlier studies with young normal children, the author noted that such studies had also found a lower than expected response rate for *yes/no* questions. Steffenson (1977), for example, in a study of two young normal children, had found that only 50% of her *yes/no* questions had received a response and that there was a strong bias toward an affirmative response. Other studies had also observed such a bias (Klima & Bellugi, 1966; Broen, 1972; Padilla & Lindbloom, 1976; Tyack & Ingram, 1977). Steffenson's explanation was based on task complexity. She concluded that young children did not as yet understand the semantics of the *yes/no* particle, although they were aware of the illocutionary force of the query. An explanation of task complexity was also offered in the above study, although the study differed from that of Steffenson because of the conflict between the linguistic and extralinguistic situation and the added dimension of contrastive stress. Task complexity in the Baltaxe study was seen as a decision-making process in which prosodic, pragmatic, semantic, and syntactic variables had to be incorporated to achieve a correct response. Interestingly, for all three subject groups, incorrect responses were limited to incorrect stress assignment in the presence of the correctly substituted lexical element. In addition, the prevalent pattern of stress misassignment for all three groups was one in which stress appeared to be shifted one stressable syllable to the right, cyclically. Thus, there was evidence that all subject groups were able to assess the negative truth value of the presupposition of the query, but had difficulty synchronizing its linguistic expression. This showed up in the slight disjunction in temporal patterning between the lexico-syntactic level and the prosodic levels of the utterance. The autistic subjects' additional error pattern of simultaneous stress assignment and stress misassignment to function words, in the face of correct lexical substitutions, also suggested that even though they could make the required judgments cognitively and pragmatically, they seemed to be at a special disadvantage in making use of prosodic markers, presumably because of more general prosodic and linguistic difficulties.

With one exception, the above results generally parallel those of Hornby and Hass (1970) in their study of normal 4-year-olds. In agreement with the present findings, these authors also found the most consistent use of contrastive stress for subject position, less for verb, and even less for object position. Hornby and Hass related their findings to word order and the importance of subject position from the perspective of a topic–comment distinction. A similar explanation is provided in the currently discussed study.

In another study of the accentual system in autistic children, Baltaxe and Guthrie (in press) examined the use of primary sentence stress in the same group of children. Although contrastive stress is an optimal element that may occur on any element placed into focus, primary sentence stress is syntactically determined and predicted by the rules of grammar (Chomsky, Halle, & Lukoff, 1956; Chomsky & Halle, 1968). In the study of primary sentence stress, neutral declarative utterances of the subject–verb–object type were collected in a play situation and analyzed, again using listener judgment. Primary sentence stress in these utterances was predicted for object position (Chomsky & Halle, 1968). In contradistinction to the contrastive stress study, the results showed that the responses for all three groups in this study were at or near criterion level. The three groups differed, however, in the number of correct responses as well as in the pattern of stress misassignment. The major finding was that, even though primary sentence stress was predicted for object position, the results did not substantiate this prediction and subject position was the most salient perceptually for all three groups. Primary sentence stress for only 15% of the normal subjects' and 5% of the aphasic subjects' responses were perceived on object position, whereas the autistic group did not mark object position at all. Further analysis showed that, in approximately 25% of the normal subjects' responses, stress was perceived equally on subject and object positions, whereas only a very few instances of such simultaneous stress assignment occurred for the aphasic group. However, both the aphasic and the autistic groups misassigned stress to verb position. As in the contrastive stress study, the autistic subjects further misassigned stress to function words. Based on these findings, the authors concluded that frequency of occurrence may be a better criterion for correctness in judging primary sentence stress and that subject position should probably be considered the target for sentence stress in the utterances studied. Our findings that primary sentence stress for all three groups occurred mostly in subject position are in agreement with Bresnan's topical stress rule (1972), which predicts stress on subject position; however, subject position in our case also seemed to receive major sentence accent even when it was not specifically marked as the topic of the sentence. Since the topical stress rule is a pragmatic rule, the authors suggest that one explanation for their findings might be that, with regard to prosody, young children are governed more by pragmatic rules than by grammatical rules, at least in the early stages of language development. The incidence of simultaneous stress assignment by the normal subjects, together with the limited degree to which stress is assigned to object position, may then be interpreted as evidence of the normal children's awareness of grammatical rules with regard to which the two language-delayed groups lag behind. Although all three groups showed an ability for accent placement, the aphasic and autistic groups performed more poorly than the normal subjects, and the autistic group performed the worst in that autistic subjects frequently also failed to make the distinction between stressable and non-stressable elements.

The above review reflects the limited extent of prosodic studies with autistic as well as language-delayed (aphasic) children. Although prosodic disturbances represent an integral aspect of the autistic language disorder, such disturbances have not been reported for language-delayed (aphasic) children, although an indication for such deficits may already be present in studies relating to production and perception characteristics in such populations. For example, Stark and Tallal (1979), in a study of stop consonant production errors by these children, proposed, based on acoustic analysis, that the voicing errors seen in their subjects were related to a lack of precise control over the timing of speech events. Our own work in progress on the durational characteristics of autistic and aphasic children, although only discussed to a limited extent with respect to an autistic population (Baltaxe, 1981), also provides evidence for poor timing control in both groups of children. Future studies with children with developmental language disorders will undoubtedly shed further light on the extent of prosodic involvement in such populations.

In summary, then, prosodic studies in autism appear to indicate that autistic children may not be as globally abnormal in their use of prosody as suspected from early studies and observations. Deficits may depend on the parameter of prosody studied. They may vary depending on whether fundamental frequency, intensity, or timing characteristics are examined and whether the *linguistic use* of these parameters is considered. On the one hand, the autistic child may have a fundamental frequency range that is judged as too narrow or too wide in comparison with that of a normal control. Nevertheless, within that range, from a linguistic perspective, the stress and intonation contour may be expressed appropriately, at least in part. On the other hand, the autistic child's frequency range may be close to normal, yet the linguistic information expressed within that range by prosodic markers may be inaccurate. The more usual case in the above studies was that deficiencies were found along both these dimensions. As in the normal subjects studied, correctness and/or appropriateness depended on the individual prosodic markers studied. Although our results show considerable heterogeneity, expecially for the autistic subjects, both delay features and specific abnormalities could be identified when compared to the normal children. Surprisingly, a number of the aphasic children who served as controls in three of the above studies appeared prosodically similar in some respects to several of the autistic children. These similarities included a narrowed frequency range. However, the autistic subjects were generally more extensively impaired in their use of prosody. The aphasic subjects also took an intermediary position between the normal group and the autistic group and were generally more similar in prosodic patterning to the normal subjects. Mean length of utterance, which in the past has been used as a basis of comparison for normal and language-delayed populations, was not a valid predictor of level of prosodic development for the language-deficient groups. As in earlier studies with normal children, there also seems to be an indication that control of pragmatically based prosodic markers may be achieved ahead of those based on purely syntactic considerations.

## CONCLUSIONS AND DIRECTIONS FOR FUTURE RESEARCH

The review of the literature underscores the intricate nature of prosody, both as a separate area of study and in terms of its complex interaction with other levels of language in the production as well as in the perception of speech. It also supports the important role of prosody in language acquisition. Earlier studies focused on the acquisition of phonology, syntax, and semantics and showed that language unfolds in a series of stages. Similarly, the picture that emerges from developmental studies of normal and impaired prosody also shows that the development of prosodic abilities is one of a gradual unfolding. Prosodic characteristics and markers for such stages have just begun to be identified, and current findings suggest that some of these markers develop earlier than others. Studies to date also support the notion that children reach some degree of prosodic stability by the age of 4, but do not reach adult-like competence until the beginning of puberty. The development of prosody thus emerges as a result of a continuing and complex interaction between the prosodic level of language, general maturational progression, and continued linguistic, cognitive, and pragmatic development.

Research evidence has also underscored the facilitative and early organizational role of prosody with regard to other levels of language. A basic prosodic impairment, regardless of its etiology, would thus appear to significantly influence these functions as well. The interaction of prosodic development with other levels of language development also appears well documented. Consequently, it would also be reasonable to assume that an impairment or delay in any of these levels would affect prosody, or at least its fine tuning. Nevertheless one must consider the possibility that impairment and/or delay in prosody and impairment and/or delay in other linguistic areas can occur independently in the same individual, as studies from adult aphasia have amply demonstrated (Monrad-Krohn, 1947, 1957, 1963; Goodglass, Fodor, & Schulhoff, 1967; Jakobson, 1968; Cole, 1971; Goodglass, 1973). The mutual effects of such impairments could then be additive. When such deficits also exist in the areas of perception and/or comprehension, the ultimate effect on language acquisition can be devastating. One disorder that may demonstrate this is infantile autism, which has been characterized as a pervasive impairment in several developmental areas, including those of speech and language. Perceptual as well as comprehension deficits have been identified as part of the overall diagnostic picture (Ornitz & Ritvo, 1976; Baltaxe & Simmons, 1975). In addition, most levels of language function are affected by disturbances (for comprehensive reviews, see Baltaxe & Simmons, 1975, 1981). It may well be that the peculiar constellation of linguistic deficits, characterized both by delay and specific abnormalities, is also reflective of prosodic impairment. Some of the language difficulties seen in autism, such as problems in distinguishing between different grammatical categories, could also impair the "linguistic" use of prosody.

In studies to date and in contrast to the normal and the aphasic subjects, the autistic subjects seemed to attend less to the more "linguistic" signals in their use of prosody. The lack of a systematic differential effect of content and function words on their prosodic use would be such an example. In our ongoing work concerning the durational characteristics of speech production, there is evidence that autistic children often neglect the use of temporal cues in signaling grammatical information, in contradistinction to normal and aphasic subjects. Differences that relate to the temporal processing of meaning-carrying elements (stressed elements) were also seen in our 1981 study where these had been related to different models of speech production. Autistic children seemed to function surprisingly well, however, when pragmatic distinctions were required, as in the contrastive stress task that represented an interface between cognitive, linguistic, and social abilities. Still, when one compares the findings of all these studies as they relate to prosodic abilities in aphasic and autistic subjects, it would appear that the autistic subjects also suffer from a more pervasive deficit in prosody than do the aphasic subjects. Thus, the apparently constructive use of echolalia in autistic children who develop more adequate language function may reflect the autistic child's inability to use prosody in speech perception and comprehension. The autistic child, unable to break down the flow of speech into its component parts, may then adopt alternate strategies in language acquisition. Larger linguistic units, including entire utterances in the form of echolalia, may initially be used in an attempt to communicate (Baltaxe & Simmons, 1973, 1975, 1981; Prizant, 1983). Baltaxe and Simmons (1973) considered such an alternate strategy in terms of right hemisphere functioning, claiming that it presented a "gestalting" of the linguistic signal in its prosodic envelope. Prizant (1983) presented a similar view. It could be suggested that echolalia, in that sense, can be compared to the early prosodic "frames," "envelopes," "matrices," or "protowords" described by Bruner (1975), Dore (1975), Menn (1976), Crystal (1979), and others.

When prosody is viewed from the perspective of hemispheric specialization, experimental and pathological evidence has shown that, subject to some limitation, its more properly linguistic use is controlled by the left, language-dominant hemisphere (Monrad-Krohn, 1947, 1957, 1963; Cole, 1971; Danly, deVilliers & Cooper, 1979; Swinney, Zurif, & Cutler, 1980; Baum, Kelsch, Daniloff, Daniloff, & Lewis, 1982; Danly & Shapiro, 1982; Buxton, 1983; Danly, Cooper, & Shapiro, 1983; Joanette, Lecours, Lepage, & Lamoureux, 1983). On the other hand, when prosody is used in terms of its affective or "emotional" function, more recent evidence has shown that it may be a function of the right hemisphere (Haggard & Parkinson, 1971; Heilman, Scholes, & Watson, 1975; Schlanger, Schlanger, & Gerstman, 1976; Safer & Leventhal, 1977; Ross & Mesulam, 1979; Weintraub, Mesulam, & Kramer, 1981). Prosody presumably also is right hemisphere controlled when it is used pragmatically (Weintraub, Mesulam, & Kramer, 1981).

Studies in the early use of prosody support the notion that its prelinguistic use is exclusively affective in nature (Tonkava-Yampolskaya, 1969, 1973; Murry, Amundson, & Hollien, 1977) and that its subsequent linguistic use evolves from its initial affective status (Crystal, 1979). One could thus hypothesize that, in the prelinguistic stages and perhaps through the early stages of language development, all children are right-hemisphere processors when it comes to prosody. With the gradual unfolding of linguistic abilities, prosodic function begins to interact increasingly with more specifically linguistic function. In that context, prosodic abilities may then also shift to the language-dominant hemisphere. Autistic children may not be equipped to make an adequate switch, either because of deficits that directly or indirectly affect the dominant hemisphere or because of a possible maturational lag at the cortical level or both. In contrast, aphasic (language-delayed) children may show a lesser degree of difficulty in making such a switch and/or may be influenced by a different set of maturational variables.

With regard to the above speculation, it is of interest that, although autistic individuals have almost universally been noted to be deficient in prosody, many have been reported to have good musical ability (Applebaum, Egel, Koegel, & Imhoff, 1979). In some individuals, this has been so noteworthy that it has been labeled "idiot-savant" in quality (Sherwin, 1953; Rimland, 1964, 1978; Viscott, 1970). The same acoustic features used in the perception and production of prosody are also used in the perception and production of music. Musical ability, subject to some qualifications, is recognized as a dominantly right hemisphere function (Damasio & Damasio, 1977; Gates & Bradshaw, 1977; Kellar & Bever, 1980).

The idea of an impairment in the specialization of the dominant hemisphere and/or a maturational lag at the cortical level in the autistic individual has also been suggested by other investigators looking at the problem from different perspectives. These include psychological testing (Lockyer & Rutter, 1970; Tymchuk, Simmons, & Neafsey, 1971), specific studies designed to test for such hemispheric specialization as monoaural, binaural, and dichotic listening studies (Blackstock, 1978; Prior & Bradshaw, 1979; Dawson, Warrenburg, & Fuller, 1982), electrophysiological and anatomical studies (Hauser, DeLong, & Rosman, 1975; Tanguay, 1976; Hier, LeMay, & Rosenburger, 1979; Damasio, Maurer, Damasio, & Chiu, 1980) of autistic individuals using a variety of control subjects. These studies have been reviewed in depth by McCann (1981). It is obvious from McCann's review, as well as from the assessment of an increasing body of subsequent studies (Maurer & Damasio, 1982; Arnold & Schwartz, 1983; Gillberg, Rosenhall, & Johansson, 1983; Gillberg & Svendsen, 1983; James & Barry, 1983), that the issue of brain dysfunction in autism is far from settled. Thus, because of its specialized status with respect to hemispheric function, prosody may also be an especially fruitful area for continued investigation with respect to the basic brain dysfunctions seen in autism.

ACKNOWLEDGMENTS

This research was supported by MCH Grant 927-13-1, DD Grant OHD-59-T-45192-13, and NINCDS Grant NS 16479-2.

# REFERENCES

Allen, G., & Hawkins, S. (1980). Phonological rhythm: Definition and development. In G. Yeni-Komshian, J. Kavanagh, & C. Ferguson (Eds.), *Child phonology* (pp. 227–256). New York: Academic Press.

Applebaum, E., Egel, A., Koegel, R., & Imhoff, B. (1979). Measuring musical abilities of autistic children. *Journal of Autism and Developmental Disorders, 9,* 279–285.

Arnold, G., & Schwartz, S. (1983). Hemispheric lateralization of language in autistic and aphasic children. *Journal of Autism and Developmental Disorders, 13,* 129–139.

Atkinson-King, K. (1973). Children's acquisition of phonological stress contrasts. *Working Papers in Phonetics, Vol. 21.* Los Angeles: University of California.

Bagshaw, N. (1978). *An acoustic analysis of fundamental frequency and temporal parameters of autistic children's speech.* Unpublished master's thesis, University of California at Santa Barbara, Santa Barbara, CA.

Baltaxe, C. (1981). Acoustic characteristics of prosody in autism. International Congress for the Scientific Study of Mental Deficiency. In P. Mittler (Ed.), *New frontiers of knowledge in the scientific study of mental deficiency,* (pp. 223–233). Baltimore, MD: University Park Press.

Baltaxe, C. (1984). The use of contrastive stress in normal, aphasic and autistic children. *Journal of Speech and Hearing Research, 27,* 97–105.

Baltaxe, C., & Guthrie, D. (in press). The acquisition of primary sentence stress in normal, aphasic and autistic children. *Journal of Autism and Developmental Disorders,* (in press).

Baltaxe, C., & Simmons, J. Q. (1973). *Echolalia and language acquisition in autism.* Paper presented at the American Speech and Hearing Association, Chicago, IL.

Baltaxe, C., & Simmons, J. Q. (1975). Language in childhood psychosis. *Journal of Speech and Hearing Disorders, 40,* 439–458.

Baltaxe, C., & Simmons, J. Q. (1977). Language patterns of German and English autistic adolescents. In P. Mittler (Ed.), *Proceedings of the International Association for the Study of Mental Deficiency* (pp. 223–233). Baltimore, MD: University Park Press.

Baltaxe, C., & Simmons, J. Q. (1981). Disorders of language in childhood psychosis: Current concepts and approaches. In J. Darby (Ed.), *Speech evaluations in psychiatry,* (pp. 285–325). New York: Grune & Stratton.

Baltaxe, C., & Simmons, J. Q. (1983). Communication deficits in the adolescent and adult autistic. *Seminars in Speech and Language, 4,* 27–41.

Baltaxe, C., Simmons, J. Q., & Zee, E. (1984). Intonation patterns in normal, autistic and aphasic children. In A. Cohen & M. van de Broecke (Eds.), *Proceedings of the Tenth International Congress of Phonetic Sciences* (pp. 713–718). Dordrecht, The Netherlands: Foris Publications.

Bates, E., & MacWhinney, B. (1979). A functionalist approach to the acquisition of grammar. In E. Ochs & B. Schieffelin (Eds.), *Development pragmatics* (pp. 167–211). New York: Academic Press.

Baum, S., Kelsch, Daniloff, J., Daniloff, R., & Lewis, J. (1982). Sentence comprehension in Broca's aphasics: Effects of some supresegmental variables. *Brain and Language, 17,* 261–271.

Blackstock, E. (1978). Cerebral asymmetry and the development of infantile autism. *Journal of Autism and Childhood Schizophrenia, 8,* 339–353.

Blasdell, R., & Jensen, P. (1970). Stress and word position as determinates of imitation in first-language learners. *Journal of Speech and Hearing Research, 13,* 193–202.

Bolinger, D. L. (1964). Around the edge of language. *Harvard Educational Review, 34,* 282–293.

Bonvillian, J. D., Raeburn, V. P., & Horan, E. A. (1979). Talking to children: The effects of rate, intonation and length on children's sentence imitation. *Journal of Child Language, 6,* 459-467.

Branigan, G. (1979). Some reasons why successive single word utterances are not. *Journal of Child Language, 6,* 411-421.

Bresnan, J. Q. (1972). Stress and syntax: A reply. *Language, 48,* 326-342.

Broen, P. (1972). *The verbal environment of the language learning child.* American Speech and Hearing Association Monograph, Vol. 17.

Brown, R., & Bellugi, R. (1964). Three processes in the child's acquisition of syntax. *Harvard Educational Review, 54,* 133-151.

Brown, R., & Fraser, D. (1963). The acquisition of syntax. In C. Cofer & B. Musgrave (Eds.), *Verbal behavior and learning* (pp. 158-197). New York: McGraw-Hill.

Bruner, J. (1975). The ontogenesis of speech acts. *Journal of Child Language, 2,* 1-19.

Butterworth, B. (1980). Some constraints on models of language production. In B. Butterworth (Ed.), *Language production, Vol. 1. Speech and talk* (pp. 432-459). London: Academic Press.

Buxton, H. (1983). Auditory lateralization, an effect of rhythm. *Brain and Language, 18,* 249-259.

Chomsky, N., & Halle, M. (1968). *The sound patterns of English.* New York: Harper & Row.

Chomsky, N., Halle, M., & Lukoff, F. (1956). On accent and juncture in English. In M. Halle (Ed.), *For Roman Jacobson* (pp. 65-80). The Hague, The Netherlands: Mouton Press.

Cole, M. (1971). Dysprosody due to posterior fossa lesions. *Transactions of the American Neurological Association, Vol. 96,* 151-154.

Cooper, W., & Sorensen, J. (1977). Fundamental frequency contours at syntactic boundaries. *Journal of Acoustic Society of America, 62,* 683-692.

Cooper, W., & Sorensen, J. (1981). *Fundamental frequency in sentence production.* New York: Springer-Verlag.

Crystal, D. (1973). Non-sequential phonology in language acquisition: A review of the issues. *Lingua, 32,* 1-45.

Crystal, D. (1979). Prosodic development. In P. Fletcher & M. Garman (Eds.), *Language acquisition,* (pp. 33-48). Cambridge, England: Cambridge University Press.

Cutler, A. (1983). Semantics, syntax, and sentence accent. *Abstracts of the Tenth International Congress of Phonetic Sciences* (pp. 85-91). Utrecht, The Netherlands.

Cutler, A., & Foss, D. J. (1977). On the role of sentence stress in sentence processing. *Language and Speech, 20,* 1-10.

Cutler, A., & Isard, S. D. (1980). The production of prosody. In B. Butterworth (Ed.), *Language production, Vol. 1.* London: Academic Press.

Cutler, A., & Swinney, P. A. (1980). *Development of the comprehension of semantic focus in young children.* Paper presented at the *Fifth Boston University Conference on language Development,* Boston, MA.

Damasio, A., & Damasio, H. (1977). Musical faculty and cerebral dominance. In M. Critchley & R. A. Henson (Eds.), *Music and the brain* (pp. 141-154). London: W. Heinemann Medical Books.

Damasio, H., Maurer, R. G., Damasio, A. R., & Chiu, H. C. (1980). Computerized tomographic scan findings in patients with autistic behavior. *Archives of Neurology, 37,* 504-510.

Danly, M., & Shapiro, B. (1982). Speech prosody in Broca's aphasia. *Brain and Language, 16,* 171-190.

Danly, M., deVilliers, J. G., & Cooper, W. G. (1979). The control of speech prosody in Broca's aphasia. In J. J. Wolf & D. H. Klatt (Eds.), *Proceedings from the 97th Annual Meeting of the Acoustic Society of America* (pp. 259-263). New York: Acoustic Society of America.

Danly, M., Cooper, W. E., & Shapiro, E. (1983). Fundamental frequency processing and linguistic structure in Wernicke's aphasia. *Brain and Language, 19,* 1-25.

Darwin, C. J. On the dynamic use of prosody in speech perception. In A. Cohen & S. G. Noteboom (Eds.), *Structure and process in speech perception* (pp. 178-194). Berlin: Springer-Verlag.

Dawson, G., Warrenburg, S., & Fuller, P. (1982). Cerebral lateralization of individuals diagnosed as autistic in early childhood. *Brain and Language, 15,* 353-367.

DeMeyer, M., Barton, S., DeMeyer, W. E., Norton, J. A., Allen, J., & Steele, R. (1973). Prognosis in autism: A follow-up study. *Journal of Autism and Childhood Schizophrenia, 3,* 199-246.

DiSimoni, F. G. (1974a). Influence of sound environment on the duration of consonants in the speech of three-, six-, and nine-year-old children. *Journal of the Acoustic Society of America, 56,* 360-361.

DiSimoni, F. G. (1974b). Influence of consonant environment on the duration of vowels in the speech of three-, six-, and nine-year-old children. *Journal of the Acoustic Society of America, 56,* 362-363.

DiSimoni, F. G. (1974c). Some preliminary observations on temporal compensation in the speech of children. *Journal of the Acoustic Society of America, 56,* 697-699.

Dore, J. (1975). Holophrases, speech acts and language universals. *Journal of Child Language, 2,* 21-40.

Eilers, R. Suprasegmental and grammatical control over telegraphic speech in young children. *Journal of Psycholinguistic Research, 4,* 227-239.

Ervin-Tripp, S. (1966). Imitation and structural change in children's language. In E. Lenneberg (Ed.), *New directions in the study of Language* (pp. 163-189). Cambridge, MA: M.I.T. Press.

Fairbanks, G. (1942). An acoustic study of the pitch of infant hunger wails. *Child Development, 13,* 227-232.

Fairbanks, G., Herbert, R. L., & Hammond, J. M. (1949). An acoustical study of vocal pitch in seven- and eight-year-old girls. *Child Development, 20,* 71-78.

Fairbanks, G., Wiley, J. H., & Lassman, F. M. (1949). An acoustical study of focal pitch in seven- and eight-year-old boys. *Child Development, 20,* 63-69.

Flege, J. E. (1982). *Timing in the speech of children and adults.* Paper presented at the 103rd Meeting of the Acoustical Society of America, Chicago, IL.

Fletcher, C. (1976). *A comparison of pitch patterns of normal and autistic children.* Unpublished master's thesis. University of California at Santa Barbara.

Fromkin, V. (1983). The independence and dependence of syntax, semantics, and prosody. In A. Cohen & M. van de Broecke (Eds.), *Abstracts of the Tenth International Congress of Phonetic Sciences* (pp. 93-97). Utrecht, The Netherlands.

Fry, H. (1955). Duration and intensity as physical correlates of linguistic stress. *Journal of the Acoustical Society of america, 27,* 765-768.

Fry, H. (1958). Experiments in the perception of stress. *Language and Speech, 1,* 126-152.

Garding, E. (1982). Prosodic expression and pragmatic categories. *Working Papers, Department of Linguistics and Phonetics.* Lund University, Sweden, 22, 117-135.

Garding, E. (1983). Intonation units and pivots, syntax and semantics. In *Abstracts of the Tenth International Congress of Phonetic Sciences* (pp. 99-103). Utrecht, The Netherlands.

Garnica, O. V. (1977). Some prosodic and paralinguistic features of speech to young children. In C. E. Snow & C. A. Ferguson (Eds.), *Talking to children: Language input and acquisition* (pp. 63-88). Cambridge: Cambridge University Press.

Gates, A., & Bradshaw, J. (1977). The role of cerebral hemispheres in music. *Brain and Language, 4,* 403-431.

Gillberg, C., & Svendsen, P. (1983). Childhood psychosis and computed tomographic brain scan findings. *Journal of Autism and Developmental Disorders, 13,* 19-32.

Gillberg, C., Rosenhall, U., & Johanson, E. (1983). Auditory brainstem responses in childhood psychosis. *Journal of Autism and Developmental Disorders, 13*, 181-194.

Goldfarb, W., Braunstein, P., & Lorge, I. (1956). A study of speech patterns in a group of schizophrenic children. *American Journal of Orthopsychiatry, 26*, 544-555.

Goldfarb, W., Goldfarb, N., Braunstein, P., & Scholl, H. (1972). Speech and language faults of schizophrenic children. *Journal of Autism and Childhood Schizophrenia, 2*, 219-233.

Goodglass, H. (1973). Studies on the grammar of aphasics. In H. Goodglass and S. Blumstein (Eds.), *Psycholinguistics and aphasia* (pp. 185-215). Baltimore, MD: Johns Hopkins University Press.

Goodglass, H., Fodor, I., & Schulhoff, C. (1967). Prosodic factors in grammar—evidence from aphasia. *Journal of Speech and Hearing Research, 10*, 5-10.

Haggard, M., & Parkinson, A. (1971). Stimulus task factors as determinants of ear advantages. *Quarterly Journal of Experimental Psychology, 23*, 168-177.

Hauser, S., DeLong, G., & Rosman, M. (1970). Pneumoencephalographic findings in the infantile autism syndrome. *Brain, 98*, 667-688.

Heilman, K. M., Scholes, R., & Watson, R. T. (1975). Auditory affective agnosia. *Journal of Neurology, Neurosurgery and Psychiatry, 38*, 69-72.

Hicks, J. (1972). Language disabilities of emotionally disturbed children. In J. Irwin & M. Marge (Eds.), *Principles of childhood language disabilities* (pp. 137-158). Englewood Cliffs, NJ: Prentice-Hall.

Hier, D., LeMay, N., & Rosenberger, P. (1979). Autism and unfavorable left-right asymmetries of the brain. *Journal of Autism and Developmental Disorders, 9*, 137-158.

Hornby, P., & Haas, W. (1970). Use of contastive stress by preschool children. *Journal of Speech and Hearing Research, 13*, 395-399.

Huggins, A. W. (1972). On the perception of temporal phenomena in speech. *Journal of Acoustic Society of America, 51*, 1279-1290.

Jakobson, R. (1968). Child language, and phonological universals. In A. R. Keiler (Trans.), *Kindersprache, Aphasie und allgemeine Lautgesetze*. The Hague, The Netherlands: Mouton.

James, A. L., & Barry, R. J. (1983). Developmental effects in the cerebral lateralization of autistic, retarded, and normal children. *Journal of Autism and Developmental Disorders, 13*, 43-56.

Joanette, Y., Lecours, A. R., Lepage, Y., & Lamoreux, M. Language in right-handers with right-hemisphere lesions: A preliminary study including anatomical, genetic, and social factors. *Brain and Language, 20*, 217-248.

Kanner, L. (1946). Irrelevant and metaphorical language in early infantile autism. *American Journal of Psychiatry, 103*, 242-246.

Kanner, L. (1971). Follow-up study of eleven autistic children, originally reported in 1943. *Journal of Autism and Childhood Schizophrenia, 2*, 119-145.

Kanner, L., & Eisenberg, L. (1956). Early infantile autism. *American Journal of Orthopsychiatry, 26*, 556-564.

Kaplan, E. (1970). Intonation and child language acquisition. *Papers in Research in Child Language Development, 1*, 1-21.

Keating, P., & Buhr, R. (1978). Fundamental frequency in the speech of infants and children. *Journal of the Acoustic Society of America, 63*, 567-571.

Kellar, K., & Bever, T. (1980). Hemispheric asymmetries in the perception of musical cords as a function of musical experience and family handedness. *Brain and Language, 10*, 24-39.

Kent, R. D., & Forner, L. L. (1980). Speech segment durations in sentence recitations by children and adults. *Journal of Phonetics, 8*, 157-168.

Kirk, L. (1973). Analysis of speech imitations by Gã children. *Anthropological Linguistics, 15*, 267-275.

Klatt, D. G. (1975). Vowel lengthening is syntactically determined in connected discourse. *Journal of Phonetics, 3*, 129-140.

Klatt, D. (1976). Linguistic uses of sequential duration in English: Acoustic and perceptual evidence. *Journal of Acoustic Society of America, 59,* 1208–1221.

Klima, E. S., & Bellugi, U. (1966). Syntactic regularities in the speech of children. In J. Lyons & R. J. Wales (Eds.), *Psycholinguistic papers* (pp. 183–208). Edinburgh: Edinburgh University Press.

Kozhevnikov, V. A., & Chistovich, L. A. (1965). *Speech: Articulation and perception, Vol. 30* (p. 543). Washington, DC: Joint Publication Research Service, Department of Commerce.

Kubaska, C. A., & Keating, P. A. (1981). Word duration in early child speech. *Journal of Speech and Hearing Research, 24,* 615–621.

Kutik, E., Cooper, W., & Boyce, S. (1983). Declination of fundamental frequency in speakers' production of parenthetical and main clauses. *Journal of Acoustic Society of America, 73,* 1731–1738.

Ladd, D. R. (1983). Phonological features of intonational peaks. *Language, 59,* 721–759.

Lashley, K. (1951). The problem of serial order in behavior. In L. A. Jefress (Ed.), *Cerebral mechanisms of behavior* (pp. 112–136). New York: Wiley.

LeHiste, I. (1970). *Suprasegmentals.* Cambridge, MA: M.I.T. Press.

LeHiste, I. (1972). The timing of utterances and linguistic boundaries. *Journal of Acoustic Society of America, 51,* 2018–2024.

LeHiste, I. (1973a). Phonetic disambiguation of syntactic ambiguity. *Glossa, 7,* 107–122.

LeHiste, I. (1973b). Rhythmic units and syntactic units in production and perception. *Journal of Acoustic Society of American, 54,* 1228–1234.

LeHiste, I. (1977). Isochrony reconsidered. *Journal of Phonetics, 5,* 252–263.

LeHiste, I. (1978). Temporal organization and prosody-perceptual aspects. Paper presented at the *Joint Meeting, Acoustic Society of America and Japan.* Honolulu, Hawaii.

LeHiste, I. (1982). The role of prosody in the internal structuring of a sentence. Preprints of the *Plenary Session Papers of the Thirteenth International Congress of Linguistics, Tokyo* (pp. 189–198).

LeHiste, I. (1983a). Signaling of syntactic structure in whipsered speech. *Folia Linguistica, 7,* 239–245.

LeHiste, I. (1983b). Semantics, syntax, and prosody. In *Abstracts of the Tenth International Congress of Phonetic Sciences* (pp. 69–74). Utrecht, The Netherlands.

LeHiste, I., Olive, J. P., & Streeter, L. A. (1976). Role of duration in disambiguating syntactically ambiguous sentences. *Journal of the Acoustic Society of America, 60,* 1199–1202.

Lenneberg, E. (1967). *Biological foundation of language.* New York: Wiley.

Liberman, M. Y. (1983). In favor of some uncommon approaches to the study of speech. In P. F. MacNeilage (Ed.), *The production of speech* (pp. 265–274). New York: Springer-Verlag.

Lieberman, P. (1968). *Intonation, perception and language.* Cambridge, MA: M.I.T. Press.

Lieberman, P. (1975). *On the origin of language.* New York: MacMillan Co.

Lockyer, L., & Rutter, M. (1970). A five to fifteen year follow-up study of infantile psychosis: IV. Patterns of cognitive ability. *British Journal of Social and Clinical Psychology, 9,* 151–163.

Lovaas, O. I., Schreibman, L., Koegel, R., & Rehm, R. (1970). Selective responding by autistic children to multiple sensory input. *Journal of Abnormal Psychology, 77,* 211–222.

Martin, J. (1972). Rhythmic vs. serial structure in speech and other behavior. *Psychological Review, 79,* 487–509.

Martin, J. (1975). Rhythmic expectancy in continuous speech perception. In A. Cohen & S. Nooteboom (Eds.), *Structure and process in speech perception* (pp. 161–177). New York: Springer-Verlag.

Martin, J. (1979). Rhythmic and segmental perception are not independent. *Journal of Acoustic Society of America, 65,* 1286–1297.

Martin, Ph. (1977). A theory of English intonation. *R. A. Institut de Phonetique Bruxelles, 11*, 83–96.

Martin, Ph. (1982). Phonetic realization of prosodic contours in French. Speech Communication, 1, 3–4.

Martin, Ph. (1983). Semantics, syntax, and intonation. In *Abstracts of the Tenth International Congress of Phonetic Sciences* (pp. 75–83). Utrecht, The Netherlands.

Maurer, R. G., & Damasio, A. R. (1982). Childhood autism from the point of view of behavioral neurology. *Journal of Autism and Developmental Disorders, 12*, 195–205.

McCann, B. S. Hemispheric asymmetries and early infantile autism. *Journal of Autism and Developmental Disorders, 11*, 401–411.

Menn, L. (1976). *Pattern, control, and contrast in beginning speech: A case study in the development of word form and word function.* Unpublished doctoral dissertation, University of Illinois at Urbana-Champaign, IL.

Miller, W., & Erwin, S. (1964). The development of grammar in child language. *Monographs of the Society for Research in Child Development, 29*, 9–33.

Monrad-Krohn, G. (1947). Dysprosody or altered "melody of language." *Brain, 70*, 405–415.

Monrad-Krohn, G. (1957). The third element of speech: Prosody in the neuropsychiatric clinic. *Journal of Mental Science, 103*, 326–333.

Monrad-Krohn, G. (1963). The third element of speech and its disorders. In L. Halpern (Ed.), *Problems of dynamic neurology* (pp. 101–118). Jerusalem: Rothschild Hadassah University Hospital and Hebrew University Hadassah Medical School.

Morse, P. (1974). Infant speech production: A preliminary model and review of the literature. In *Experimental Child Psychology, 14*, 477–492.

Morese, P. (1974). Infant speech production: A preliminary model and review of the literature. In R. Schiefelbusch and L. Lloyd (Eds.), *Language perspectives—acquisition, retardation and intervention* (pp. 19-54). Baltimore, MD: University Park Press.

Murry, T., Amundson, P., & Hollien, H. (1977). Acoustic characteristics of infant cries. *Journal of Child Language, 4*, 321–328.

Nakatani, L., & Schaffer, J. (1978). Hearing "words" without words. Prosodic cues for word perception. *Journal of Acoustic Society of America, 63*, 234–245.

O'Hala, J. (1977). The physiology of stress. In L. M. Hyman (Ed.), *Studies in stress and accent. Los Angeles: Southern California Occasional Papers in Linguistics, Vol. 4.*

O'Hala, J. (1978). Production of tone. In *Tone: A linguistic survey.* New York: Academic Press.

Ornitz, E., & Ritvo, E. (1976). Medical assessment. In E. Ritvo (Ed.), *Autism diagnosis, current research and management* (pp. 7–26). New York: Spectrum Publications.

O'Shaughnessy, D. (1979). Linguistic features in fundamental frequency patterns. *Journal of Phonetics, 7*, 119–145.

Paccia, J., & Curcio, F. (1982). Language processing and forms of immediate echolalia in autistic children. *Journal of Speech and Hearing Research, 25*, 42–47.

Padilla, A. M., & Lindbloom, K. (1976). Development of interrogative, negative, and possessive forms in the speech of young Spanish–English bilinguals. *The Bilingual Review/La Revisa Bilingua, 3*, 122–152.

Petersen, G. E., & Barney, H. L. (1952). Control methods used in a study of the vowels. *Journal of the Acoustic Society of America, 24*, 175–184.

Petersen, G. E., & LeHiste, I. (1960). Duration of syllabic nuclei in English. *Journal of the Acoustic Society of America, 32*, 693–703.

Pierrehumbert, J. (1979). The perception of fundamental frequency declination. *Journal of the Acoustic Society of America, 66*, 363–369.

Prior, M., & Bradshaw, J. (1979). Hemispheric functioning in autistic children. *Cortex, 15*, 73–81.

Prizant, B. (1983). Gestalt language and gestalt processing in autism. *Topics in language Disorders, 3,* 16–23.

Pronovost, W., Wakstein, M., & Wakstein, P. (1966). A longitudinal study of the speech behavior and language comprehension of fourteen children diagnosed atypical or autistic. *Exceptional Children, 33,* 19–26.

Rimland, B. (1964). *Infantile autism.* New York: Appleton-Century-Crofts.

Rimland, B. (1978). Inside the mind of the autistic savant. *Psychology Today, 12,* 68–80.

Ross, E. D., & Mesulam, M. M. (1979). Dominant language function of the right hemisphere. Prosody and emotional gesturing. *Archives of Neurology, 59,* 721–759.

Rutter, M. (1966). Prognosis: Psychotic children in adolescence and early adult life. In J. K. Wing (Ed.), *Early childhood autism: Clinical, educational, and social aspects* (pp. 83–100). London: Pergamon Press.

Rutter, M., & Lockyer, L. (1967). A five to fifteen year follow-up study of infantile psychosis. I: Description of sample. *British Journal of Psychiatry, 113,* 1169–1182.

Safer, M., & Leventhal, H. (1977). Ear differences in evaluating emotional tones of voice and verbal content. *Journal of Experimental Psychology, Human Perception and Performance, 3,* 75–82.

Scherer, K. R. (1979). Non-linguistic vocal indicators of emotions and psychopathology. In C. E. Isard (Ed.), *Emotions in personality and psychopathology* (pp. 493–529). New York: Plenum Press.

Scherer, K. R. (1981a) Speech and emotional states. In J. Darby (Ed.), *Speech evaluation in psychiatry* (pp. 189–220). New York: Grune & Stratton.

Scherer, K. R. (1981b). Vocal indicators of stress and speech production. In J. Darby (Ed.), *Speech evaluation in psychiatry* (pp. 171–187). New York: Grune & Stratton.

Schlanger, B., Schlanger, P., & Gerstman, L. (1976). The perception of emotionally toned sentences by right hemisphere damaged and aphasic subjects. *Brain and Language, 3,* 396–403.

Seashore, C., Lewis, D., & Saetit, J. G. (1956). *Manual for the Seashore Test of Musical Talents* (rev. ed.). New York: The Psychological Association.

Sedlackova, E., & Neshidalova, R. (1975). Development of autistic children with special regard to their means of verbal expression. *Folia Phoniatrica, 27,* 157–165.

Sheppard, W. C., & Lane, H. L. (1968). Development of the prosodic features of infant vocalizing. *Journal of Speech and Hearing Research, 11,* 94–108.

Sherwin, A. (1953). Reactions to music of autistic (schizophrenic) children. *American Journal of Psychiatry, 109,* 823–831.

Simmons, J. Q., & Baltaxe, C. (1975). Language patterns in adolescent autistics. *Journal of Autism and Childhood Schizophrenia, 5,* 333–351.

Simon, N. (1975). Echolalic speech in childhood autism. *Archives of General Psychiatry, 32,* 1439–1446.

Smith, B. (1978). Temporal aspects of English speech production: A developmental prospective. *Journal of Phonetics, 6,* 37–68.

Smith, B. K., Sugarman, M., & Long, S. (1983). Experimental manipulation of speaking rate for studying temporal variabilities in children's speech. *Journal of the Acoustic Society of American, 74,* 744–749.

Spring, D., & Dale, P. (1977). The discrimination of stress in early infancy. *Journal of Speech and Hearing Research, 20,* 224–32.

Stark, R., & Tallal, P. (1979). Analysis of stop consonant production errors in developmentally dysphasic children. *Journal of the Acoustic Society of America, 66,* 1703–1712.

Steffenson, M. S. (1977). Satisfying inquisitive adults: Some simple methods of answering yes/no questions. *Journal of Child Language, 5,* 221–236.

Swinney, D., Zurif, E., & Cutler, A. (1980). Effects of sentential stress and word class upon comprehension on Broca's aphasia. *Brain and Language, 10,* 132–145.

Tanguay, P. (1976). Clinical and electrophysiological research. In E. R. Ritvo, B. J. Freeman, E. M. Ornitz, & P. E. Tanguay (Eds.), *Autism: Diagnosis, current research and management* (pp. 75–84). New York: Spectrum Publications.

Tingley, B., & Allen, G. (1975). Development of speech timing control in children. *Child Development, 46,* 186–194.

Tonkava-Yampolskaya, R. V. (1969). Development of speech intonation during the first two years of life. *Soviet Psychology, 7,* 48–54.

Tonkava-Yampolskaya, R. V. (1973). Development of speech intonation in infants during the first two years of life. In C. Ferguson & D. I. Slobin (Eds.), *Studies of child language development* (pp. 128–138). New York: Holt, Rinehart & Winston.

Tyack, D., & Ingram, D. (1977). Children's production and comprehension of questions. *Journal of Child Language, 4,* 211–224.

Tymchuk, A., Simmons, J. Q., & Neafsey, S. (1971). Intellectual characteristics of adolescent childhood psychotics with high verbal ability. *Journal of Mental Deficiency Research, 21,* 133–138.

Viscott, D. (1970). A musical idiot savant. *Psychiatry, 33,* 494–515.

Weintraub, S., Mesulam, M., & Kramer, L. (1981). Disturbances in prosody: A right hemisphere contribution to language. *Archives of Neurology, 38,* 742–744.

Weir, R. (1962). *Language in the crib.* The Hague, The Netherlands: Mouton Press.

Weitz, S. (1979). Paralanguage. In S. Weitz (Ed.), *Nonverbal communication: Readings with commentary* (pp. 221–231). New York: Oxford University Press.

Wieman, L. (1976). Stress patterns in early child language. *Journal of Child Language, 3,* 282–286.

Williams, C. E., & Stevens, K. N. (1981). Vocal correlates of emotional states. In J. Darby (Ed.), *Speech evaluation in psychiatry* (pp. 221–240). New York: Grune & Stratton.

# 6

# Semantic Problems in Autistic Children

## PAULA MENYUK and KATHLEEN QUILL

### INTRODUCTION

Language appears to be represented in the "adult" mind in multiple ways. Semantic storage is in terms of sensory, functional, hierarchical, and associational parameters. Thus, the word *cat* evokes visual, tactile, and other sensory images, the superordinate category animal, and objects, actions, and events (such as jump or chase a mouse) that are related to the basic category word. When the word *cat* appears in a sentence, there are additional features associated with its meaning. It may either be a subject or an object in a sentence, and more rarely, a verb or adjective. The sentence context may further define the meaning of a particular cat. For example, "the big black cat bounded into the dark alley" is a very different representation than "the white fluffy cat snuggled into her lap." When the word cat appears in a story, it can be further defined by new events and relations that are described in the story. In this way, knowledge of what cats are and what they do grows. As these multiple representations are achieved, on-line processing of language can take place with increasing rapidity and accuracy until some asymptote is achieved.

Despite the fact that a word such as *cat* can have multiple meanings, it, nevertheless, represents a basic category or primitive unity. There are lexical items, however, that describe a *relation* between other lexical items and, therefore, a relation between objects and events as they exist. For example, verbs describe a relation between subjects and objects; adjectives and other noun modifiers describe a relation between an object and other objects of that class within a set; adverbs, prepositions, and verb modifiers describe a relation be-

PAULA MENYUK and KATHLEEN QUILL • Boston University, School of Education, Boston, Massachusetts 02215.

tween an action or a state and other actions and states of that class within a set. So-called deictic terms describe a multiple set of relations, including such factors as identification (pronouns), location of objects (demonstratives), and direction of action (directional verbs). Comprehension of the meaning of such lexical items is *never* an evocation of a set of representations, even when the word is in isolation. Comprehension *is* dependent on keeping in mind and mentally manipulating more than one set of representations.

Although autistic children can have great difficulty in acquiring category names and even greater difficulty in understanding that such names can, in fact, have multiple meanings, they appear to have particular difficulty in acquiring relational lexical items. In this chapter what is known about the acquisition of categorical and relational meaning by normally developing and autistic children will be summarized. The cognitive factors that play a role in the development of categorical and relational meaning will be examined to seek an explanation for the patterns of development observed in both groups of children. Finally, the implications of this examination for future research in the semantic development of autistic children and possible avenues of intervention will be discussed.

Before summarizing and attempting to explain semantic development in the two populations it is necessary to remind the reader of two facts. First, although it is widely proposed that autistic children demonstrate a severe cognitive–semantic deficit, only a few studies have examined the specific nature of this deficit and the processes of semantic development in these children. Given this small data base, we can only suggest, in many instances, what the semantic problems of autistic children might be. Second, since autism is a label applied to a continuum of disorders (Menyuk, 1978), caution must be taken in making generalizations about the semantic problems of autistic children. Therefore, this chapter is a very preliminary view of the topic.

## DEVELOPMENT OF CATEGORICAL MEANING BY NORMAL AND AUTISTIC CHILDREN

Under this heading, the process of acquisition of the meaning of words that "stand for" categories in the environment will be discussed. These categories are existing classes to which a lexical item is applied. For example, the lexical items *chair, spoon, hat* are each applied to a class of objects that are similar to each other in terms of a number of features. The lexical item used is arbitrarily selected (and symbolic) in that there is nothing inherent in the word itself that causes it to be applied to the class of objects. The objects in the class, however, are similar in terms of a set of criterial features and differ from objects in other classes in one or more of these features.

In the normally developing child, there are several factors that appear to affect the order in which lexical items for categories are understood and produced. Further, the meaning the child has for these items changes as the child matures (Menyuk, 1977). The communicative importance of the item, the perceptual saliency of the word class or category for which the item stands, the physical parameters of the item (its phonology in sound or sign), and the frequency with which it is used in the environment appear to be the most important factors in determining order of acquisition of lexical items. Thus, for example, items that refer to self and other important persons (baby, mommy, daddy) are acquired early because of their communicative importance. Items that describe easily identifiable objects and events that are physically present are acquired before those that mark objects that are distant or obscure. For example, *truck* and *shoe* are acquired before *moon* and *life*. Words of one syllable with a simple consonant–vowel–consonant structure (cat) are acquired before multisyllabic words with complex series of consonants and vowels. Obviously, those words that are used with the greatest frequency are acquired before those that are used rarely. Each of these factors interact in determining order of acquisition.

As stated, in addition to the above factors, the child's understanding of the meaning of any particular item changes as the child matures. A developmental progression that appears to cut across lexical items has been observed. Evidence for this progression in acquisition of *categorical* meaning is largely based on the production of words at early ages rather than comprehension of these words. This developmental progression has been described as taking place in the stages listed in Table 1.

As can be seen in Table 1, the child first associates a lexical item with a particular referent or event (specificity). The application of a lexical item to a broad category (overgeneralization) then takes place before the category is narrowed in terms of so-called criterial features (differentiation). These features are both perceptual and functional. Thus, *cup* is defined by both its physical features and how it is used. Further, a word's meaning is related to other word meanings and superordinate classes are formed (generalization). What is important to further development is that there appears to be increasing flexibility in the application of words. They are more widely defined and are used across different syntactic categories and in creative language (multiple meanings).

There has been a good deal of discussion about the role of the feature acquisition in the development of the meaning of a word. Some researchers (Clark & Clark, 1977) take the position that word acquisition is dependent on observation of new and more subtle or complex features. Early word meanings are only subsets of the complete feature composition of the word. Clark and Clark propose that children acquire word meanings by gradual addition of perceptual features. For example, *dog* might first be understood as having the fea-

Table 1.   Development of the Meaning of the Word *Cup*

| Stage | Referential meaning |
|-------|---------------------|
| Specificity | One particular cup |
| Overgeneralization | All items you drink from (cup, glass, bottle) |
| Differentiation | Only items that have criterial features |
| Generalization | Member in set of items that you drink from |
| Multiple meaning | As a verb (as in ''cup your hands'') |
| | As part of a metaphor (as in ''cup of kindness'') |

tures + animal, + four legs and only later the additional features of + small, + bark. These added features would distinguish the application of the word dog from the words *horse* and *cat*. Other researchers suggest that words are understood in particular contexts at first and then in a wider range of contexts. It is not the suggested features that are crucial in development of word meaning, but rather determination from varying contexts of the intrinsic and variable meanings of a word (Carey, 1978). The question that needs to be addressed is whether or not the same or similar processes take place in the autistic child's acquisition of meanings.

The early vocabulary of autistic children is usually limited to those lexical items that refer to inanimate objects. The children demonstrate a disproportionate number of nouns. A typical profile of autistic children's vocabulary development shows that lexical items are restricted to food and inanimate object labels. Reference to common nouns, then, often extends to such terms as color names, numbers, and letter identification. Thus, it appears that aspects of the environment that are perceptually static are initially acquired. This contrasts with studies of normal word acquisition. The normal young child's first words cover a range of experiential and personal–social terms, such as *bye-bye*, *up*, *all gone*, *dirty*, and *mommy*.

As normal children expand their vocabulary, they also demonstrate an ''intuitive'' understanding of categorical relations. We infer the child's knowledge of basic relations between items of a category from his or her lexical overextension of a term to other class members (Rescorla, 1981). This is the stage of overgeneralization described in Table 1. Perceptual similarities between class members and functional commonalities among the items lead to overgeneralization *and* eventually contribute to the child's categorization skills. Such overgeneralization has not been noted in the lexical acquisition of autistic children. Indeed, there is ample evidence that the meaning of some terms never gets beyond the specificity stage. Rescorla suggests that the normal child's organization of objects and events into categories is an ability that ''approximates the adult system in internal structure . . . while lacking understanding of the logical relationships inherent in each class.'' This ability to form natural classes may be a basic difficulty for many autistic children.

Recently, Tager-Flusberg (1983) examined the ability of autistic chldren to categorize familiar objects at the basic and superordinate levels. These were children who knew the names of most task items. These items included such basic level classes as chair, fish, and house, as well as such superordinate level categories as animals, clothing, and food. She found that the autistic children's performance matched that of the retarded and normal control groups used (mental ages 3–9). For example, the children were able to match-to-sample picture stimuli of items from the same class. They also successfully selected from an array of pictures the members of a verbally named category and correctly identified items belonging to a specific class through *yes/no* question responses. These findings suggest that some autistic children can form natural classes.

Further evidence that some of these children are capable of categorical semantic organization comes from the linguistic analyses of language samples from high-functioning autistic adolescents (Simmons & Baltaxe, 1975). Although semantic errors were frequently observed, the pattern of errors involved systematic substitutions from the correct semantic field and syntactic class. This suggests lexical organization patterns similar to normal.

Schuler and Bormann (cited in Fay & Schuler, 1980) also used a match-to-sample paradigm to explore categorization of natural classes with severely impaired autistic children. However, they concluded that the children's categorization ability was limited. The children had difficulty understanding functional relations between items. The researchers determined this by teasing apart strategies used in categorizing. Their findings show that the autistic children were able to match perceptually similar and identical items, but had difficulty matching objects on the basis of functional equivalence (comb to brush) and functional complements (paper to pencil).

This variation in findings among the studies must reflect the heterogeneous nature of the autistic syndrome or, in particular, differences in skill levels between groups of these children. These differences also imply that the children may be using different strategies in categorizing items. Some autistic children may develop a category that contains a set of critical features, for example, animalness, and they learn how these features can extend. They are able to organize their visual world into categories according to perceptual features and experiences. Other autistic children may not be relying upon perceptual and experiential relations between items as a criteria for categorization and word application. Categorization, for them, may be based on a simple chaining together of items that have been explicitly organized for them by others. For example, attribute + object may be stored as a fixed whole (for example, *big box*, *small boy*, etc.) rather than as separable and recombinable items that generate phrases such as *big boy*, *small box*, etc. Thus, word application is a fixed routine or a specifically cued response. All autistic children, however, appear to lack the knowledge of functional attributes of lexical items. This information is not available to them as a criteria for categorization. They base the formation of categories on either perceptual similarities or fixed routines.

In support of the above conclusions are the findings of Waterhouse and Fein (1982). An error analysis of autistic children's naming responses on the Peabody Picture Vocabulary Test revealed different retrieval strategies from normal children. When autistic children were unable to name an item, they would respond with the name of a related object with similar perceptual qualities (pin for nail) or from the same semantic category (bird for turkey). However, a common strategy used by normal children when having difficulty naming was to describe the item's function: a hammer is "for daddy's work" and a broom is "you clean with it." The normal child might also gesture to show how you act upon the item (pretends to play the guitar). These retrieval strategies were never observed in the autistic children. Thus, it appears that autistic children have limitations in organizing categories in the environment on the basis of their functional attributes. Of course, functional attributes imply *relations* between actors, instruments, and objects. It is these relations that appear particularly difficult for autistic children in *addition* to their difficulty in categorizing in appropriate ways.

## DEVELOPMENT OF RELATIONAL MEANING BY NORMAL CHILDREN

There have been many studies of the development of relational terms by normally developing children. What is important to note is that this development takes place over a number of years but begins at a fairly early age. By about age 8 or 9, many of these relational terms are understood and used in an adult manner. Most of the terms are in the process of being acquired during the period from 2 to 5 years. The early beginnings can be observed with deictic verbs (come–go), locative prepositions (in, on, under), quantifiers (more–less), and temporal terms (before–after). In fact, relational terms, such as *more* and *no*, are found in children's early two-word utterances at ages 18 to 24 months. Wales (1970) provides evidence, that attributive terms, such as *big*, are understood as being *comparative* rather than absolute by children of 3 1/2 years. Clark and Clark (1977), in their discussion of semantic development, suggest that comprehension of dimensional terms starts at age 2 to 3 with the *big–small* contrast and then spreads to more complex terms, such as *thick–thin*, *wide–narrow*, and *deep–shallow*. In sum, despite the proposed abstractness of these terms; that is, they presumably require mental comparisons, they begin to be acquired very early on.

Despite early beginnings, there are marked changes in the way in which children understand and use these terms over the period of 3 to 9 years, and additional terms are added over the same period. This pattern of semantic development is said to be a reflection of several factors. The first of these is the conceptual base on which the term is said to rest. Later-developing concepts result in later acquisition of the terms that represent them (Slobin, 1979). An example of this is marking of verb tense. The present participle that marks ongoing action is acquired before the past tense or future tense markers. The child can, at first, only observe the fact that action is ongoing and, not until later, that action has already taken place or will occur some time in the future. Another factor is the arbitrariness of the lexical item or, in many instances, the expression. Thus, with expressions of time such as "his birthday is *on* June 9" or "...*in* June," children frequently alternate the prepositions *on* and *in*. This factor does not consistently affect the sequence of acquisition. Again, children learning languages with articles marking gender (such as *la* or *le*) appear to have little difficulty in acquiring the appropriate articles (Maratsos, 1979), despite the arbitrariness of the marking. This may be due to the strategy of learning employed. In the above case, the article and noun may be learned as one unit to begin with. The final factor, then, may be the type of learning strategies used by the child. Those strategies can lead to correct or incorrect conclusions about relational terms, depending on the exact nature of the terms and the context in which they appear. For example, in comprehension of the deictic verbs *come–go*, *come* appears to be more accurately and easily understood than *go*. There is a marked tendency for children to treat all directional terms as describing direction toward (Macrae, 1976).

Although the above factors are not mutually exclusive, each factor on the surface seems to be particularly germane to a specific class of relational terms. Nevertheless, all of these factors could be subsumed under the general heading of learning to relate relations between objects and actions to linguistic representations and, therefore, a relational learning task.

The product of this learning can be said to be a result of the information processing strategies employed by children over time: what they attend to, encode, and remember. The argument that will be made here is that there are two aspects in the acquisition of relational terms that make them particularly difficult for autistic children to acquire: first, the need to process contextual and linguistic material simultaneously for understanding of relational terms, a difficulty that severely affects many aspects of language development by autistic children; second, the gestalt or associative manner in which relations are encoded in the memory of autistic children. The acquisition of deictic terms by normally developing children will be used as the example of how these factors could be considered explanatory. The few data that are available on autistic children's acquisition of relational terms will then be discussed.

Table 2 lists category types of relational terms with examples of each type.

Table 2.  Categories of Relational Terms

| Class | Relations |
|---|---|
| | Comparisons |
| Verbs | Among subjects and objects |
| | Ex: Transitive—kiss |
| | Ex: Change of State—break |
| Determiners | Among objects within a set |
| | Ex: Size—Big |
| | Ex: Quantity—Many |
| Adverbs | Among actions and states within a set |
| | Ex: Manner—quickly |
| | Ex: Time—now |
| | Contexts |
| Prepositions | Among objects and events within contexts |
| | Ex: Place—in |
| | Ex: Direction—to |
| Deictic Terms[a] | Among *self*, objects, and events within contexts |
| | Ex: Determiner—this, that |
| | Ex: Prepositions—to, from |
| | Ex: Verb—bring, take |
| | Ex: Adverb—temporal marker |

[a]Includes all classes above.

As can be seen in Table 2, deictic terms include all types of relational terms and, in addition, *always* mark the very special relation among *self*, objects, and events. It should be noted that adverbs and prepositions are very similar in function and hard to distinguish from deictic terms.

Deixis is probably the most relevant category of relational terms to discuss in order to approach an understanding of the semantic problems of autistic children. Deictic terms function as pointers in space and time and describe relations among self, others, objects, and events. Further, in order to comprehend utterances containing these terms, the listener needs not only to understand the utterance *per se*, but also the situation or context in which it is being used.

In light of the social–cognitive problems attributed to autistic children, the factors that play a role in the processing of deictic terms make them of particular importance in understanding the semantic problems of autistic children.

The acquisition of deixis has been recently discussed and summarized by Clark and Clark (1977) and Wales (1979). In his summary, Wales briefly describes five areas of deixis: (a) *this–that, here–there*; (b) pronouns; (c) front, back, and sides; (d) *come* and *go*; and (e) temporal deixis. Only three of these areas (a, b, and d) will be discussed here.

*This–that* and *here–there* were frequently labeled as being in the Pivot class in early *Pivot-Open* descriptions of these two-word utterances (Menyuk, 1977). When they are first used, these terms are frequently accompanied by a pointing and/or handling gesture on the part of both the mother and child in communicative interaction. Thus, the attention-getting "meaning" rather than the adult contrastive locative meaning of these terms has clearly been acquired at a very early age. Further, the children contrast *this* and *here* from *that* and *there* by using the former two terms for objects appearing on the scene and the latter for those disappearing from the scene. Knowledge of the meaning of these terms rises in interactive situations in which both parties initially use these terms to direct attention. From approximately 2 years on, children increase their knowledge of the meaning of these terms in distinct ways. First, they realize that the spatial location of the speaker is involved and parcel out the location cues in particular situations with reference to the speaker. Wales describes this determination of relevant cues as a gradual process in which the child constructs a system of contrasts and learns when and how to apply this system.

The process of acquiring such directional verbs as *come* and *go* is quite similar to that described for the demonstratives and locatives. Children's "correct" interpretation of these terms is highly dependent on the particular situations in which they are being asked to perform. As children mature, correct production and interpretation becomes less dependent on particular situations. Other factors such as movement (in this case, toward) play a role in the order of acquisiton of these terms. Correct final location determines use of demonstrative and locative deictic terms. Thus, movement within observable space between self and others is an important aspect of construction of the system of contrasts.

The same set of strategies is also used in the acquisition of pronouns. There is early frequent pointing by mother and child when using the third-person pronoun, as there is for demonstratives and locatives. The personal pronouns *I* and *you*, however, are learned by the normal child simply by frequent references to persons present and without frequent pointing.

In summary, development of deictic terms takes places gradually, is initially highly dependent on interaction, begins with the indicating function, and ends with contrastive notions that are very dependent upon particular contextual events.

## DEVELOPMENT OF RELATIONAL MEANING BY AUTISTIC CHILDREN

Autistic children's language is characterized by slow acquisition and restricted use of relational word classes. They have particular problems in generalizing meaning across settings and, therefore, use certain of these word classes in an absolute rather than relational manner, even though the terms themselves are relational in nature. A similar phenomena is said to exist for a brief period in normal development. Piaget stated that young children tend to "misconstrue relations as absolute classes" (Flavell, 1977). This behavior is observed during the specificity stage of word acquisition (Table 1). However, as indicated previously, there is early knowledge of comparisons with some of these relational terms. This appears not to be the case with autistic children.

Most aspects of the determiner's meaning entail making comparisons. Attributes such as *big* (spatial), *fast* (temporal), *some* (quantifier), and *ugly* (qualitative) all require contextual comparisons for meaning. For example, one must understand the parameters of the terms *big* and *little* in order to grasp the relations between them. It is possible that for the autistic child, the attribute *big* is understood simply as a term for sets of objects that share some common feature rather than as relations holding between persons and objects within sets. *Big* is interpreted as an attribute of that object, which is represented in memory as a particular perceptual image and context, rather than as an attribute of an object that can be judged differently across contexts. The autistic child's inability to make these conceptual comparisons and judgments may then result in a narrow range of meaning assigned to each term.

Prepositions do not have a particular perceptual referent as a basis of meaning. Prepositions, like deictic terms, serve both as spatial and temporal devices that describe relations among objects and events. Prepositions, in addition, can have multiple meanings. For example, the preposition *in* can denote such multiple relations as: "put the toy *in* the cabinet," "go to lunch *in* 5 minutes," or "change *into* your pajamas." Similarly, when prepositions function as verb particles, an understanding of the relation between the particle and the verb is required. *Stand up, pick up,* and *walk up* each represent a different notion of directionality. Difficulty with assigning multiple meanings to a single lexical item is yet another aspect of the autistic child's semantic limitations and was noted in Kanner's original description of the syndrome (1943). Churchill (1972) found, in attempting to teach directional prepositions to an autistic child, that the child could use the given preposition in a specified way in the learning setting, but was unable to generalize the term to new situations. Problems with preposition errors were also noted in the language sample analyses by Simmons and Baltaxe (1975).

Verbs, deictic or otherwise, are often difficult for autistic children to acquire because verbs vary in the degree to which they are linked to events and objects. In normal development, the process of verb acquisition is slower than the development of nouns (Gentner, 1978) because the meaning of verbs is less perceptually linked than nouns. In addition, all verbs become figurative extensions of space and time and tend to be broad in their meaning and usage (Gentner, 1978). For example, the verb *turn* can be learned in the context of "turn the page," but can be extended to convey such multiple meanings as "turn the handle," "turn the key," "turn the corner," "turn over..." and, in metaphoric usage, "the Easter egg turned pink." The normally developing child's acquisition of verb meaning follows a pattern of analysis and gradual accretion of these various meaning components. This analysis requires the ability to extract similarities and identify relations conveyed by the verb across various contexts.

Although there is no exploration of verb acquisition in the literature on autism, one would expect comprehension and use to vary according to (a) degree of abstractness and (b) breadth of meaning and usage. For example, the children should acquire a gerund such as *fishing*, since gerunds are nominalized verbs and encode visually presented information. Action verbs can also be directly linked to a set of perceptual features and events and are often observed in the autistic child's vocabulary. However, the compositional analysis necessary for the flexible use of these verb classes poses difficulty for them. Each verb is often acquired and used in a very restricted manner. That is, verb usage is limited to the context within which it was acquired. Further, as previously discussed, deitic verbs entail a relation between self and objects, others and an action. The verbs *come-go, give-take* require the child to shift perspective from the point of view of the speaker in order to understand the meaning. These pose particular difficulty for the autistic child, as do the first and second person pronouns, and for much the same reasons. The processing requirements of verbs that code actions and external events are, in additional ways, different from verbs that code internal states and change of state. These latter verb classes have little surface information upon which to apply meaning and/or require the conceptualizations of changes over time. The autistic child demonstrates difficulties with understanding the meaning of such stative verbs (want, like, believe, expect) and verbs that code changes of state (find, make, change).

Thus far, the difficulties autistic children are observed to have, or that we postulate they have, with adjectives, prepositions, and verbs can be accounted for by (a) the need for mental comparisons; (b) the need to observe changes of meaning across contexts; and (c) the need to derive meanings from linguistic and situational contexts that do not make these meanings obvious. Other categories of relational terms cause difficulties for autistic children for similar reasons.

Autistic children fail to understand changes in meaning associated with morphemes. Ricks and Wing (1976) noted abnormal constructions in which the morphemes were omitted, but the main relations preserved. Bartolucci, Pierce, and Streiner (1980) analyzed the acquisition of Brown's morphemes in autistic children and matched control groups. The autistic children lacked mastery of verb tense markers and uncontracted copula and auxiliary verbs. Their atypical order of acquisition and delay in the use of these morphemes did not correlate with other measures of syntactic complexity, namely, MLU. This pattern of morpheme development demonstrates deficits in aspects of meaning that contribute to relational notions expressed in the verb phrase. For example, modification of the verb through tense markers provides temporal information about the verb and requires a shared understanding of time references in discourse.

Bartolucci and Albers (1974) systematically examined verb tense usage in autistic children. Through elicitation tasks, sentence completion tasks, and language samples, the use of present progressive and past tense by autistic children was compared to matched control groups. Although present tense use was the same as that of controls, the autistic group was significantly depressed in production of past tense. This marked discrepancy between the use of the two verb tenses was unique to the autistic children. The findings suggest that difficulties with verb tense parallel the autistic child's problems with deriving meaning from linguistic and situational contexts that do not make the meaning explicit or do not stand in a one-to-one relation with an absolute category.

When the linguistic and situational context does make clear the meaning of the morphemes, the autistic child may be more successful in varying morpheme application. Blank and Milewski (1981) made more explicit, in a systematic way, the role of morphemes that encode here-and-now experiences. Their one subject evidenced generalization in use of these morphemes across verbs.

Semantic knowledge goes beyond the meaning of individual lexical items and isolated constituents (verb phrase) and includes a range of experiences that are expressed in larger syntactic–semantic units. Structured relations among words are essential for an understanding and expression of meaning.

Comprehension of semantic relations involves a set of linguistic analyses that are nonlinear. The word order of a sentence does not always directly reflect the order in which events occur. The verb, considered the core to sentence meaning, generally sits in the middle. Semantic relations are understood by an analysis of the verb as it relates to other constituents of the sentence. Sentences, therefore, cannot simply be processed word by word. Normal children initially rely on general knowledge about the world to interpret sentences that are semantically biased. This has been called the probable-event strategy. They also utilize a word order strategy. The child interprets each subject–verb–object (SVO) construction as agent–action–object. Such SVO sentences have been found to be successfully comprehended by autistic children (Tager-Flusberg, 1981). She assessed the sentence comprehension and strategy use of 18 autistic children compared to matched normal 3- and 4-year-olds. The children were asked to act out active and passive, biased and reversible sentences. The autistic children's overall comprehension was lower. But more importantly, they did not generally use a probable-event strategy to understand the sentence. Rather, they relied upon the word order alone for comprehension. Thus, with the sentence "The boy hits the truck" they acted it out following the word order. The autistic children's strategy of acting out agent–action–object in word order for all sentences demonstrated their knowledge of the individual terms. Their lack of using a probable-event strategy demonstrates an inability to understand the logical relations and functions of the nouns and verbs of each sentence. Where the normal child's responses are affected by the probability of the event, the autistic children did not appear to have a notion of how the constituents of each sentence interact with each other to generate meaning.

Similar results were found through an assessment of more severely impaired children's comprehension of two-word intransitive phrases and three-word transitive phrases (Prior & Hall, 1979). These children also demonstrated difficulty comprehending relations between agent, action, and object. Analysis of their errors revealed that responses were often cued by the subject of the sentence. This might point to the beginnings of a word order strategy for comprehension. It might also suggest that the children did not understand the meaning of the verb and, therefore, relied upon the noun for responding.

Paccia and Curcio (1982) controlled for comprehension of the basic proposition when examining the responses to questions by five echolalic children. The frequency of echolalic responding was influenced by the type of question. A high frequency of echolalia was noted in responses to *yes/no* questions, whereas more appropriate responses were given for such questions as *who*, *what*, *where*, etc., and sentence completion questions constructions. Understanding *yes/no* questions requires more internal analysis of subject–verb relations (Searle, 1969 cited in Paccia & Curcio, 1982) than the other question forms and was most problematic for the children. These results lend support to previous findings that word order is the strategy used by autistic children to decode the semantic relations of a sentence.

In normal development, with the addition of more complicated structures as compared to the basic SVO structure, alternative strategies must be used by the child in interpreting language. Comprehension of the use of morphemes and relational terms contribute to this developmental process and lead to an understanding of, for example, passive sentences and the *yes/no* question forms. For the autistic child, it appears that no alternative strategies to the SVO strategy are adopted. It is used in an absolute way. The children have not learned the particular constraints on the use of this strategy nor developed new strategies.

The autistic child's problems with relational terms and their linguistic expression are most evident in discourse. Comprehension is an interface between understanding of semantic relations inherent in the sentence and assimilating the information into the communicative setting (Wells, 1981). Meaning is defined by rules of use. Semantic relations are highly dependent upon the context for interpretation. Conversation also requires the building of a schema to organize how propositions in each utterance are related. Building upon a topic requires memorizing and organizing, as well as monitoring the relevant information of a message. Language in context requires multiple level processing. Communication is a dynamic process in which the individual must attend to linguistic and contextual information that changes from moment to moment. Word and sentence meanings shift as a function of these contextual variables. Thus, the successful use of language involves (a) analysis of the relations expressed in a message and (b) the ability to follow the events of the conversation in both time and space. These analyses are difficult for autistic children at the sentence level. They pose even more problems at the discourse level. In a linguistic analysis of the language samples of seven autistic adolescents (Simmons & Baltaxe, 1975), semantic constraints represented the most frequent discourse violations. Errors in word selection indicated the children's difficulty both in understanding relations within the sentence and in relating previously used words to the current phrase. In a later study, Baltaxe (1977) described the major problem for autistic children in conversation as the differentiation of old from new information. The autistic child's limitations in understanding how language marks relations between people, objects, and events, and the resulting use of rigid sentence comprehension strategies, appear to underlie these observed conversation deficits.

## COGNITIVE FACTORS IN DEVELOPMENT OF CATEGORICAL AND RELATIONAL MEANING

Autistic children evidence limitations in the comprehension and production of semantic categories and relations (Prior & Hall, 1979; Tager-Flusberg, 1981; Layton & Baker, 1981). Maltz (1981) observed similar kinds of categorical deficits in the nonlinguistic domain. In an examination of the performance errors of autistic children on the Leiter International Performance Scales, he found that they did most poorly on subtests that require organizing concrete information on the basis of inherent relations among stimuli. Piaget attributes difficulty in understanding the relativity of relations to a generalized inability to encode multiple perspectives (Flavell, 1977). A similar conceptual constraint seems to exist in the nonlinguistic processing of autistic children (Hermelin, 1978). Thus, the cognitive factors that affect the ability to classify and determine relations among persons, objects, and events seem to be equally affected in the linguistic and nonlinguistic domains in autistic children.

Throughout this chapter we have tried to suggest those factors that affect semantic development. In this section, we will attempt to summarize what these factors are and indicate how they limit semantic development in autistic children.

As we have stated, autistic children differ in their underlying capacity to acquire knowledge. These differences manifest themselves first in variation among the children and differences between them and normal children in the processes used to organize input information and, then, in differences in the kinds of knowledge acquired.

Some autistic children learn ''language'' in an operant fashion (Ricks & Wing, 1976). Learning of linguistic symbols is accomplished by establishing associations between words or sentences and objects and events as unanalyzed wholes. These symbols are then chained together. This chaining of associations appears to be the only strategy available to a large majority of autistic children who develop minimal linguistic skills. The product of such a strategy is a repertoire of language behaviors restricted to specific situations. A similar type of language behavior is the Pledge of Allegiance produced by the children in the primary grades. The situation and the behavior are irrevocably tied together and there is, therefore, nothing *generative* in the language knowledge.

Other autistic children are able to observe perceptual similarities and differences between objects and events and assign meaning on the basis of this analysis. Their ability to analyze input information distinguishes them from the autistic children described above. The depth and the width of this analysis varies within this group and, therefore, they achieve different levels of semantic knowledge. Some of these children can only label a specific array of objects, whereas other children are able to generalize to other members of a category. It is possible that the rate at which information is processed affects the number of distinguishing features that can be observed and encoded as part of meaning. The slower the processing, the more limited the number of features that can be observed. This may lead to overspecification in meaning.

In addition to rate, the manner in which information is processed has an effect on development of semantic knowledge. This development is not only dependent upon the ability to detect criterial features and make associations between bundles of features and linguistic symbols, it also requires the ability to perform compositional analyses. These analyses, in turn, require multiple representations of the meanings of lexical items. As indicated in the beginning of this chapter, words are thought to be stored in terms of the structural roles they play, as members of hierarchical and associational sets of other words, and as perceptual features. There is little evidence that autistic children achieve these multiple representations. Because of this, they are unable to decompose information within the sentence into related parts that are crucial to derivation of meaning in sentences that differ in structure from SVO. In this latter type of sentence, a word-by-word analysis sometimes leads to corrrect interpretation.

This same limitation leads, of course, to difficulties in discourse processing in which analysis of meaning entails processing of linguistic, paralinguistic, and contextual information simultaneously.

It appears, then, that the range of semantic problems in autistic children parallels the degree to which these analyses are impaired. Analysis of the composition of the word, sentence, and/or conversation is absent, limited, or qualitatively different. This results in the constrained behaviors observed at one or all of these linguistic levels. For the large proportion of autistic children who learn language in an operant fashion, the ability to decompose information at the word level is impaired. Those children that develop strategies for sentence comprehension and use have skills in classifying lexical items, but are unable to perform analyses at the sentence level because their classifications are limited. This results in rigid approaches to interpreting sentence meaning. For the high-functioning autistic child, discourse poses the greatest difficulty. The multidimensional composition of information in discourse imposes processing demands beyond the capacities of all autistic individuals.

## IMPLICATIONS FOR FUTURE RESEARCH AND INTERVENTION

This discussion of the development of categorical and relational meaning and the cognitive factors that contribute to its development is an attempt to obtain a clearer understanding of the semantic patterns of autistic children. Using this kind of information as a framework, future investigations should be aimed at answering two basic questions: What is the precise nature of the semantic knowledge in autistic children; specifically, what word classes and sentence relations are comprehended and used by the children, and under what conditions? and, What are the learning strategies available to autistic children that influence the acquisition of semantic information? When addressing each of these questions, there are important factors to consider. First, we must determine what aspects of the linguistic information and situational context the child is processing for meaning in general. Second, we need to outline the scope of application of these meanings across contexts. Third, we need to provide the child with multiple response mode options, verbal and nonverbal.

What appears evident from the semantic patterns of autistic children is that the acquisition process is different from the process in normal children, and this is probably due to the limited learning strategies available to them. Therefore, we need to examine the development of specific semantic patterns, that is, word class and semantic relations knowledge. Under what conditions does comprehension and use of this linguistic material appear? For example, we could investigate the comprehension of directional prepositions, varying the linguistic and situational contexts and the response mode to determine the specific parameters that influence the child's understanding and use. Is it the case that the child understands the word *through* when shown a picture of a child walking through a tunnel, but is unable to comprehend the meaning of the utterance *walk through the tunnel* in a real context. Does the use of contextual cues facilitate comprehension, or is it the case that multiple stimuli in context make processing of the message more difficult? By highlighting less salient aspects of a sentence (e.g., grammatical morphemes), will the child's understanding of subtle meaning distinctions be facilitated?

Fourth, how do the strategies available to autistic children influence these patterns of semantic development? This question may be answered by examining what strategies the children use in acquiring new linguistic symbols. If, for example, you present an unfamiliar object with a novel term and introduce the object's perceptual and functional features, how will the child extend the use of the term to additional objects that are either the same or similar in one or more of these features? The strategies the children use to assign meaning might be inferred from those features that they select as criterial for defining the term. Based on this information, alternative or additional strategies could be taught.

Semantic development is dependent upon an environment that facilitates the capacities to perceive, organize, and observe relations within and across settings. If we assume that autistic children have problems interpreting multiple information simultaneously and are limited in their capacity to analyze the composition of the information in order to infer relations, then approaches to intervention need to account for *each* of these factors to derive methods of teaching categorical and relational meaning to them. The goal is to facilitate the children's understanding of the multidimensional aspects of the linguistic and contextual environment upon which meaning is built. We need to systematically assist the child in analyzing the features of word classes and the composition of sentences, using the natural environment as a means to co-actively engage the child in the mapping of language onto experiences. We must move beyond vocabulary building and expand the child's understanding of relations that exist between objects and events, and these relations may need to be taught to autistic children in a systematic manner. Networks of associations should be explicitly presented with each concept. For example, the child's identification of *cat* must be associated with what cats eat, how cats play, etc. In light of this knowledge, the child can then examine the plausibility of "catness" in various semantic relations and across linguistic contexts.

The objective of research and intervention is then twofold: to identify the capacities intrinsically available to autistic children and to determine which aspects of the linguistic and contextual environment can be modified to facilitate the use of additional learning strategies.

In summary, our understanding of autism raises more questions than it clearly answers. Still, in our developmental understanding of the "meaning of autism,'' we are like the young child. Today, each of us perceives the gestalt of the syndrome, assigning a similar but somewhat different meaning to the term "autism." However, through our continued pursuit of an understanding of the composition of the autistic child, we will gain a refined definition. It is hoped that we will soon be able to converse about autism with shared meaning.

# REFERENCES

Baltaxe, C. A. M. (1977). Pragmatic deficits in the language of autistic children. *Journal of Pediatric Psychology, 2,* 176–180.

Bartolucci, G., & Alberts, R. J. (1974). Deictic categories in the language of autistic children. *Journal of Autism and Childhood Schizophrenia, 4,* 131–141.

Bartolucci, G., Pierce, S. J., & Streiner, D. (1980). Cross-sectional studies of grammatical morphemes in autistic and mentally retarded children. *Journal of Autism and Developmental Disorders, 10,* 39–50.

Blank, M., & Milewski, J. (1981). Applying psycholinguistic concepts to the treatment of an autistic child. *Applied Psycholinguistics, 2,* 65–84.

Carey, S. (1978). The child as a word learner. In M. Halle, J. Bresnan, & G. Miller (Eds.), *Linguistic theory and psychological reality* (pp. 443–456). Cambridge, MA: M.I.T. Press.

Churchill, D. (1972). The relation of infantile autism and early childhood schizophrenia to developmental language disorders of childhood. *Journal of Autism and Childhood Schizophrenia, 2,* 182–197.

Clark, H., & Clark, E. (1977). *Psychology and Language.* New York: Harcourt Brace Jovanovich.

Fay, W., & Schuler, A. (1980). *Emerging language in autistic children.* Baltimore, MD: University Park Press.

Flavell, J. (1977). *Cognitive development.* Englewood Cliffs, NJ: Prentice-Hall.

Gentner, D. (1978). On relational meaning: The acquisition of verb meaning. *Child Development, 49,* 988–998.

Hermelin, B. (1978). Images and languages. In M. Rutter & E. Schopler (Eds.), *Autism: A reappraisal of concepts and treatment* (pp. 141–154). New York: Plenum Press.

Kanner, L. (1943). Autistic disturbances of affective contact. *Nervous Child, 2,* 217–250.

Layton, T. L., & Baker, P. S. (1981). Description of semantic–syntactic relations in an autistic child. *Journal of Autism and Developmental Disorders, 11,* 385–399.

Macrae, A. (1976). Movement and location in acquisition of deictic verbs. *Journal of Child Language, 3,* 191–204.

Maltz, A. (1981). Comparison of cognitive deficits among autistic and retarded children on the Arthur Adaptation of the Leiter International Performance Scales. *Journal of Autism and Developmental Disorders, 11,* 413–426.

Maratsos, D. (1979). Learning how and when to use pronouns and determiners. In P. Fletcher & M. Garman (Eds.), *Language Acquisition* (pp. 225–240). Cambridge, England: Cambridge University Press.

Menyuk, P. (1977). *Language and maturation.* Cambridge, MA: M.I.T. Press.

Menyuk, P. (1978). The language of autistic children: What's wrong and why. In M. Rutter & E. Schopler (Eds.), *Autism: A reappraisal of concepts and treatment* (pp. 105–116). New York: Plenum Press.

Paccia, J. M., & Curcio, F. (1982). Language processing and forms of immediate echolalia in autistic children. *Journal of Speech and Hearing Research, 25,* 42–47.

Prior, M. R., & Hall, L. C. (1979). Comprehension of transitive and intransitive phrases by autistic, mentally retarded and normal children. *Journal of Communication Disorders, 12*, 103–111.

Rescorla, L. (1981). Category development in early language. *Journal of Child Language, 8*, 225–238.

Ricks, D. M., & Wing, L. (1976). Language, communication and the use of symbols. In L. Wing (Ed.), *Early childhood autism* (2nd ed.). Oxford: Pergamon Press.

Simmons, J. Q., & Baltaxe, C. (1975). Language patterns of adolescent autistics. *Journal of Autism and Childhood Schizophrenia, 5*, 333–351.

Slobin, D. (1979). *Psycholinguistics*. Glenview, IL: Scott, Foresman.

Tager-Flusberg, H. (1981). Sentence comprehension in autistic children. *Applied Psycholinguistics, 2*, 5–24.

Tager-Flusberg, H. (1983, April). *Structure and use of semantic knowledge in autism*. Paper presented at the Boston Univerity Psychology Colloquium, Boston, MA.

Wales, R. (1979). Deixis. In P. Fletcher & M. Garman (Eds.), *Language acquisition* (pp. 241–260). Cambridge: Cambridge University Press.

Waterhouse, L., & Fein, P. (1982). Language skills in developmentally disabled children. *Brain and Language, 15*, 307–333.

Wells, G. (1981). *Learning through interaction*. Cambridge: Cambridge University Press.

# 7

# The Expressive Language Characteristics of Autistic Children Compared with Mentally Retarded or Specific Language-Impaired Children

LINDA SWISHER and M. J. DEMETRAS

## DEFINITION OF SYNDROMES

For purposes of this chapter, the three developmental disorders of autism, mental retardation, and specific language impairment will be defined as follows:

*Autism*: A developmental disorder characterized by four criteria: (a) impaired social development that has a number of special features and that is inappropriate for the child's intellectual level; (b) delayed and/or deviant language development that also has certain defined features and that is inappropriate for the child's intellectual level; (c) insistence on sameness as shown by stereotyped play patters, abnormal preoccupations, or resistance to change; and (d) onset of the above before the age of 30 months (Rutter, 1978). Synonyms for autism have included *psychosis* and *childhood schizophrenia*.

*Mental retardation*: A developmental disorder characterized by significant subaverage general intellectual functioning (operationalized as two or more standard deviations below the mean on a norm-referenced intelligence test) that exists concurrently with deficits in adaptive behavior (that

LINDA SWISHER and M. J. DEMETRAS • Early Childhood Language Research Laboratory, Department of Speech and Hearing Sciences, University of Arizona, Tucson, Arizona 85721.

is, the degree and efficiency with which the individual meets "the standards of personal independence and social responsibility expected of his age and cultural group") with both occurring within the developmental period (from birth to age 18) (Grossman, 1977, p. 11).

*Specific language impairment* (SLI): A developmental disorder characterized by a specific failure of the normal growth of language relative to other levels of functioning. It cannot readily be ascribed to deafness, mental retardation, motor disability, or severe personality disorder (Benton, 1964). Synonyms for SLI have included developmental aphasia, congenital aphasia, and dysphasia.

## INTRODUCTION

The most frequently asked questions in the literature relevant to the expressive language of children with autistic behaviors, mental retardation, or specific language impairment pertain to the issue of delay or aberrancy. That is, is a component of expressive language similar to younger, normal children, and thus delayed, or different from normal children of any age, and thus aberrant? The issue of delay versus aberrancy may not be resolvable. The most frequently used procedure for matching autistic, mentally retarded, and SLI children to normal controls is by a measure of nonverbal intelligence. This procedure typically results in the experimental group being older than the controls. Another procedure is to match the experimental groups to normal children with a measure of syntactic development. This also results in the experimental group being older than their controls. Children with more experience with the world and more experience talking cannot be expected to be simply delayed. A fine enough sieve might find developmental differences due to the experience difference alone.

Having acknowledged that we are addressing an unresolvable issue, we will proceed to emphasize that those expressive language domains that can be studied alone (e.g., syntax and morphology) appear delayed. However, when the interaction of two domains is considered (i.e., syntax and semantics or syntax and pragmatics), the expressive language of autistic children appears aberrant.

This chapter will focus on two features of the expressive language of autistic children: superficial form and form–context mismatch. When these two features are considered together, they differentiate the expressive language of autistic children from that of normal children and also from that of children with mental retardation or specific language impairment. Some of the utterances of many autistic children appear to have weak cognitive underpinnings. These utterances are constructed of strings of words that are syntactically correct, but that are either immediate echoes of what has just been said to the child or chunks of words that do not show up separately in more creative utterances. There is little recombination of the words in the "chunk" into other phrases. Wing (1976, p. 111) is apparently referring to this same characteristic when she refers to the "store of phrases" used by many autistic children. We will refer to this feature in which the syntax of an utterance is weakly attached to its semantic base as *superficial form.*

Some utterances spoken by autistic children are often perceived to be inappropriate for a given context. They do not appear to communicate to the listener what other children of the same developmental level usually mean when speaking similar words in similar contexts. As a consequence, when the context is not provided, an utterance may be assumed, incorrectly, to be appropriate. A failure to realize that the match between the form of what the child says and the context in which it is spoken is idiosyncratic may lead clinicians to conclude that the child's expressive language is more advanced than it actually is. We will refer to this second feature, in which syntax is poorly attached to its pragmatic base, as a *form–context mismatch.*

Neither feature alone is unique to children with autistic behavior. Superficial form is seen, for example, in children with hydrocephalus who are considered hyperverbal (Swisher & Pinsker, 1971; Schwartz, 1974). A form–context mismatch is characteristic of some children diagnosed as psychotic who do not meet the criteria of autism (Cunningham, 1968). Each feature may vary in level of severity between and within the subgroups of autistic children that have been described (cf. Swisher, Reichler, & Short, 1976; Rapin & Allen, 1983).

Investigations of syntax, morphology, semantics, or pragmatics that compared autistic children with another group will be reviewed in relation to the two features described above. Initially, only those studies that provided a normal control group were chosen for review, so that a judgment of delay or aberrancy could be considered when comparing the three disability groups. Very few studies, however, provided these controls. Consequently, additional studies were chosen so that comparisons between at least two of the three disability groups could be made. Since the focus of this chapter is on group comparative studies, what we are emphasizing must be understood as overall trends rather than as an inevitability for any one child.

## NORMAL DEVELOPMENT OF EXPRESSIVE LANGUAGE

A normally developing child's utterances evolve over time into adult-like sentences in terms of three language domains—syntax (word order), semantics (word, phrase, and sentence meaning), and pragmatics (the use of language in context). Initially, children say only one word in each utterance and thus word order is not a consideration. At approximately 18 months of age, children quite frequently say more than one word within each utterance. Then they begin to change the word order within their sentences to cue part of the meaning being conveyed. For example, a 24-month-old might say "dog bite man" or "man bite dog." The difference in meaning between these two utterances containing the same words is obvious not only to the man, but also to the listener. Next, the somewhat simple sentences expressed by 3-year-olds develop into the complete, complex sentences expressed by 5-year-olds within which one clause can modify another.

The meanings being expressed in words become more complex as the child's thinking becomes more sophisticated. This development of cognitive complexity is reflected in the type, variety, and number of words the child uses in each utterance. For example, a child of 10 months may say *daddy*, with little awareness of the word's meaning. This same child, at 14 months, may overgeneralize the word to refer to all men, and then at age 18 months use the word only to refer to the original referent—presumably with a more adult-like meaning being expressed.

As the semantics and syntax become more complex and interdependent, a child also develops a greater variety of ways to obtain the objects and information he seeks. He increasingly chooses his words in relation to the information needs of his listener and the sentence type in relation to the politeness rules of society. For example, a child of 3½ may be regarded as charmingly direct when he asks, "Do you love my mommy?" of his mother's new suitor. An older child, however, is expected to be more indirect and might use a statement to declare that he, in fact, loves his mommy. By being indirect, he provides an opportunity for the suitor to respond but does not request that the information be given to him.

In summary, the level of development in syntax, semantics, or pragmatics fairly easily predicts the level of development in the other domains for normally developing children. For example, a child at the telegraphic stage of sentence development who has not yet used an auxiliary verb would not be expected to express causal relationships. When the level of development in one domain does not predict the level in another, the mismatch usually indicates some type of impairment.

## EVIDENCE FOR SUPERFICIAL FORM IN AUTISTIC CHILDREN

The following two dialogues are typical examples of evidence for superficial form in autistic children (Shapiro, Roberts, and Fish, 1970, pp. 425 and 427).

EXAMINER: Look at me? What's my name?
CHILD: What's my name?

EXAMINER: (aside) He's touching the letters like he's reading them.
CHILD: The letters touch read, read, read.

## Syntax

The most extensive investigation that compared the syntax of autistic children to at least one other group of children was conducted by Pierce and Bartolucci (1977). They collected spontaneous speech samples from three groups of subjects (10 autistic, 10 mentally retarded, and 10 normal children) selected for nonlinguistic mental age (NLMA) on the Arthur Adaptation of the Leiter International Performance Scale (Leiter) (Arthur, 1952). All subjects were required to have an NLMA on the Leiter of approximately 6 years. Two measures of syntax were used to analyze 50 different spontaneous utterances—the Developmental Sentence Scoring system (DSS) (Lee, 1974) and a transformational analysis system based on the work of Chomsky (1957, 1965). Both analyses measure syntactic complexity with no reference to either the meanings represented or the context in which the utterances are expressed. The DSS indicated that the autistic children had significantly poorer $(p < .05)$ scores on this measure than did the other two groups of children. The transformational analysis indicated that the grammatical systems of all three groups were similar in being rule-governed, but that only the autistic group used significantly less $(p < .05)$ complex language.

Bartak, Rutter, and Cox (1975) compared two groups of boys (19 autistic and 23 "dysphasic") on a wide variety of measures. The Reynell Developmental Language Scales, a spontaneous language sample, a parent interview, and a standardized test of language skills developed by the investigators were used to assess the subjects' linguistic skills. The groups were matched for performance intelligence (IQ) on the Wechsler Intelligence Scale for Children (WISC) (Wechsler, 1949). The mean performance IQs for the autistic and dysphasic groups were 93.0 and 92.3, respectively. The mean age for the autistic group was 7 years, 0 months; the mean age for the dysphasic group was 8 years, 2 months. The authors found that both groups had a similar mean length of utterance (MLU) of four to five words and did not differ in the grammatical complexity of their speech.

Twenty-four of the children (12 autistic, 12 dysphasic) in the Bartak *et al.* (1975) study were reevaluated two years later by Cantwell, Baker, and Rutter (1978). The mean ages for the autistic and dysphasic group were 9 years, 2 months and 9 years, 11 months, respectively. The WISC performance IQ scores were 93 for the autistic group and 96 for the dysphasic. Ninety-minute language samples were obtained from an audiotape recorded session in each child's own home at a time when the mother was free to be with the child. Analyses were then made of phrase structure and transformational rules for the child's nonecholalic utterances. No significant differences were found between the two groups for either syntactic analysis.

With one exception (Pierce & Bartolucci, 1977), these studies suggest that when the DSS, MLU, phrase structure, or transformational rules are used to measure level of syntax, autistic children are significantly delayed with respect to normal controls, but not with respect to children with mental retardation or specific language impairment. The one exception is the finding that the autistic group had significantly lower scores than the mentally retarded group's performance on the DSS in Pierce and Bartolucci's study (1977). This finding could reflect the fact that not all mentally retarded children are language impaired. The matching of subjects by nonverbal mental age did not ensure that they would have similar levels of language functioning, since some of the mentally retarded children may have language skills appropriate for their level of performance skills. By definition the autistic children (and SLI, for that matter) would not.

## Morphology

Several investigators have analyzed the production of morphemes in the language of autistic children as compared with other groups with developmental disabilities. By definition, a morpheme is the smallest recurring unit of the syntax of a language that, in and of itself, has meaning (e.g., *dog, -ed, -ing,* or *-s*).

Cantwell *et al.* (1978) analyzed the usage of morpheme rules in the 22 subjects described in the Bartak *et al.* (1975) study (11 autistic and 11 dysphasic matched for nonverbal IQ). Nine morphemes were chosen for this analysis (e.g., *ing,* plural *s, -ed,* and possessive *'s*). The occurence of each morpheme in the language samples of the children was scored on a 0 to 3 scale (0, no usage; 1, frequently omitted; 2, infrequent error; and 3, no error). The two groups differed (*p* < .05) only on the production of one morpheme—third person present tense *s*. Consequently, they concluded that no noteworthy differences existed in usage of morpheme rules between the autistic and dysphasic groups.

Bartolucci, Pierce, and Streiner (1980) investigated the production of morphemes in the same subjects studied by Pierce & Bartolucci (1977) (10 autistic, 10 mentally retarded, and 10 normal children matched for nonverbal IQ). Fourteen morphemes studied by Brown (1973) and de Villiers and de Villiers (1973) were chosen for the analysis. First, the frequency of occurrence of these morphemes in obligatory contexts, that is, where an adult would use a certain morpheme, was analyzed for the three groups. This analysis revealed a significant difference ($p < .05$) between the autistic and normal groups, with the autistic children omitting more morphemes. No significant difference was found between either the autistic and mentally retarded groups or the mentally retarded and normal groups. In the second analysis, the authors compared the rank-ordering of correct usage of the morphemes by the autistic and the mentally retarded children with the normal data reported by de Villiers and de Villiers (1973). No significant correlations were found between the results of any of the three groups. The authors then suggested that the development of morphological features in the autistic group was "atypical," that is, aberrant. Two factors warrant consideration before this conclusion may be drawn from their data. The mean and standard deviation for correct production of morphemes for the three groups varied markedly (autistic: $X=89\%$, $s=6.2$; mentally retarded: $X=97\%$, $s=3.8$; normal: $X=59\%$, $s=24$). First, there was less variability in the correct production of the morphemes for both the autistic and mentally retarded groups than for the normal group described in the de Villiers' data. Second, the high percentage of correct usage (as evidenced by the means) for both the mentally retarded and autistic group resulted in a ceiling effect. This effect indicates that the task was not of equal difficulty for all groups.

These two studies suggest that the morphological development of autistic children's expression of morphemes in their spontaneous language is delayed, compared with normal controls. No difference was found when they were compared with children with mental retardation or specific language impairment matched on nonverbal IQ measures. Thus, as was true for syntax, autistic children appear to be delayed with respect to normal controls, but not with respect to children with mental retardation or specific language impairment.

## Semantics

In spite of the numerous reports that autistic children do not always use meaningful speech, Tager-Flusberg (1981) noted that there are no systematic studies of semantic development in autistic children comparable to the current body of research on semantic development in normal children (e.g., Bowerman, 1978). Furthermore, no studies have directly investigated the relationship of expressive semantic skills in different populations of disordered children. The most pertinent evidence comes from investigations of verbal memory skills.

Hermelin and O'Connor (1967) investigated the recall skills of 12 psychotic children (who met the criteria for autism) and 12 mentally retarded children in two separate experiments. The ages for the children ranged from 8 years to 14 years, 5 months ($X=10$ years, 8 months). They were individually matched on a receptive vocabulary measure (Peabody Picture Vocabulary Test, Dunn, 1959) and an immediate memory span for digits. The mental age scores on the Peabody ranged from 2–6 to 10–8 ($X=4$–3) and the digit span ranged from 2 to 7 ($X=4.5$). No standard deviations were reported. In the first experiment, the sentences presented had (a) words frequently used by children in an order appropriate for English; (b) frequently used words in an agrammatical order; or (c) infrequently used words in a grammatical order. Three analyses of variance were carried out. No statistically significant differences were found between the groups for recall of frequent words when compared with infrequent word sentences. Both groups recalled more frequent words than infrequent words. However, the psychotic children recalled more words ($p < .025$) in both conditions than the mentally retarded children. Similarly, the comparison of recall for sentences of infrequent words with random arrangements of frequent words did not result in a significant difference between groups, but the psychotic children did better ($p < .001$) than the controls in both instances. An analysis of the difference between scores from sentences and randomly arranged sequences of words matched for frequency resulted in a groups by conditions interaction ($p < .025$). Although the mentally retarded children did significantly better with sentences than with random sequences, no significant difference was found for the psychotic children. Thus, the effect of meaningful language on recall was less marked for the psychotic group than for the mentally retarded group. Overall, it appeared that the psychotic group had better recall skills than the mentally retarded, but they made less use of the aid to recall provided by meaning in sentence structure.

In the second experiment, Hermelin and O'Connor (1967) investigated recall of agrammatical sentences of eight words apiece, a span chosen deliberately to be beyond the digit memory span of both groups (e.g., "blue, three, red, five, white, six, green, eight"). No differences were found between the two groups in terms of number of items recalled. A further analysis compared the clustering of similar items—clustering being defined as the sequential reordering of any items that conceptually belonged to a similar category (colors, numbers, animals, etc.). They found that the mentally retarded group reordered their responses significantly more ($p < .05$) than did the psychotic group. An additional test that analyzed the placing of items into categories resulted in similar differences ($p < .01$) with the psychotic children making less use of the conceptual information. The psychotic subjects tended to repeat the exact order of the words as they were presented, suggesting that they did not reorganize the material according to its meaning. Thus, the psychotic group did not appear to use the conceptual categories inherent in the word lists to aid their recall as much as did the mentally retarded group.

In summary, these studies of recall skills may indicate that autistic children do not take as much advantage of the semantic information presented to them as do normal controls or mentally retarded children. Another possibility is that they did not comprehend what was said to them and, as a consequence, did not process the semantic information. Thus, we cannot conclude that their development of semantic skills is aberrant, but rather that, until proven otherwise, it is delayed.

## EVIDENCE FOR FORM–CONTEXT MISMATCH IN AUTISTIC CHILDREN

The following utterance is a classic example of form–context mismatch in autistic children (Kanner, 1946, p. 242).

CHILD: Don't throw the dog off the balcony.

*Nonlinguistic Context*: several instances when the child was tempted to throw an object.

*Linguistic Context*: Mother had said these words to the child after repeatedly retrieving a toy dog he threw off the balcony of their hotel room.

### Pragmatics: A Behavioral Assessment of Meaning

Semantics and pragmatics would seem to be closely related. How could a child be expected to appropriately use words for which he does not have a meaning base? In fact, observation of the use of words relative to the context in which they are used is a way to behaviorally define meaning. A child who uses—by adult standards— a given word in appropriate contexts, but not in inappropriate contexts, e.g., "dog" to refer to a small dog, a big dog, but not a horse, would be considered to have more of the meaning of "dog" than a child who speaks the word in the presence of a cat, a horse, or a cow. In fact, any example that would serve as an illustration of an utterance with little meaning would also serve as an example of one that is not tied normally to the context in which it was spoken.

The pragmatic approach to the study of meaning, however, involves a serious methodological limitation. The degree to which an utterance has meaning—that is, is appropriate for the context in which it was spoken—is a judgement made by a listener. Consequently, the process involves one person's opinion and another's intent. In this case, the opinion is generally that of an adult, and the intent that of a child.

### Investigations of Pragmatics

Many researchers and clinicians have pointed out that one of the major deficits in autistic children is in the area of communicative competence. Most of these studies have focused only on the autistic population (cf. Baltaxe, 1977; Baltaxe & Simmons, 1975; Shapiro, Chiarandini, & Fish, 1974; Shapiro, Huebner, & Campbell, 1974; Shapiro & Fish, 1969) and, thus, will not be reviewed. The following two studies provide evidence that autistic children differ significantly from other disordered groups because of their deficient amount of spontaneous verbal expression and their deficient communication skills. In the study that included a normal group, the author concluded that the autistic group appeared "deviant."

Ball (1978) analyzed speech acts (the intentions a speaker wants a listener to recognize) and discourse rules in the spontaneous speech obtained from five autistic, five developmental aphasic (who met the criteria for specific language impairment), and five normal children. The children were individually matched for receptive vocabulary on the PPVT (Dunn, 1959), and the mean age for each group was autistic, 4-6; aphasic, 4-2; and normal, 4-3. No standard deviations were reported, but the range was from 3-3 to 5-7 years. The Leiter International Performance Scale (Leiter, 1969) was administered to the autistic and aphasic children. All children in these two groups scored 70 or greater (range, 70 to 98). The means and standard deviations were not reported for either group, and no performance measure was reported for the normal group. An analysis of expressive language skills indicated that the aphasic and normal groups had similar mean length utterances (MLU), as did the autistic group when compared to the aphasic group. In contrast, the MLU for the autistic group was significantly lower ($p < .01$) than the normal group. The mean chronological age for each group was autistic, 8-2; aphasic, 6-0; and, normal, 4-0. The two year gap in ages between groups represented a significant difference in all cases ($p < .001$).

The analysis of speech acts was based on a broad classification developed by Bloom (1974), and the language samples were then analyzed according to an adapted version of the functional code formulated by McNeill and McNeill (1975). The results for the analysis of speech acts indicated that the autistic children used the two functions of "informing" and "regulating" their listeners significantly less than ($p < .05$) both the normal and aphasic groups. No significant differences were reported between the aphasic and normal groups for this analysis. The results for the analysis of discourse rules indicated that a greater amount ($p < .01$) of inappropriate utterances was found only in the speech of the autistic group when compared to either of the other two groups.

Ball concluded that the autistic children were functioning at a less advanced level of pragmatic development than their aphasic and normal counterparts. She also concluded that the process of pragmatic development of the autistic children is "deviant." Careful analysis of the subject characteristics, however, is warranted before this second conclusion can be drawn. When the difference in expressive language skills and the wide variability in Leiter scores is taken into account, this "deviant" pattern may, indeed, represent a delay in development.

Cantwell *et al.* (1978) analyzed three main types of functional language usage in the 12 autistic and 12 dysphasic subjects matched for nonverbal IQ originally studied by Bartak *et al.* (1975): socialized speech (i.e., spontaneous remarks, directions, and appropriate echoes), abnormal and "egocentric" speech (inappropriate immediate and delayed echoes, thinking aloud, metaphorical speech), and automatic and nonverbal speech. The dysphasic children used significantly more ($p < .01$) socialized speech, with the noteworthy difference ($p < .002$) being that the dysphasic group made twice as many spontaneous remarks than the autistic children. The groups did not differ in their usage of appropriate or prompted immediate echoes, which accounted for 10% of the utterances spoken by both groups. However, "abnormal" or egocentric usage was very much more common ($p < .01$) in the autistic group, accounting for over 18% of utterances compared with less than 3% in the dysphasic group. Delayed echoes were rare for the dysphasic children, whereas they accounted for some 5% of autistic utterances ($p < .05$). When individual children were considered in each group, none of the dysphasic children showed more than 1% usage of abnormal speech, whereas seven of the twelve autistic children did ($p < .01$). Of the five who did not show this type of speech, four were noteworthy for their low rate (less than 30%) of spontaneous remarks. In summary, at both the individual and group levels, there were marked differences between autistic and dysphasic children in their functional usage of language, with the former showing less "socialized" speech, more "abnormal, egocentric" speech, and more delayed echolalia.

## ECHOLALIA

When the domains of syntax and morphology are viewed alone, there is no direct evidence for aberrancy in the expressive language of autistic children as compared with that of the two other disordered groups. However, when we combine two domains, either syntax and semantics or syntax and pragmatics, we find that there is a mismatch in skills in the autistic children that does not exist in children with mental retardation or specific language impairment. This mismatch is most evident in the phenomenon of echolalia, in which children are able to repeat long utterances that do not appear to be attached to a semantic base.

Past a certain point in a child's development, the presence of echolalia is often associated with language impairment, as is shown in the speech of autistic, mentally retarded, and SLI children (Baltaxe & Simmons, 1975; Fay, 1980; Schuler, 1979). It is found in normally developing children beginning at approximately 9 months and continuing until 2 or 3 years of age. As normal children's language skills become more complex, the frequency of the echolalia decreases (Prutting & Connolly, 1976; Menyuk, 1977). Howlin (1982) demonstrated that echolalia in autistic children also decreases in frequency as their language skills become more complex. What aspect of echolalia, then, accounts for it being described as aberrant?

Without clear differentiation of which form of echolalia (e.g. immediate, mitigated, or delayed) is being studied (Schuler, 1979; see also Chapter 8 by Schuler & Prizant), it is difficult to draw valid conclusions. However, two studies reported that autistic children use significantly more echolalia than their controls. Shapiro *et al.* (1970) reported greater ($p < .03$) immediate echolalia in the 4-year-old autistic children than three groups of normal controls of different ages (2, 3, and 4 years). Contrarily, Cantwell *et al.* (1978) reported no significant difference in immediate echolalia for their autistic subjects when compared with dysphasic children matched for nonverbal IQ. They did, however, report a difference for delayed echolalia between the two groups. The immediate echolalia would be most characteristic of superficial form, and the delayed echolalia of form–context mismatch.

The conflicting views regarding echolalia are not surprising, considering the difference in matching procedures. When chronological age is used, the autistic children, by definition, will be more language impaired than their controls. In line with the results of Howlin (1982), Prutting and Connolly (1976), and Menyuk (1977), they would be expected to have more echolalia. Similarly, if nonverbal IQ is used as the matching criterion for autistic children and mentally retarded children, the autistic children will more than likely have a greater language impairment than their controls. Consequently, the issue of echolalic speech in autistic children, as compared with children with other developmental disabilities, cannot be solved until more elaborate designs are used to account for the developmental level of both nonverbal IQ and language skills.

## DISCUSSION

At present, the evidence for superficial form is indirect from both verbal recall experiments and studies of echolalia. The verbal recall experiments indicate that either the meaning carried by the input was not comprehended or utilized or both. Compared to nonmeaningful strings of words, meaningful strings of words (i.e., sentences) did not facilitate recall as much for the autistic children as for the mentally retarded children. The experiments also indicated that the autistic children were better able than the retarded children to recall all verbal material presented to them. In another experiment, the responses of autistic children did not show as much of a clustering effect related to word categories as did the responses of the mentally retarded children. The inference is that meaning is not solidly connected to the words used in the spontaneous utterances of autistic children.

The studies reviewed for form–context mismatch suggest that autistic children appear to use language in a manner that is different from both normal children and children with mental retardation or specific language impairment matched for normal nonverbal IQ. This finding is in line with parental reports cited by Bartak *et al.* (1975, 1977). Pierce and Bartolucci (1977) and Bartolucci *et al.* (1980) reached similar conclusions after finding no differences between their experimental groups on measures of syntax and morphology. These conclusions of aberrant use of language may be accounted for by the mismatch between the form that autistic children produce and the contexts in which the words are spoken.

Examples of immediate and delayed echolalia were given at the beginning of the superficial form and form–context mismatch sections, respectively. In both instances, the semantic underpinnings may be weak relative to the memory components. It appears that autistic children can remember words better than they can connect them to a cognitive base. A result of these discrepant skills appears to be the storage of the syntactical structure of an utterance without the meaning accompanying it. Immediate echolalia, then, becomes a case of a remembered, poorly analyzed utterance spoken immediately after the event; and delayed echolalia becomes a remembered, poorly analyzed utterance spoken as a chunk of words a long time after the utterance was presented to the child by someone else. The major difference between immediate and delayed echolalia may simply be the amount of time the child holds onto a heard utterance before recalling it in a poorly analyzed form.

In conclusion, the issue of delay versus aberrancy cannot be addressed by analyzing individual domains of expressive language skills of autistic children. Until proven otherwise, we must conclude that the development of these individual domains in these children is delayed. When an interaction of domains is viewed, however, we find that there is a mismatch in skills in the autistic children that does not exist in children with mental retardation or specific language impairment. It is this mismatch that must be addressed when we develop facilitation programs for individual children.

## CLINICAL IMPLICATIONS FOR AUTISTIC CHILDREN

Several implications for assessment and intervention can be drawn from the two features of expressive language we have discussed. The presence of superficial form indicates that an autistic child may be very much at risk for being started in intervention at too difficult a level. Thus, both the examiner and language facilitator must be well versed in developmental sequences of language and cognition. They must understand the developmental stages through which children move in the process of becoming more and more efficient in communicating with others through words. Clinicians with this knowledge can more easily and accurately find the growing edge of the child's meaningful, appropriately used utterances and, therefore, can more easily and accurately determine what language-learning task usually comes next in development.

One consequence of intervening at the child's growing edge is that the frequency of echolalic speech may decline. Once the appropriate level for the child is found, the language facilitator will adjust what he says to the child accordingly. Echolalia is more common, for example, following stimuli such as *wh-* questions or utterances that are beyond the child's level of comprehension (Fay, 1980; Paccia & Curcio, 1982). A further benefit of using more appropriate levels of input will be a potential growth in the child's level of language comprehension.

With regard to form–context mismatch, as pointed out by Prizant (1983), we have no evidence to suggest that children do not *want* to communicate conventionally to others. We can only say that they do not communicate well with words. We could interpret this feature as indicating that a child might be attempting to communicate, but that the listener does not have the appropriate referent. Consequently, when a child utters a sentence that appears to be totally inappropriate to the listener, the listener must remember that he was not present to observe all past communicative exchanges that might have a bearing on the present one. Kanner's (1946) example of delayed echolalia quoted at the beginning of the form–context mismatch section illustrates this point.

Procedures for assessing the expressive language of autistic children must provide a means of separating those utterances that are more complex in syntax than in their semantic underpinnings from those that have a more normal tie to their semantic base. Standardized tests may not provide this information. Tests of expressive language that rely heavily on the direct, immediate imitation of words may overestimate the child's level of meaningful, communicative expressive language. Regardless of modality, the use of standardized tests focuses on too limited a context—usually pointing to or talking about pictures. Because of both superficial form and form–context mismatch, repeated observations of the child's expressive language in a variety of communicative settings may be the most useful information for formulating expressive language objectives. Standardized tests of comprehension can be useful, however, in leading the examiner to use appropriate levels of language input to the child.

A focus for intervention should be the development of a semantic base for words, phrases, and sentences spoken in appropriate contexts. Forms already spoken by the child when therapy began could be elicited in a variety of contexts in order to facilitate the development of more in-depth semantic underpinnings. Should expressive tasks become too difficult, listening to the same words used appropriately by others would also be encouraged. Although comprehension was not a focus of the present review, poor comprehension would be expected to accompany both superficial form and form mismatched to context.

Many of the clinical strategies for autistic children will be similar to those appropriate for any child with a language impairment. We stress beginning and maintaining language facilitation at appropriate developmental levels for both comprehension and expression so that the child will have a chance to learn and thus succeed. Children who are successful will seek more opportunities to learn. If we are at too high a level, we frustrate them and, as a result, discourage them from seeking these opportunities. Check to see if the topics and activities are of interest to the child. Autistic children, at least as frequently as normal children, prefer to talk about their own interests rather than those of the language facilitator. Most importantly, check the level of language spoken to the child, and if it is at too high a level in relation to the semantic underpinnings, a cutback to a lower semantic level is in order.

# REFERENCES

Arthur, G. (1952). *The Arthur adaptation of the Leiter international performance scale.* Washington, DC: Psychological Service Center Press.

Ball, J. (1978). *A pragmatic analysis of autistic children's language with respect to aphasic and normal language development.* Unpublished doctoral dissertation, Melbourne University, Melbourne, Australia.

Baltaxe, C. A. (1977). Pragmatic deficits in the language of autistic adolescents. *Journal of Pediatric Psychology, 2,* 176–180.

Baltaxe, C. A., & Simmons, J. Q. (1975). Language in childhood psychosis: A review. *Journal of Speech and Hearing Disorders, 40,* 439–458.

Bartak, L., Rutter, M., & Cox, A. (1975). A comparative study of infantile autism and specific developmental receptive language disorder: I. The children. *British Journal of Psychiatry, 126,* 127–145.

Bartak, L., Rutter, M., & Cox, A. (1977). A comparative study of infantile autism and specific developmental receptive language disorders. III. Discriminant Function Analysis. *Journal of Autism and Childhood Schizophrenia, 7,* 383–396.

Bartolucci, G., Pierce, S. J., & Streiner, D. (1980). Cross-sectional studies of grammatical morphemes in autistic and mentally retarded children. *Journal of Autism and Developmental Disorders, 10,* 39–50.

Benton, A. L. (1964). Developmental aphasia and brain damage. *Cortex, 1,* 40–52.

Bloom, L. (1974). Talking, understanding and thinking. In R. L. Schiefelbusch & L. L. Lloyd (Eds.), *Language perspectives, acquisition, retardation and intervention* (pp. 285–311). Baltimore, MD: University Park Press.

Bowerman, M. (1978). Semantic and syntactic development: A review of what, when, and how in language acquisition. In R. L. Schiefelbusch (Ed.), *Bases of language intervention* (pp. 97–190). Baltimore, MD: University Park Press.

Brown, R. (1973). *A first language: The early stages.* Cambridge, MA: Harvard University Press.

Cantwell, D., Baker, L., & Rutter, M. (1978). A comparative study of infantile autism and specific developmental receptive language disorder. IV. Analysis of syntax and language function. *Journal of Child Psychology and Psychiatry, 19,* 351–362.

Chomsky, N. (1957). *Syntactic structures.* The Hague, The Netherlands: Mouton Press.

Chomsky, N. (1965). *Aspects of a theory of syntax.* Cambridge, MA: M.I.T. Press.

Cunningham, M. A. (1968). A comparison of the language of psychotic and non-psychotic children who are mentally retarded. *Journal of Child Psychology and Psychiatry, 9,* 229–244.

de Villiers, J., & de Villiers, P. (1973). A cross-sectional study of the aquisition of grammatical morphemes in child speech. *Journal of Psycholinguistic Research, 2,* 267–278.

Dunn, L. (1959). *Peabody Picture Vocabulary Test.* Circle Pines, MN: American Guidance Service, Inc.

Fay, W. H. (1980). Aspects of language. In W. H. Fay & A. L. Schuler (Eds.), *Emerging language in autistic children* (pp. 51–85). London: Edward Arnold.

Grossman, H. J. (Ed.). (1977). *Manual on terminology and classification in mental retardation.* Washington, DC: American Association on Mental Deficiency.

Hermelin, B., & O'Connor, N. (1967). Remembering of words by psychotic and subnormal children. *British Journal of Psychology, 58,* 213–218.

Howlin, P. (1982). Echolalic and spontaneous phrase speech in autistic children. *Journal of Child Psychology and Psychiatry, 23,* 281–293.

Kanner, L. (1946). Irrelevant and metaphorical language in early infantile autism. *American Journal of Psychiatry, 103,* 242–246.

Lee, L. (1974). *Developmental sentence analysis.* Evanston, IL: Northwestern University Press.

Leiter, R. G. (1969). *Leiter international performance scale.* Chicago: Streelting Co.

McNeill, N., & McNeill, D. (1975). *Linguistic interactions among children and adults.* Committee on Cognition and Communication, University of Chicago, Chicago, IL.

Menyuk, P. (1977). *Language and maturation.* Cambridge, MA: M.I.T. Press.

Paccia, J. M., & Curcio, F. (1982). Language processing and forms of immediate echolalia in autistic children. *Journal of Speech and Hearing Research, 25,* 42–47.

Pierce, S., & Bartolucci, G. (1977). A syntactic investigation of verbal autistic, mentally retarded, and normal children. *Journal of Autism and Childhood Schizophrenia, 7,* 121–134.

Prizant, B. M. (1983). Language acquisition and communication behavior in autism: Toward an understanding of the "whole" of it. *Journal of Speech and Hearing Disorders, 48,* 296–307.

Prutting, C. A., & Connolly, J. E. (1976). Imitation: A closer look. *Journal of Speech and Hearing Disorders, 41,* 412–433.

Rapin, I., & Allen, D. A. (1983). Developmental language disorders: Nosologic considerations. In U. Kirk (Ed.), *Neuropsychology of language, reading, and spelling* (pp. 155–184). New York: Academic Press.

Rutter, M. (1978). Diagnosis and Definition. In M. Rutter & E. Schopler (Eds.), *Autism: A reappraisal of concepts and treatment* (pp. 1–25). New York: Plenum Press.

Schuler, A. L. (1979). Echolalia: Issues and clinical applications. *Journal of Speech and Hearing Disorders, 44,* 411–434.

Schwartz, E. R. (1974). Characteristics of speech and language development in the child with myelomeningocele and hydrocephalus. *Journal of Speech and Hearing Disorders, 4,* 465–468.

Shapiro, T., & Fish, B. (1969). A method to study language deviation as an aspect of ego organization in young schizophrenic children. *Journal of the American Academy of Child Psychiatry, 8,* 36–56.

Shapiro, T., Roberts, A., & Fish, B. (1970). Imitation and echoing in young schizophrenic children. *Journal of the American Academy of Child Psychiatry, 9,* 548–567.

Shapiro, T., Chiardini, I., & Fish, B. (1974). Thirty severely disturbed children. *Archives of General Psychiatry, 30,* 819–826.

Shapiro, T., Huebner, H., & Campbell, M. (1974). Language behavior and hierarchic integration in a psychotic child. *Journal of Autism and Childhood Schizophrenia, 4,* 71–90.

Swisher, L., & Pinsker, J. (1971). Language characteristics of hyperverbal hydrocephalic children. *Developmental Medicine and Child Neurology, 13,* 746–755.

Swisher, L., Reichler, R. J., & Short, A. (1976). Language development history and change in autistic children. In S. K. Hirsh, D. H. Eldredge, I. J. Hirsh, & S. R. Silverman (Eds.), *Hearing and Davis: Essays honoring Hallowell Davis* (pp. 323–331). Saint Louis, MO: Washington University Press.

Tager-Flusberg, H. (1981). On the nature of linguistic functioning in early infantile autism. *Journal of Autism and Developmental Disorders, 11,* 45–56.

Wechsler, D. (1949). *Wechsler Intelligence Scale for Children.* New York: Psychological Corp.

Wing, L. (Ed.). (1976). *Early childhood autism.* New York: Pergamon Press.

# 8

# Echolalia

ADRIANA L. SCHULER and BARRY M. PRIZANT

## KANNER'S EARLY OBSERVATIONS

In his first publication describing characteristics of the autistic syndrome, Leo Kanner (1943) noted that "the children's inability to relate themselves in the ordinary way to people and situations" (p. 33) and an obsessive insistence on sameness were the most prominent features of the syndrome. Yet, as one reads Kanner's early detailed clinical descriptions, it becomes evident that his great fascination and interest in his clients was due, to a large extent, to their specific patterns of speech and language behavior. In his second published article on autism, Kanner (1946) stated that "among numerous other features, the peculiarities of language present an important and promising basis for investigation" (p. 45).

In this chapter, Kanner's early observations will provide the starting point for examining and reevaluating our understanding of echolalia in autism. Since Kanner's observations, considerable new knowledge has accumulated. This new knowledge, which reflects contributions from a number of academic disciplines, will be reviewed critically in discussions of a number of pertinent topics. The classification of echolalic behaviors on the basis of their functional properties will be discussed in relation to matters of definition and intervention. This perspective will also provide a means to reexamine the extent to which autistic echolalia differs from other types of echolalia and from speech repetition, as, for example, observed in the context of normal language acquisition. Differences between more rote and automatic versus more functional

---

ADRIANA L. SCHULER • Department of Special Education, San Francisco State University, San Francisco, California 94132. BARRY M. PRIZANT • Speech and Language Department, Emma Pendleton Bradley Hospital, 1011 Veterans Memorial Parkway, East Providence, Rhode Island 02915.

forms of echoes will be discussed in reference to neurolinguistic considerations. Finally, echolalia will be reappraised from a broader developmental and biological perspective in an attempt to explain autistic echolalia in the context of the developmental and, particularly, the cognitive discrepancies associated with the syndrome.

Kanner's attention to speech and language symptomatology was dominated by his interest in echolalic behaviors, defined briefly as the rote and literal repetition of the speech of others. Kanner's (1943, 1946) examples of echolalic behavior in autism demonstrate that such utterances took many forms, occurred across many situations, and were used for a variety of purposes. His first use of the term "echolalia" appeared in a description of an affirmative response by his first case, Donald T.; "Don expressed his agreement by repeating the questions literally, echolalia-like" (p. 5) (Kanner, 1943). Later in the same article, Kanner distinguished between utterances repeated immediately, as in the example above, and utterances repeated at a later time, for which he coined the term *delayed echolalia.*" Kanner noted that the utterances of others "are sometimes echoed immediately, but they are just as often 'stored' by the child and uttered at a later date. One may, if one wished, speak of *delayed echolalia* (p. 35). Currently, this distinction between delayed and immediate echolalia is acknowledged and discussed frequently in the literature on autism (Schuler, 1976; Fay & Schuler, 1980; Prizant, 1983; Schuler, 1979). The essential similarity between immediate and delayed echolalia is that whole utterances, or parts of utterances, are repeated verbatim; however, differences in memory processing possibly underlie these two types of echolalia (Fay & Schuler, 1980).

In citing the occurrence of immediate echolalia, Kanner (1943) wrote "her [Case 11] reactions to questions—after several repetitions—was an echolalia-type reproduction of the whole question or, if it was too lengthy, of the end portion" (p. 31). Kanner (1943) added that "affirmation is indicated by literal repetition of a question" (p. 35). Although many researchers have come to regard immediate echolalia as a result of an inability to comprehend language (Fay, 1969; Shapiro, 1977), Kanner emphasized that such behavior reflects a more general profile of obsessive and repetitive behavior in autism, alluding to cognitive differences.

Kanner's (1943, 1946) discussions and examples of delayed echolalia produced by his clients comprise his most detailed and enthusiastic account of language behavior in autism. He seemed to imply that delayed echolalia provides a window through which one can observe how individuals with autism process information, organize their experiences, conceive of language, and in some cases, attempt to participate in social exchanges.

Kanner's obervations on echolalic patterns included the use of "metaphorical language," or language with private meanings, and pronominal reversal, in which "personal pronouns are repeated just as heard, with no change to suit the altered situation" (p. 35) (1943). Pronominal reversal was thus viewed by Kanner as an artifact of delayed echolalia.

Kanner (1943) first used the term "verbal rituals" to describe how Donald T. [Case 1] produced utterances such as "say, 'eat it or I won't give you tomatoes, but if you don't eat it, I will give you tomatoes' " (p. 4). Kanner stated that this utterance "had obviously been said to him [Donald T.] often" (p. 4). In highlighting pronominal problems, which he later referred to as pronominal reversal, Kanner gave the following examples from Donald T.: "When he wanted his mother to pull his shoe off, he said: 'Pull off your shoe.' When he wanted a bath, he said: 'Do you want a bath?' "(p. 4).

Other examples of delayed echolalia given by Kanner demonstrate the diversity in meaning and use of such "memorized" utterances. Kanner spoke of utterances that "were clearly connected with actions," such as one child who sang "cutting paper" while he cut paper, and stated "the engine is flying" while he "ran around the room holding it up high" (p. 14) (1943). Kanner noted that this same child produced complex utterances that "could not be linked up with immediate situations...[but]...could be definitely traced to previous experiences" (pp. 14–15). Another child, Charles N. [Case 9], produced the utterance "I'll give it to you!" when some blocks were taken away from him. Kanner interpreted this as meaning "you give it to me." Probably the example cited most frequently is that of Paul G. [Case 4], who produced the utterance "don't throw the dog off the balcony," which was "used to check himself" from throwing objects (Kanner, 1946, p. 46). According to Kanner, the child had been scolded by his mother for throwing a toy dog off a hotel balcony and he continued to produce the utterance for many years after when he was tempted to throw an object.

Despite Kanner's varied examples of delayed echolalia, his statements as to their significance reflect inconsistencies and, in some cases, contradictions. For example, in comparing the abilities of his original 11 subjects, Kanner (1943) stated that "as far as the communicative functions of speech are concerned, there is no fundamental difference between the eight speaking and the three mute children" (p. 35) and "in none of the eight 'speaking' children has language over a period of years served to convey meaning to others" (p. 34). Yet in Kanner's examples, some of which are cited above, there is clear evidence of echolalic forms functioning communicatively and being used to convey meaning. (It should be noted that all of Kanner's eight "speaking" children were reported as being echolalic.)

Regarding delayed echolalia, this apparent contradiciton is softened in Kanner's 1946 discussion of the concept of metaphorical language in which "the autistic child has his own private, original, individualized references" (p. 47) resulting in language forms that may not be communicative because the meanings are not conventional or shared by a community (Bates, 1979). After giving ample examples of metaphoric use of whole phrases as well as of single words, Kanner went on to indicate that "once the connection between experience and metaphorical utterance is established...does the child's language become meaningful"(p. 49). In other words, such utterances may function communicatively if a listener can interpret their meaning based on shared experience with the child or can refer to accompanying nonverbal behaviors or situational features. The apparent contradictions and confusions on communication, language, and meaning are most likely the result of unclear, or rather, private use of these terms, as Kanner at that point in time could not refer to an established literature dealing with normal speech, language, and communicative development and disorders thereof. In fact, the term echolalia was never clearly defined and has, up to this point, remained a source of confusion. (For a detailed review, see Schuler, 1979.) Another source of confusion on Kanner's writings pertains to the sample of autistic individuals described, which did not include the more severely retarded. Consequently, many instances of more automatic and meaningless echoing were not described, which may have obscured the continuum that exists along the dimensions of communicativeness and intentionality; this will be discussed in greater detail later in the chapter.

The significance of Kanner's contribution was due to his rich descriptions and clinical insights into the speech and language behavior and, specifically, echolalic behavior of his clients. Not only did he carefully describe the speech and language behaviors observed, he also hypothesized and speculated about the unobservable cognitive and linguistic processes underlying echolalic behavior. Kanner's extensive clinical expertise and his intuitive understanding of language use, speech development, and development in general could have been the source of an invaluable and fruitful line of research. Yet over the past four decades, few systematic research efforts have followed up on Kanner's provocative speculations. Recent changes in methodological and philosophical approaches to the study of communicative development in normal children promise to clarify and extend many of Kanner's valuable and, in some cases, extraordinary insights into language behavior in autism. The next section of this chapter will describe how a systematic functional analysis of echolalia may serve to clarify the extent to which the behaviors involved may be communicative and/or meaningful.

## DIMENSIONS AND FUNCTIONS OF ECHOLALIA

The complexity and diversity of echolalic behavior was amply demonstrated in the examples of echoic utterances as provided by Kanner (1943, 1946). At this point, it would be useful to consider how echoic utterances may vary by referring to the many dimensions of echolalic behavior. In fact, we are suggesting that a unidimensional approach that considers language structure alone (e.g., number of words repeated, exactness of repetition) has contributed little to our understanding of echolalia. Unfortunately, many researchers in both theoretical and applied disciplines have focused primarily on language structure, which has led to misleading and erroneous assumptions about echolalic behavior (e.g., it is *only* meaningless parroting, it is a nonfunctional behavior).

In recent years, changes in both underlying philosophies and research methodologies have had great influence on the study of language and communicative behavior of normal children. For example, it is now considered essential to account for social aspects of language production (e.g., purposes, and functions of utterances), cognitive aspects (e.g., underlying meaning, conceptual underpinnings) as well as structural aspects (e.g., the observable form of utterances) when studying language acquisition and use (Bloom & Lahey, 1978; Lund & Duchan, 1983; McLean & Snyder-McLean, 1978). In reference to echolalia, issues analogous to social, cognitive, and linguistic dimensions noted above would include (a) whether an an utterance is repeated for any specific purpose or function (i.e., is it produced with or without communicative intent); (b) whether there is any comprehension of the utterance that is repeated; and (c) whether any structural changes are made in repetition that are indicative of mediating linguistic processes. A consideration of language structure alone, which until recently was the predominant approach to studying echolalia in autism, provides little information regarding issues of social use and language comprehension. A common research strategy exemplary of this approach is the presentation of a list of stimulus sentences for repetition that have no relevance to the situational or communicative context (Buium & Steucher, 1974; Schreibman & Carr, 1978). Furthermore, because researchers were not interested in studying the occurrence of echolalia in natural interactions, there were no attempts to record or document extra-linguistic and situational factors associated with the production of echolalia.

In recent years, ethological approaches to the study of child language have stressed the importance of studying language behavior in dynamic and natural contexts, which demands accounting for such extra-linguistic features as gestures, gaze behavior, and body orientation and objects, people, and events in the situation. Such approaches emphasize that any particular behavior can only be understood in its context of occurrence and that "context-stripping" or context-controlling approaches result in invalid assumptions when attempts are made to generalize findings to naturally occurring behaviors (Mishler, 1979). In order to make judgments regarding the purpose or function of echolalia, and the extent of comprehension underlying echoing behavior, it becomes apparent that research procedures should account for such behavior in more natural interactions and across communicative contexts (Schuler, 1979).

Kanner's (1943, 1946) discussions and examples of echolalic behavior, as well as examples from echolalia in other clinical populations (Prizant, 1978; Schuler, 1979), alluded to a variety of forms and functions of echolalia. Furthermore, informal parental and teacher interviews further substantiated clinicians' anecdotal accounts that pointed to the diversity of echolalic behavior (Prizant & Duchan, 1981). For both immediate and delayed echolalia, the salient dimensions include degree of comprehension of the repeated utterance, whether an utterance is produced interactively or noninteractively, and whether any structural changes are imposed in repetition. For delayed echolalia, an additional factor is the relevance of an utterance to the situational or conversational context.

By the mid-1970s, there appeared to be two schools of thought regarding echolalic behavior in autism. The first position stated that echolalia is aberrant, nonfunctional behavior or a communicative disorder symptomatic of childhood psychosis. Because of its undesirability, efforts should be made to eliminate echoing or at least reduce its frequency of occurrence. The alternative approach viewed echolalia to be a consequence of a severe communicative impairment, which, at the very least, should be viewed as a child's strategy to maintain social contact, thus serving a primitive "phatic" or social facilitation function (Caparulo & Cohen, 1977; Fay, 1969; Shapiro, 1977). Because clinical observations and anecdotal accounts suggested a broader range of echolalic behavior than implied by these two positions, more in-depth, ethological studies of echolalic behavior were called for (Schuler, 1979).

With this impetus, a series of studies were undertaken to attempt to delineate patterns of usage of immediate and delayed echolalia by individuals with autism (Prizant, 1978; Prizant & Duchan, 1981; Prizant & Rydell, 1984). Pragmatic research, or studies of language use in context (Dore, 1975; Halliday, 1975), provided a methodological foundation for studying the use of immediate and delayed echolalia by autistic individuals. In examining the production of echolalic utterances in these studies, determinations of interactiveness and comprehension of the utterances were made by analyzing and documenting such factors as body orientation, gaze, gesture, and actions upon objects, as well as objects and events in the immediate context. The timing of the production of the echoic utterances in relation to any actions or gestures was also documented for each utterance. Based upon these analyses, a variety of functional categories of echolalia were derived.

In the immediate echolalia study (Prizant, 1978; Prizant & Duchan, 1981), seven functional categories were derived from a videotaped analysis of 1,009 echoes produced by four autistic children over an 8-month period. The inital breakdown resulted from analyzing the echoes and accompanying nonverbal and situational features in the dimensions of interactiveness and comprehension evidence. This yielded four *structural categories:*

1. Echolalia produced noninteractively with no evidence of comprehension
2. Echolalia produced interactively with no evidence of comprehension
3. Echolalia produced noninteractively with evidence of comprehension
4. Echolalia produced interactively with evidence of comprehension

With further consideration of the timing of nonverbal behavior in relation to the production of the echoic utterances, seven *functional* categories were derived from the initial breakdown including: (a) nonfocused (from category 1); (b) turn-taking (from category 2); (c) rehearsal and (d) self-regulatory (from category 3); and (e) declarative, (f) *yes*-answer, and (g) request (from category 4).

From a functional perspective, the *nonfocused* category included echoes that were extremely automatic, that were often produced during states of high arousal (e.g., pain, anxiety), and that sometimes appeared to be self-stimulatory. *Turn-taking* echoes enabled the children to fill their turn in dyadic interaction when they did not comprehend utterances directed to them. *Declaratives*, *yes answers*, and *requests* served the respective functions of directing others' attention through labeling, affirming a prior utterance, and requesting specific objects or actions. *Rehearsal* and *self-regulatory* echolalia served the cognitive functions of repetition of utterances for further processing and regulations of body actions, respectively. In all, the categories represent behavior ranging from nonintentional and highly automatic repetition (e.g., nonfocused) to clearly intentional communicative behavior (e.g., request). The significant features of the categories are summarized in Table 1.

The results of the delayed echolalia study (Prizant & Rydell, 1984), based on an analysis of 387 delayed echoes of three autistic individuals, revealed a greater variety of use across the subjects than in the immediate echolalia study. As in the immediate echolalia study, the functions ranged from relatively automatic and nonintentional utterances (i.e., *nonfocused* and *situation-association* functions) through utterances serving turn-filling or conversational functions (i.e., *turn-taking*, and *verbal completion*), and cognitive functions (i.e. *rehearsal, self-directive*, and *non-interactive labeling*) to echolalia serving communicative functions (i.e. *protest, request, interactive labeling, calling, providing information, directive*, and *affirmation*). For a summary of the significant features of these categories, see Table 2.

These studies demonstrated a wide range of functional use of immediate and delayed echolalia. Further research is needed to determine how functional use of echolalia varies across individuals with a wider range of cognitive and linguistic abilities and how functional profiles may change over time. The findings of these studies actually reaffirm many of Kanner's early clinical observa-

Table 1. Features of the Functional Categories in Immediate Echolalia

| Echo category | Evidence of attention | Echo directed to person | Degree of change | Timing of echo: Behavioral change | Evidence of comprehension | Expectation of response from adult | Comments |
|---|---|---|---|---|---|---|---|
| Nonfocused | No[a] | No[a] | Minimal | — | No[a] | No | |
| Turn-taking | Yes[a] | Yes | Minimal | — | No[a] | No | |
| Declarative | Yes[a] | Yes | Variable | During or subsequent to | Yes[a] | Checking gaze possible | Demonstrative gesture indicating object, location[a] |
| Self-regulatory | Yes[a] | No, with exceptions | Variable | During[a] | Yes[a] | No | |
| Rehearsal | Yes[a] | No, with exceptions | Selective; high information segmentals | Prior to[a] | Yes[a] | No | Delay[a] between echo and verbal or nonverbal behavior |
| Yes answer | Yes[a] | Yes[a] | Minimal | — | Yes[a] | Yes[a] | Verbal or nonverbal evidence of affirmation[a] |
| Request | Yes[a] | Yes[a] | Variable; usually elements are added | — | Yes[a] | Yes | Verbal or nonverbal evidence of child's desire to obtain an object or have action performed[a] |

[a]Core attributes.

Table 2.   Fourteen Functional Categories of Delayed Echolalia and Core Attributes of Each Category

| Echo categories | Relevance to linguistic or situational context | Evidence of interactiveness | Evidence of comprehension | Other core features | Comments |
|---|---|---|---|---|---|
| Nonfocused | No | No | No | Not accompanied by meaningful behaviors | Does not appear to serve any apparent purpose. May be self-stimulatory |
| Situation association | Yes | No | No | Utterance triggered by object, person, situation, or activity | |
| Rehearsal | Yes | No | Yes | Practice of linguistic form for subsequent interactive response | Utterance usually spoken in low, soft tone |
| Self-directive | Yes | No | Yes | Utterance produced prior to or in synchrony with activity, often with low volume | Appears to serve cognitive function of regulating own actions |
| Label (noninteractive) | Yes | No | Yes | Label in reference to action or object | Similar to label (interactive), but labels to self |
| Turn-taking | Yes/no | Yes | No | Utterance used as turn filler in alternating verbal exchange | No evidence of communicative intent |
| Verbal completion | Yes | Yes | No | Completion of verbal routine | Response to verbal routine initiated by other |

*(continued)*

Table 2. (Continued)

| Echo categories | Relevance to linguistic or situational context | Evidence of interactiveness | Evidence of comprehension | Other core features | Comments |
|---|---|---|---|---|---|
| Label (interactive) | Yes | Yes | Yes | Label in reference to action or object (demonstrative gesture) | No further intentions indicated other than to point out referent |
| Providing information | Yes | Yes | Yes | Offers new information to listener | Utterance may be initiated or in response to other's initiation |
| Calling | Yes | Yes | Yes | Call attention to oneself or to establish/maintain interaction | Persistence often demonstrated if child does not get listener's attention |
| Affirmation | Yes | Yes | Yes | Affirmative response to prior utterance | Subsequent behavior indicates affirmative attitude (e.g., takes object) |
| Request | Yes | Yes | Yes | Requesting in order to obtain object | Focus on object desired. Persistence until goal is achieved |
| Protest | Yes | Yes | Yes | Protests actions of others | May also be used to prohibit others' actions |
| Directive | Yes | Yes | Yes | Used to direct others' actions | Goal is to instigate others' actions, rather than obtain object (see Request) |

tions, and dispel the belief that echolalic behaviors in autism are cognitively and communicatively insignificant.

The functionality of at least some forms of echoing invites speculation on similarities between autistic echolalia and speech repetition, which occurs in the context of normal language acquisition. It also demands a critical examination of the status of autistic echolalia as compared to similar behaviors observed in other conditions, which raises definitional issues.

## AUTISTIC ECHOLALIA, LANGUAGE ACQUISITION, AND COGNITIVE CONSIDERATIONS

Marked differences between more automatic and more intentional forms of echoing, which may cover a whole range of communicative and cognitive functions, explain why controversies regarding definition and terminology are not easily settled. Precise operational criteria, separating echolalia from more normal speech repetition, as observed in the context of normal language acquisition, for example, are not readily imposed upon continuum phenomena. With regard to these matters, autistic echolalia has often been described as deviant. For instance, DeHirsch (1967) suggested that "the echolalic speech of schizophrenic children with its mechanical, birdlike quality carries a feeling entirely different from that of the occasional echolalic utterances of children with severe and specific language deficits." Fay (1969) used the term "parasitic fidelity" in reference to autistic echolalia. He also commented on the monotonous vocal delivery of autistic echoes, as well as on their often indiscriminate and automatic nature.

Claims regarding the deviant status of autistic echolalia are often coupled with speculations on the associated causes. Various explanations have been posited. Baltaxe and Simmons (1981) implied a basic perceptual deficit with regard to the prosodic features of speech. The memorization of "unanalyzed chunks" is viewed as the result of an inability to segment speech sequences on the basis of prosodic cues.

Differentiations between echolalia and more normal forms of literal speech repetition are becoming increasingly muddled, as the prevalence of such behavior in the speech of normal 2-year-olds is becoming more and more apparent (Weir, 1962; Clark, 1973; Crystal, 1975; Keenan, 1977). Utterances produced by young children are not necessarily the product of creative linguistic processes, but rather literal repetitions and/or slight modifications and expansions of previous adult utterances. This becomes particularly clear when language samples are analyzed in context and more extensive samples of both child and adult speech are collected over time. Analogues of delayed echolalia are easily missed if the researcher analyzes utterances out of context without being sufficiently familiar with the child being studied.

With regard to the prevalence of rote speech in normal children, researchers of normal language development have recently reported on so-called "gestalt language styles" (Clark, 1977; Ferrier, 1978; Peters, 1977) and have emphasized that such styles are probably much more prevalent in young children than has been realized previously. Such children acquire language by memorized multiword units, which are eventually segmented to allow for an appreciation of constituent language structure and the induction of productive linguistic rules (see Nelson, 1981, for a review). A "gestalt" mode contrasts with an analytic mode, which has been accepted by researchers as being the most common approach to language acquisition (Bloom & Lahey, 1978). In an analytic mode, a child progresses in language through movement from single to two- to three-word utterances and beyond, by the acquisition and application of productive linguistic rules. An analytic approach in early language development allows for greater creativity and flexibility than is apparent in the early language of "gestalt" children. Other chldren who demonstrate "gestalt" strategies include second-language learners (Fillmore, 1979) and some blind children, especially those blinded by retrolental fibroplasia (RLF) (Prizant & Booziotis, in press).

In autism, it is the extreme nature of "gestalt" processing that may account for the extensive use of echolalia (Prizant, 1983). Normal children who demonstrate an early "gestalt" style need to shift to a more analytic made in development. In fact, Bates (1979) and Peters (1977) suggested that normal children who begin with a "gestalt" style may be slower to develop language due to their processing mode. Autistic children appear to remain primarily "gestalt" processors and are truly at a disadvantage. Accumulated clinical observations of autistic students persisting in elaborate phrases, once they have learned them, or producing a chain ("juice," "want," "cookie," "eat," "more") illustrate the applied ramifications of the "gestalt" language processing concept. Autistic students failing to generalize because taught phrases were part of the contextual "gestalt" in which they were originally produced illustrate this concept in a broader instructional context. The "gestalt" notion also helps to clarify the interrelations between cognitive and communicative peculiarities. Echolalia and related behaviors have been associated with cognitive rather than perceptual peculiarties (Prior, 1979; Prizant, 1983), cognitive style, in which experiences are "processed" and retained in a rather superficial and holistic manner in close association with one particular contextual cue. Information is "taken in" simultaneously with little further analysis or depth of processing (Fay, 1983). An analytic mode, however, allows for a sequential analysis of constituent components and part/whole relationships, resulting in an appreciation of hierarchical, nonsequential structure, as exemplified in language and symbolic play. The gestalt processing style is clearly not language-specific; visual information tends to be analyzed in terms of its spatial organization, with little appreciation of its temporal qualities (Hermelin, 1976; DeMyer, 1976; Schuler, 1979; Schuler & Bormann, 1983). The pervasive problems with not only verbal, but also nonverbal aspects of communication, such as gesture and gaze, and the reliance on spatially coded information testify to this point. Such an extreme gestalt mode, confounded by the presence of cognitive deficiency in over 80% of the autistic population, may account for the high incidence of echolalic behavior, both immediate and delayed, in verbal autistic individuals, and the lack of language development in approximately 50% of the autistic population (Ritvo & Freeman, 1977).

Some autistic persons, however, do move out of primarily echolalic language to more productive and flexible language. For these individuals, language acquisition appears to involve movement to a more analytic mode allowing for rule induction and resulting in the analysis and segmentation of gestalt forms, with linguistic rule induction (Baltaxe & Simmons, 1977; Prizant, 1978; Schuler, 1979), as well as other rules pertaining to, for example, symbolic play and social interaction. Echolalia may play an important role in this process, for the first indication of flexibility and linguistic rule governance usually takes the form of the substitution of elements within previously memorized patterns. Such mitigated echolalia (i.e., echolalia with structual change) may be the bridge between primarily echolalic language and true creative language. For example, one child we observed generalized the memorized form "Do you want a cookie?" to requests for other items. At first, he used this exact intact utterance to request a cookie and, later, a drink of water, etc. His nonverbal behavior indicating regard toward environmental referents and his persistence in his requests clarified his actual intent. He eventually segmented this utterance into two primary units, a request frame ("Do you want a _____?) and a slot to specify the object of desire ("cookie," "water," etc.). This early productive rule (i.e., request frame + desired object/activity) was used to generate such utterances as "*Do you want a* water?" "*Do you want a* build the tower?" "*Do you want a* time to go home?" Such patterns appear to represent the beginning of generativity, governed by simple combinatorial rules. Further linguistic growth may depend, to some extent, on further analysis and segmentation of such gestalt forms (Prizant, 1983; Schuler, 1979). However, immediate and delayed echolalia may remain a part of the verbal repertoire of even relatively higher functioning autistic adolescents and adults.

For communicative growth and language acquisition, immediate and delayed echolalia may provide a means by which many autistic children learn how they can affect the behavior of others, manipulate their environment, and use specific forms to accomplish specific goals. Furthermore, echolalia may provide the requisite tools for many autistic children to be active participants in social interaction and conversational exchange, which provides the structure and framework for further communicative growth. For individuals with greater cognitive potential, echolalia may provide the raw linguistic material that will serve as the basic ingredients in the construction of a more generative and flexible rule system. Clearly, detailed longitudinal research is needed to prove or disprove these hypotheses by documenting the progression from early echolalic behavior to more creative language. This would provide much needed guidance for language remediation and would help to delineate differences between autistic and nonautistic echoing.

## THE AUTOMATICITY–INTENTIONALITY CONTINUUM: NEUROLINGUISTIC CONSIDERATIONS

So far, the more functional forms of echoing have been emphasized. At this point, the discussion will be shifted toward more automatic and non-discriminate forms of echoing that seem to lack communicative intentions and contextual sensitivity. The occurrence of so-called "nonfocused" echoing, as discussed earlier, as well as clinical reports on more "pathological" forms of echoing, which often occur in the context of other self-stimulatory behavior, require further examination.

Occasionally, nonfunctional echolalia persists despite relatively more advanced knowledge of the structure of language. In other words, the persistence of echolalic behavior is not always accounted for by limited comprehension or expressive skills. A brief case summary may help to illustrate this point. We studied the echoing behavior of a 14-year-old girl diagnosed as autistic. She typically echoed anything that "caught" her ear, exhibiting a rich repertoire of both delayed and immediate echolalia. Some common functions served by the echoing were requesting and turn-taking. Although the majority of the delayed echoes were of the situation-association type, a number of them appeared nonfocused. Spoken instructions, which are commonly repeated for rehearsal purposes, were echoed in a highly erratic, nonfunctional manner. For instance, when asked to pick up a comb, a cup, and a brush, the whole instruction was repeated verbatim. Meanwhile, the girl's manual response was completely at odds with the concurrent verbalization. She would almost always pick up the brush first, followed by the comb and the cup in variable order. What was most striking about her performance was the baffling lack of synchrony between verbal and motor behavior. As far as the girl's hand motions were concerned, a recency effect may have accounted for the last-named object being picked up first. Such extreme isolation between verbal and motor behavior may be indicative of a primitive, nonintegrated speech reflex, and it raises questions as to the neuropsychological organization of such behavior. The ability to repeat speech, or any sound for that matter, is implied without any conscious analysis and/or awareness of the speech produced.

Another illustration of the discrepancies between structural knowledge of language and rote echoing may be found in the clinical observations of isolated grammatical abilities within otherwise extremely automatic and noncommunicative echoing. In her detailed case description of a case of echolalia not associated with autism, but rather with presenile dementia, Whitaker (1976) postulated the notion of a "grammatical filter." The subject of Whitaker's study was observed to correct utterances that were wrong from a syntactic or morphophonological point of view while she was echoing them. Yet, she would leave semantically erroneous utterances unaltered, being apparently unable to make the relevant conceptual judgments. Although overall cognitive performance was severely impaired, in conjunction with an overall lack of initiation and volitional behavior, an automatic level of reflex-like speech had been retained. In this case, discrepancies among speech, language, and cognition were clearly attributable to acquired organic damage. Such extreme discrepancies due to acquired loss of function are not readily observed in cases of developmental echolalia. Nevertheless, a recent case description of echolalic behvior in an autistic-like girl does suggest that grammatical performance may be divorced from cognitive and communicative performance. Tomlinson (1982) reported on the presence of relatively advanced syntactic and morphonological abilities despite extreme limitations in communicative and semantic development and severe retardation, as evidenced by a pervasive absence of goal-directed behavior. Despite the fact that at least 90% of utterances sampled were of the nonfunctional type, some grammatical judgment could be inferred from the ways in which pieces of speech were correctly interconnected or conjugated.

With regard to the interpretation of the observed discrepancies, one might speculate that the urge to mimic speech may initially be a product of primitive reflex-like mechanisms, not unlike parroting reflexes in birds. An automatic rudimentary ability to mimic words and phrases *along* with some "gut" knowledge of morphological and syntactic mechanisms may be in operation, even if these speech reproduction skills are not used for communicative purposes and are not integrated with other perceptual and cognitive processes.

In discussing the observed discrepancies with regard to the neuropsychological organization of echoing behavior, we will not limit our discussion to echolalia in autism. Echolalia has been observed in a number of other conditions, including developmental disorders as well as acquired pathologies. (For an extensive review, see Schuler, 1979.) Given the response latencies involved, and the link with acquired cortical damage, it could be argued that lower brain, that is, subcortical, mechanisms may be responsible for the more automatic forms of echoing. Such a position would be in line with other evidence for the subcortical organization of automatic aspects of speech. (For a detailed review, see VanLancker, 1975.) Reports on echolalia in the context of documented cortical damage also suggest that more primitive echoing responses reappear when more volitional propositional speech abilities are lost. In humans, increased cortical organization of behavior is associated with increased volitional control and more formalized knowledge. More primitive echoing responses have been reported in the context of altered states of consciousness, and drowsiness, as well as specific brain lesions. (See Schuler, 1979, for a review.) In this context, the more volitional inhibition of such responses may be disrupted. The latter conditions, as well as cases of more generalized brain damage, including the frontal lobe, may trigger a more generalized recurrence of primitive reflexes, including both echolalia and echopraxia, which is defined as the automatic imitation of the actions of others.

The occurrence of echolalia only, combined with well-preserved motor initiation and planning, may reflect more specific damage to the speech areas, as intact echoing mechanisms are used intentionally and communicatively. As far as developmental echoing (echoing not associated with specific organic damage and/or sudden loss of speech) is concerned, persistence of echoing may result from developmental stagnations and discrepancies. For instance, the ability to reproduce purposefully the speech of others may lag behind, as behavior in other domains (e.g., gesture) may become increasingly intentional. Although increased cortical control is acquired over other behaviors, speech may remain largely mediated by lower brain mechanisms.

Inferences about brain mechanisms underlying echoing behavior, based on anecdotal, single-case reports, remain highly speculative. If echoing and its neuropsychological correlates are to be truly understood, it is imperative that careful functional, as well as structural, analyses of echolalia, as described in this chapter, are carried out and that echolalic behavior is examined in conjunction with other aspects of communicative behavior and with linguistic and cognitive status.

Notwithstanding the lack of clinical and empirical knowledge, the next section of this chapter will present a reappraisal of echolalia, based on what has been learned about autistic echolalia in reference to normal cognitive and linguistic development. The analogies between the automaticity–intentionality continuum and the gradual substitution of reflexive behavior by increasingly intentional behavior, as observed in normal development, invite such an endeavor.

## ECHOLALIA REAPPRAISED

The concurrent analysis of echolalia along the dimensions of both form and function allows for a closer reexamination of the status of echolalia, of the relationships between autistic and nonautistic echolalia, and of speech repetition mechanisms in general, including their neurological organization and evolutionary history. The comprehensive framework provided by such a multidimensional analysis explains how primitive echo reflexes become increasingly internalized and integrated with unfolding communicative and cognitive abilities. Preintentional and automatic vocal mimicry, as observed when sounds are indiscriminately repeated solely for sound effect and repetition's sake, become gradually replaced by increasingly discriminate and intentional mechanisms, characterized by increased response latencies. This process seems analogous to the emergence of goal-directed behavior in the context of merely repetitive sensorimotor behavior as described by Piaget (1962). Based on our preliminary observations, it seems that more automatic, reflex-like echoing is followed by echoing that is situation-specific. This type of echoing, described as "situation-association," is in turn followed by increasingly intentional and functionally diversified communicative acts. Along with the emergence of more generative speech alternatives, inhibitory control is acquired over more primitive echoing, limiting its occurrence to socially sanctioned contexts.

Regression to more automatic forms may result from disruptions in cortical control mechanisms, as may be observed in cases of brain damage, extreme fright, and altered states of consciousness. (See Schuler, 1979.) More primitive forms of rote repetition of others' speech may also occur if socially sanctioned, such as in the context of choral singing, or the telling of a joke. We can only speculate about the precise course of development from automatic vocal mimicry to intentional and functionally diversified speech repetition and to propositional and grammatical speech. Yet some tentative claims can be made, based on (a) funtional analysis of autistic echolalia, as described above, (b) the role of speech repetition in normal language acquisition, and (c) analogies with vocal behaviors in other species.

Nondiscriminative echoing void of communicative intent, such as the echoing of TV commercials in states of agitation, is most likely mediated by older, lower brain structures. These more primitive forms of echoing appear closely affect-related, analogous to, for example, many types of animal vocalization. Although no specific semantic content is being conveyed, meaning may be derived in terms of emotional state. More complex levels of neurological organization may be indicated in those more discriminative echoes that are tied to particular contextual cues, which indicate a form of learning not unlike what has been described as the classical conditioning paradigm. Yet more sophisticated cortical mechanisms appear involved in intentional forms of echoing serving a range of communicative and cognitive functions. The gradual differentiation of vocal mimicry mechanisms into complex verbal behavior may reflect the increased involvement of relatively newer cortical structures, as well as the inhibition of more primitive vocal reflexes indicative of the increased encephalization of the human brain (for further neurolinguistic considerations, see Wetherby, 1984).

As pointed out earlier, detailed analyses of echolalia, as described in this chapter, serve to clarify the status of autistic echolalia with regard to other forms of echoing. Echolalic behavior in autism bears a striking resemblance to many other forms of speech repetition, such as those observed in normal language acquisition. Yet claims of differences, mostly being a matter of degree, fail to do justice to the clinical picture. Observed differences regarding length and persistence of echoing responses, their "parasitic" vocal quality, and their relation to more analytic segmented speech are not merely explained as developmental delay or extremism at the end of the normal continuum. Instead, differences between autistic and nonautistic echolalia may be viewed as a conglomerate of (a) normal variation along the "gestalt–analytic" continuum, (b) disturbances in affective development, and (c) related developmental imbalances and discontinuities. In contrast to more advanced object cognition (Schuler, 1979; Wing, 1981) and relatively normal, or even superior, perceptual-motor and memory skills, conceptual limitations in social cognition and related areas appear to be the core of the autistic syndrome. This discrepancy explains some aspects of autistic echoing as preintentional communication patterns are coupled with more mature, relatively sophisticated speech imitation and memory skills. Normal infants between approximately 15 and 29 months might exhibit considerably more echoing behavior if their vocal and memory mechanisms would allow them to do so. When they finally are "allowed" to do so, their preintentional communication patterns have been replaced by more advanced communication skills, including gesture and gaze, as well as propositional speech. In fact, the literal repetition of other's speech may be observed quite commonly in normal infants if one listens closely enough to early word and intonation approximations that are not clearly enunciated.

Disturbances in affective and social development might explain the vocal peculiarities and the prevalence of echoing behaviors in at least two ways. First, vocal and nonsegmental variation are directly linked to affect. The communication of affective states is disrupted in autism; autistic individuals fail to understand facial expression, tone of voice, etc., and they also fail to use them for self-expression. Second, the lack of joint attention and focus inherent in deficiencies in social interaction thwarts the attribution of meaning and the segmentation of utterances into their constituent parts. Whole utterances are not readily broken down into their constituent parts if referents of individual words are not recognized and if no or limited attention is paid to the contextually relevant cues. Lack of joint attention and joint action, so typical of autism, will severely impede the recognition of words and the learning of what words mean, and how they can be combined.

The reactions of adults and peers should also be examined if differences between autistic and nonautistic echoing are to be understood. The nonconventional appearance of autistic echolalic utterances may prevent others from reacting in ways that might make echolalic utterances more meaningful. Even when echolalic utterances take on communicative functions, this may not be apparent, the meaning of these utterances remaining nonconventionalized and "private." In addition, the type of adult feedback, such as expansions and mitigations that serve to crack the constituent structure, take place in an interactive context, characterized by joint action and joint attention. Those types of interactions are not easily arranged for with autistic individuals. Because such utterances do not become segmented into separate words and restructured, a gestalt mode may arise, with utterances that fail to be decontextualized. "Communication" through borrowed nonconventionalized phrases tied to specific contextual, often spatial cues illustrate this. Echolalia, idiosyncratic reference, and "metaphoric" language are the net result of limited communicative knowledge and relatively sophisticated speech production and memory skills. Echolalia, as well as gestalt processing, might stem from disorders of social interaction and affect. These matters may well be clarified through future research. The role of the early communication of affect in the language acquisition process deserves further investigation, as the meaning derived may serve as a catalyst for further semantic exploration.

Many questions remain. On the normal end, too little is known about gestalt versus analytic learning styles, particularly pertaining to child-rearing styles, developmental discontinuity, etc. On the autistic end, the nature of social and attentional anomalies needs to be clarified. Which biological deficiencies prevent autistic children from being socially responsive and, ultimately, socially competent? Also, specific breakdowns within the higher auditory processing mechanisms have not been ruled out. The segmentation of speech into its constituent parts requires sophisticated auditory analyses, which at some point of development are carried out without reliance on contextual cues. Controversies about right versus left versus bilateral brain involvement also pertain to this issue, since the ability for temporal analysis is typically attributed to the left hemisphere. Nevertheless, autistic speech idiosyncrasies do not appear quite as deviant if the interrelationships between communicative, social, cognitive, and linguistic behaviors are considered, as well as normmal speech repetition strategies.

To determine whether autistic echolalia could indeed be the product of discrepancies between verbal imitation and social and communicative knowledge, as well as of subsequent caregiver responses, rather than of identifiable pathology, much more needs to be learned about normal "echolalia." For instance, Do some of the early prespeech vocalizations of normal children resemble the echoes of autistic children? and What types of functions are served by the "echoing" of normal children? Longitudinal data, documenting changes in proportions and types of echoes over time in relation to other cognitive and

communicative measures, caretaker responses, and personality and tempera-
ment variables, are needed. For instance, What are the differences between
children who echo, and children who don't? and Which children show primarily delayed echolalia as opposed to immediate echolalia, and how does that relate to communicative functions most prevalent in their repertoire, and ultimately communicative style? The idiosyncracies of speech and language in
autism promise to contribute to the understanding of normal language learning
mechanisms and their biological underpinnings.

## REFERENCES

Baltaxe, C. A. M., & Simmons, J. Q. (1977). Bedtime soliloquies and linguistic competence in
    autism. *Journal of Speech and Hearing Disorders, 42*, 376–393.
Baltaxe, C. A. M., & Simmons, J. Q. (1981). Disorders of language in childhood psychosis: Cur-
    rent concepts and approaches. In J. Darby (Ed.), *Speech evaluation in psychiatry* (pp. 285–
    329). New York: Grune & Stratton.
Bates, E. (Ed.). (1979). *The emergence of symbols: Cognition and communication in infancy.* New
    York: Academic Press.
Bloom, L., & Lahey, M. (1978). *Language development and language disordes.* New York:
    Wiley.
Buium, N., & Steucher, H. (1974). On some language parameters of autistic echolalia. *Language
    and Speech, 17*, 353–357.
Caparulo, B., & Cohen, D. (1977). Cognitive structures, language, and emerging social compe-
    tence in autistic and aphasic children. *Journal of the American Academy of Child Psychiatry,
    15*, 620–644.
Clark, R. (1975). Performance without competence. *Journal of Child Language, 1*, 1–10.
Clark, R. (1977). What's the use of imitation? *Journal of Child Language, 4*, 341–358.
Crystal, D. (1976). *Child language, learning and linguistics.* London: Arnold.
DeHirsch, K. (1967). Differential diagnosis between aphasic and schizophrenic language in chil-
    dren. *Journal of Speech and Hearing Disorders, 32*, 3–10.
DeMyer, M. K. (1976). Motor, perceptual-motor and intellectual disabilities of autistic children.
    In L. Wing (Ed.), *Early childhood autism* (pp. 169–193). London: Pergamon Press.
Dore, J. (1975). Holophrases, speech acts, and language universals. *Journal of Child Language, 2*,
    21–40.
Fay, W. H. (1969). On the basis of autistic echolalia. *Journal of Communication Disorders, 2*,
    38–47.
Fay, W. (1983). Verbal memory systems and the autistic child. In B. M. Prizant (Ed.), *Seminars
    in Speech and Language, Vol. 4* (pp. 17–26). New York: Thieme-Stratton.
Fay, W., & Schuler, A. L. (1980). *Emerging language in autistic children.* Baltimore, MD:
    University Park Press.
Ferrier, L. (1978). Word, context, and imitation. In A. Lock (Ed.), *Action, gesture, and symbol.*
    London: Academic Press.
Fillmore, L. (1979). Individual differences in second language acquisition. In C. Fillmore, D.
    Kempler, & W. Wang (Eds.), *Individual differences in language ability and language be-
    havior* (pp. 203–229). New York: Academic Press.
Halliday, M. A. K. (1975). *Learning how to mean.* New York: Elsevier/North Holland.
Hermelin, B. (1976). Coding and the sense modalities. In L. Wing (Ed.), *Early childhood autism*
    (pp. 135–168). London: Pergamon Press.

Kanner, L. (1943). Autistic disturbances of affective contact. *Nervous Child, 2,* 217–250.

Kanner, L. (1946). Irrelevant and metaphorical language in early infantile autism. *American Journal of Psychiatry, 103,* 242–246.

Keenan, E. O. (1977). Making it last: Repetition in child's discourse. In: S. Ervin-Tripp and C. Mitchell-Kernan (Eds.), *Child discourse* (pp. 125–138). New York: Academic Press.

Lund, N., & Duchan, J. F. (1983). *Assessing children's language in naturalistic contexts.* Englewood Cliffs, NJ: Prentice-Hall.

McLean, J., & Snyder-McLean, L. (1978). *A transactional approach to early language training.* Columbus, OH: Merrill.

Mischler, E. (1979). Meaning in context: Is there any other kind? *Harvard Educational Review, 49,* 1–21.

Nelson, K. (1981). Individual differences in languae development: Implications for development and language. *Developmental Psychology, 2,* 170–187.

Peters, A. (1977). Language learning strategies: Does the whole equal the sum of the parts? *Language, 53,* 560–573.

Piaget, J. (1962). *Play, dreams and imitation in childhood.* New York: Norton.

Prior, M. (1979). Cognitive abilities and disabilities: A review. *Journal of Abnormal Child Psychology, 2,* 357–380.

Prizant, B. M. (1978). *An analysis of the functions of immediate echolalia in autistic children.* Unpublished Ph.D. dissertation. State University of New York. Buffalo, NY.

Prizant, B. M. (1983). Echolalia in autism: Assessment and intervention. In B. M. Prizant (Ed.), *Seminars in speech and language, Vol. 4* (pp. 63–77).

Prizant, B. M. (1984). Language acquisition and communicative behavior in autism: Toward an understanding of the "whole" of it. *Journal of Speech and Hearing Disorders.*

Prizant, B. M., & Booziotis, K. (in press). Toward an understanding of language symptomatology of visually impaired children. *Proceedings of the Fifth Canadian Interdisciplinary Conference on the Visually Impaired Child.* Canadian National Institute for the Blind.

Prizant, B. M., & Duchan, J. F. (1981). The functions of immediate echolalia in autistic children. *Journal of Speech and Hearing Disorders, 46,* 241–249.

Prizant, B. M., & Rydell, P. (1984). An analysis of the functions of delayed echolalia in autistic children. *Journal of Speech Hearing Research, 27,* 183–192.

Ritvo, E., & Freeman, B. J. (1977). National Society for Autistic Children definition of the syndrome of autism. *Journal of Pediatric Psychology, 2,* 146–148.

Schreibman, L., & Carr, E. (1978). Elimination of echolalic responding to questions through the training of a generalized verbal response. *Journal of Applied Behavior Analysis, 11,* 453–464.

Schuler, A. L. (1976). Speech and language characteristics of autistic children. In A. Donnellan (Ed.), *Teaching makes a difference.* Santa Barbara, CA: Santa Barbara County Schools.

Schuler, A. L. (1979). Echolalia: Issues and clinical applications. *Journal of Speech and Hearing Disorders, 44,* 411–434.

Schuler, A. L., & Bormann, C. (1983). The Interrelations between cognitive and communicative development; some implications of the study of a mute autistic adolescent. In C. L. Thew & C. E. Johnson (Eds.), *Proceedings of the Second International Congress on the Study of Child Language* (Volume 2, pp. 269–282). Washington, DC: University Press of America.

Shapiro, T. (1977). The quest for a linguistic model to study the speech of autistic children. *Journal of the American Academy of Psychiatry, 16,* 608–619.

Tomlinson, C. (1982). *The application of a normal language model to a case study of echolalia.* Unpublished Manuscript, Department of Speech, University of California, Santa Barbara.

VanLancker, D. (1975). Heterogeneity in language and speech: Neurolinguistic studies. *Working Papers in Phonetics, Vol. 29* (pp. 1–220). Department of Linguistics, University of California, Los Angeles.

Weir, R. (1962). *Language in the crib.* The Hague, The Netherlands: Mouton.

Wetherby, A. (1984). Possible neurolinguistic breakdown in autistic children. *Topics in Language Disorders, 4,* 39–58.

Whitaker, H. (1976). A case of the isolation of the language function, In H. Whitaker & H. Whitaker (Eds.), *Study in neurolinguistics, Vol. 2* (pp. 1–59). New York: Academic Press.

Wing, L. (1981). Language, social, and cognitive impairments in autism and severe retardation. *Journal of Autism and Developmental Disorders, 2,* 31–45.

IV

Approaches to Intervention

# 9

# The TEACCH Communication Curriculum

## LINDA R. WATSON

## PHILOSOPHY

### A Concern for Individualization

The curriculum described in this chapter is being developed at Division TEACCH (Treatment and Education of Autistic and related Communication-handicapped CHildren), a statewide program serving autistic and communication-handicapped persons and their families in North Carolina (Reichler & Schopler, 1976). Through a network of five regional centers, TEACCH provides diagnostic, evaluation, and treatment services, working with individual families to develop teaching programs focusing on the areas of the handicapped child's behavior and development that are of most concern to the family. In addition, TEACCH provides staff training and consultation to local programs serving autistic persons throughout the state and around the country. These local programs include group homes, vocational settings, and classrooms.

Presently in North Carolina, there are 50 classrooms serving over 250 children identified as autistic or having related communication and/or behavioral deficits. This statewide system of classrooms, the first of its type in the country, began in 1972 when parents petitioned the North Carolina legislature to make such services a permanent part of the state educational structure. Each classroom is administratively part of a local educational agency; program direction, teacher training and consultation, diagnostic services, and parent training, are provided by the TEACCH centers.

LINDA R. WATSON • Division TEACCH, University of North Carolina, Chapel Hill, North Carolina 27514. This work was supported in part by funds supplied to Division TEACCH under Special Education Programs Contract Number 300-80-0841.

In the fall of 1980, Division TEACCH contracted with the Department of Education, Office of Special Education, to develop classroom curricula for use with autistic students in public school programs. These curricula were to cover the areas of social skills, language and communication, and prevocational skills. Although all of these areas had been emphasized previously in teacher training and classroom consultation provided by TEACCH, the program had not, up to that point, developed or adopted any systematic curricula.

Since its inception, TEACCH has emphasized the importance of individualized assessment and programming. A series of publications describe this process. The first volume is the manual for the Psychoeducational Profile (PEP), which was developed at TEACCH in response to the need for an assessment instrument appropriate to the developmental levels, skills, and behavioral characteristics of autistic children (Schopler & Reichler, 1979). The second volume describes the way in which the information obtained through the PEP, extensive parent interviews, and other sources is used to develop individualized teaching objectives and strategies (Schopler, Reichler, & Lansing, 1980). The third volume is a compendium of individualized programs, organized by skill area and developmental age, which were implemented with clients at the TEACCH centers (Schopler, Lansing, & Waters, 1983).

This emphasis on individualized programming arose from a consideration of the characteristics and needs of autistic children. Among persons diagnosed as autistic, there is a wide variation not only in the level of skills, but in the profile of skills as well. Unidimensional sequences of teaching objectives do not allow for the multidimensional variation in development. At the time the curriculum project began at TEACCH, available communication curricula, as well as curricula in other skill areas, did not provide for the individualized programming we felt was necessary in the education of autistic students.

The communication curriculum that has evolved out of this concern for individualization is intended to serve educators as a guide to assessment and programming; similar to the series cited above, it offers a process by which teachers can assess students' communication abilities and generate appropriate objectives and activities for individual students, rather than offering preestablished sequences of instruction. The curriculum is based, in part, on recent work by O'Neill and Lord (1982).

## Communication and the Autistic Person

Communication is an act of getting a message across to another person. These messages may serve a variety of functions or purposes, such as getting someone's attention, asking someone to do something, giving information, seeking information, and expressing one's feelings. Although communication often involves the use of a language, such as English, Chinese, or American Sign Language, it does not depend solely on language. For instance, by pointing to an object, we can get someone else to look at it; by raising her arms, a small child can ask to be picked up; or by smiling, a person can communicate feelings of pleasure.

Autistic children are characterized by deficits in the ability to communicate. These deficits include difficulties with learning language, but they are much more pervasive than difficulties with language alone. For instance, it has been observed that although autistic children at the nonverbal level may use demand-like acts to get another person to do something ("proto-imperative" acts), they do not use statement-like acts, which serve to point out or show things to other people ("proto-declarative" acts) (Curcio, 1978). Both types of acts are commonly seen in normally developing children.

The impaired social relationships of autistic children are evidenced by infrequent attempts to initiate contact with other people, a failure to use eye contact normally in interaction with others (Howlin, 1978; Wing, 1978), and limited or abnormal displays of affect (Ricks & Wing, 1975), as well as limited response to the affect of others (Ricks & Wing, 1975). These problems carry over in an obvious and direct way to communication, which, by definition, involves interaction with other people.

The ability to communicate also requires an understanding of the world—the relationships among people, actions, and objects—because these are the basic concepts encoded by a young child learning language. Impaired object relationships are apparent in the routinized or stereotyped play behaviors of autistic children, such as spinning objects, or lining them up in fixed patterns. Because the autistic child's understanding of the world is limited or unconventional, there is a limited common basis for communication with other people.

A third area of difficulty for autistic people, which has severe consequences for learning to communicate, is a failure to generalize readily from one situation or context to another. For instance, an autistic child may learn to respond "cow" when his teacher shows him a toy cow and asks "What is this?" But it is unlikely that he will excitedly point and say "cow" when he is riding in the car with his parents and sees a cow in a field beside the road. Furthermore, he may not even be able to respond appropriately if his father asks "What is that?" This contrasts with the behavior of young nonhandicapped children who seem both eager and able to use their newly acquired words in a great many situations. The difficulty for the autistic child may arise from a change in the referent, the setting, the person asking the question, the wording of the question, or some other factor that operated as a cue for the child in learning the original response. Fay and Schuler (1980) have attributed this failure to the tendency of autistic children to attend to only one dimension of a multidimensional stimulus (Koegel & Wilhelm, 1973; Lovaas, Schriebman, Koegel, & Rehm, 1971; Reynolds, Newsom, & Lovaas, 1974) or to attend to irrelevant dimensions of a task (Donnellan-Walsh, Gossage, LaVigna, Schuler, & Traphagen, 1976; Hermelin & O'Connor, 1970). Thus, even when rules are acquired, they are specific to the situation in which they were originally learned (Frith, 1971).

## Communication and the Curriculum

During the early phases of development, the curriculum described in this chapter was referred to as the "language curriculum." We began to realize, however, that calling it a "communication curriculum" would more accurately reflect our belief that the highest priority of education in this area should be to improve the autistic student's ability to communicate in everyday situations and not to teach "correct" language or even necessarily language at all.

This philosophy reflects our understanding of the nature of the deficits of autistic persons, as described in the section above. Further, we were motivated to design a curriculum that would serve the needs of nonverbal autistic students. It has been observed that a large proportion of the autistic population is mute, with various studies reporting incidences ranging from 28 to 61% (Fish, Shapiro, & Campbell, 1966; Lotter, 1967; Wolff & Chess 1965). We feel that many mute children who are not developmentally ready to learn language can nevertheless learn some communication skills at a preverbal or nonverbal level.

The curriculum is not designed solely for nonverbal children, however. Our observation of children who do have some language skills, either speech or sign language, confirms that these skills often are not used by the children for spontaneous communication, even though appropriate responses can be elicited by teachers, therapists, or parents who ask the right questions or give the right cues in particular contexts. That is, the children are only able to "communicate" with people who have foreknowledge of what the child "wants to" or "should" say, which can hardly be considered communication. Such children have as great a need as mute autistic children to learn communication skills.

More globally, we desire to educate autistic children in ways that will have the most impact on their abilities to function more successfully in everyday life. Whatever system of expression is taught—spoken language, sign language, gestures, motoric acts, picture cards, or some other system—should be taught to the autistic child as a means for conveying messages in everyday situations. The criterion for success of the program is the spontaneous use of new communication skills by the student under the most ordinary of conditions.

## A Multidimensional Approach

Development is a multidimensional process. The importance of considering various dimensions of development in the assessment of autistic children is reflected in the organization of the PEP, which yields developmental scores in seven areas: imitation, perception, gross motor skills, fine motor skills, eye–hand integration, cognitive performance, and cognitive verbal skills. Normally developing children would be expected to show a relatively even profile across the skill areas, whereas autistic children are characterized by an uneven pattern of skills (American Psychiatric Association, 1980; Rutter, 1978).

The uneven profile across various developmental dimensions is characteristic not only of the overall development of autistic children, but also of their development within particular skill areas. For instance, reviewing studies of the language development of autistic children, Tager-Flusberg (1981) concludes "what we see, then, is a picture of asynchronous language acquisition. This pattern of language development suggests that the various aspects of language that are functioning at different levels in autism are relatively independent of one another and may be based on different underlying skills" (p. 53).

Because this uneven pattern of development carries over to the area of communication skills, a suitable curriculum for autistic children must allow for multidimensional assessment and programming. In the TEACCH curriculum, we include five dimensions: (a) the *functions* or purposes of communication (e.g., requesting, commenting, expressing feelings); (b) the *contexts* or situations in which communication occurs (e.g., place, people, activities involved); (c) the categories of meaning or *semantic categories* that a student expresses (e.g., talks about objects, actions, people doing things); (d) the specific *words* that are used; and (e) the *form* that communication takes, whether it is a nonverbal system of gestures, pictures, etc., or a verbal system that may be used at a simple level of single words or at an advanced level of complicated sentences (or at a variety of levels in between). These dimensions were selected for their value in helping teachers consider the various aspects of communication, and also because they reflect areas of limitation for autistic students that can be improved with appropriate assessment and programming.

## Developmental Appropriateness

The developmental focus that has characterized the view and treatment of autism at TEACCH is increasingly accepted, as evidenced, for instance, by the incorporation of this concept into the definition of autism used by the National Society for Autistic Children (NSAC, 1978), the inclusion of autism under the Developmental Disabilities Act of 1975, and the removal of autism from the emotionally disturbed category by the U. S. Office of Education (Martin, 1980). The concept of autism as a developmental disability is important at TEACCH, not only in helping to explain the behavioral handicaps seen in autistic children, but also in helping to arrive at appropriate educational objectives. Using information from the PEP, developmentally appropriate objectives in the various skill areas can be approximated by considering the child's overall level of development in that area and refined by looking at specific skills that are emerging in the child's behavior.

The communication curriculum maintains the concern that objectives be developmentally appropriate for the individual child. We made extensive use of our knowledge and understanding of the normal development of communication in designing the curriculum. At the same time, our experience with autistic children indicated that we should avoid the assumption that our students would follow a normal developmental sequence. The focus of assessment in this curriculum, then, is on identifying the individual student's existing abilities to communicate spontaneously in everyday situations. Subsequent programming for the student involves building on these "old" skills rather than selecting totally new behaviors to teach.

Using the dimensions of communicative behavior described in the previous section, each student's individual pattern of communicative development is assessed—What are the functions of the student's spontaneous communication? What are the meanings expressed? What words and forms are used, and in what contexts? Once this information is gathered, teaching objectives are set up that, insofar as possible, teach only one new dimension of communication at a time. For example, if a teacher wishes to teach a child a new word, the word selected should be one which (a) comes from the same category of meaning as one he already knows; (b) can be used for a communication function he already expresses; (c) is taught in a form of communication he already uses; and (d) is taught in a context in which he knows how to communicate. Although the sequence of teaching objectives thus derived will not necessarily reflect a *normal* developmental sequence, it will be adapted to the student's own developmental pattern.

## Parent–Professional Collaboration

A final principle of the curriculum is that the assessment and education of the student should be a collaborative effort of the educator and the student's family. In 1966, when Dr. Eric Schopler and Dr. Robert Reichler began the research project that evolved into the TEACCH program, the prevailing psychogenic theories viewed autism as a form of withdrawal from pathological parenting (Bettelheim, 1967), and in the view of some behaviorists, autism resulted from a history of inappropriate reinforcement by the child's parents (Ferster, 1961). Based on their extensive clinical experience with autistic children and their families, however, Schopler and Reichler agreed with other theorists (e.g., Rimland, 1964) that autistic children suffered from some type of neurological abnormality. Parents, far from being viewed as causal agents in the autism, were viewed as being the best potential agents for improving the child's behavior. Thus, TEACCH adopted a "co-therapist" model of treatment whereby parents and professionals worked together in developing and implementing the treatment program for an individual child. The process by which such collaboration may be achieved is described more fully by Schopler *et al.* (1980).

This treatment model was based on the belief that a child's parents are the people who have the most extensive knowledge of the abilities and deficits that affect the everyday functioning of their particular child. The TEACCH communication curriculum reflects this belief as well. The assessment portion of the curriculum involves not only gathering information through classroom observations, but also gathering information from parents on their observation of the child's behavior at home.

A further premise at TEACCH is that parents are highly motivated to act in their child's best interests. Therefore, the implementation of this curriculum involves discussing the concerns and priorities parents have for improving their child's skills and selecting objectives that are not only developmentally appropriate, but that also have the potential for improving the child's ability to function as a member of the family and the community. It is important to recognize that the priorities of the family and of the teacher for improving the child's communication may differ. Parents and teachers need to clarify for each other (and themselves) what their priorities are and why they have these priorities. Coordination between home and school is essential if any generalization is to be achieved as a result of the programming. This depends upon an attitude of mutual respect between parents and professionals as they initially collaborate in identifying goals for improving the child's communication and, subsequently, in implementing the teaching programs.

## DESCRIPTION OF THE CURRICULUM

### Assessment

The crux of the assessment procedures for the TEACCH communication curriculum lies in obtaining a communication sample for each student. In taking the sample, the teacher, clinician, or other observer writes down only those utterances (or signs, gestures, etc.) that are spontaneous and serve a communicative purpose. "Spontaneous" refers here to communication that is initiated by the student or that is in response to true requests from others for information. It excludes communication that is prompted or that is in response to "test" questions (i.e., questions to which the questioner already knows the right answer). This focus on spontaneous communication during assessment does not imply that we believe elicited responses are unimportant. Effective teaching of autistic students and students with related communication handicaps is dependent on the teacher's ability to elicit targeted responses from students. The skills do not become useful to the student, however, until the student no longer has to rely upon someone else to elicit the behavior. During the assessment phase, we wish to identify those communicative behaviors that have reached the point of usefulness for the student so that we can build upon these skills in our programming.

In addition to writing down the utterance or other communicative act of the student, the observer makes notes on the context in which the communication occurs. Later, the observed communicative acts are coded for their functions and for the meanings expressed. Table 1 lists communicative functions and Table 2 lists the categories of meaning we have used in the curriculum. Although these categories are not exhaustive, we have found them to be adequate for describing most of the communication by students in our classrooms.

We suggest that the teacher try to obtain a sample of at least 50 communicative acts from a student. If this is not feasible because of an extremely low rate of communication, we suggest that the student be observed in everyday situations for at least 2 hours. A page from a coded sample for one student (Doug) is shown in Figure 1.

The information obtained from the communication sample is supplemented by two other types of information. First, an interview with the parents is con-

Table 1.  Communicative Functions

- Requesting
   Requests an object
   Requests an action
   Requests attention
   Requests permission
- Refusing/Rejecting
- Commenting
   Comments on objects
   Comments on self
   Comments on others
- Giving information
- Seeking information
- Expressing feelings
- Engaging in a social routine

Table 2.  Semantic Categories

*Object* that is wanted, is being acted on, or is being described
*Action* of a person or an object
*Actor* or the person doing something
*Location* of a person or a thing
*Attribute* of a person or a thing
*State* or experience of a person or thing
*Social Words* used in routine greetings, farewells, apologies, etc.
*Experiencer* or the person feeling something
*Possessor* or the person having or owning something
*Recipient* or the person being given something
*Person Called* or addressed
*Recurrence* of an object or event
*Negatives* used to refuse, reject, deny, or talk about disappearance or nonexistence
*Agreement Words* used to agree with another person or to affirm something
*Time* or duration of an event
*Manner* in which an action is carried out

ducted to determine how the student communicates at home and in the community. Parents are asked to describe what the student communicates, how it is communicated, and in what contexts. Parents are also asked for general information about the student's likes and dislikes, which can be used in setting up motivating teaching activities.

The other type of information obtained during the assessment is an evaluation of the priorities that the student's teacher and parents have for improving the student's communication. This evaluation is facilitated by the use of a priorities rating form. In filling it out, the teacher and parents are asked to keep two issues in mind—first, what changes will result in the most improvement in the student's ability to communicate in everyday life and second, what changes are realistic to expect in the student within a year's time.

## Selecting Instructional Objectives

### Procedures

Once the assessment is completed, the next step is to select initial teaching objectives that are as consistent as possible with the student's present skills and that reflect as much as possible the overall goals for that student as determined by the priorities the parents and the teacher have identified.

Through the assessment, the teacher has identified some behaviors that the student finds useful for communication with other people. Furthermore, the assessment has broken the behaviors down into a variety of dimensions—the

Client's name: Doug
Date: 9/2/81
Time began: 9:10
Time ended: 11:10

Observer: Martin

| Context | What client said/did | Request | Reject | Comment | Give information | Seek information | Other | Object | Action | Actor | Location | Attribute | State | Social words | Other |
|---|---|---|---|---|---|---|---|---|---|---|---|---|---|---|---|
| | | | | | | | | | | | | | | | Other |
| | | Functions | | | | | | Semantic Categories | | | | | | | |
| 1. Looks at toast on plate, then T | "Cake" | | | Obj | | | | ✓ | | | | | | | ✓ |
| 2. Sees volunteer enter; looks at T | "Mom" | | | Other | | | | | | | | | | | |
| 3. Looks at numbers on milk carton | "Six" | | | Obj | | | | ✓ | | | | | | | |
| 4. Looks at numbers on milk carton | "Twenty" | | | Obj | | | | ✓ | | | | | | | |
| 5. T: "Want bathroom?" Grabs T's hand | "Pee-pee" | Per | | | | | | | ✓ | | | | | | |
| 6. Washes hands; gets towel | "Towel" | | | Self | | | | ✓ | | | | | | | |
| 7. Looks at picture of Jerry | "Jerry" | | | Other | | | | | | | | | | | ✓ |
| 8. Lunch choice; T: "What do you want?" | "Sandwich" | | | | ✓ | | | ✓ | | | | | | | |
| 9. Picks up chair | "Chair" | | | Self | | | | ✓ | | | | | | | |
| 10. Snack | Reaches for peanut butter | Obj | | | | | | | | | | | | | |

Figure 1. Excerpt from a communication sample.

functions, contexts, semantic categories, words, and forms of the student's communication. In order to ensure that the objectives for a student are appropriate to the student's current level of skills, the teacher should endeavor to teach only one new dimension of behavior at a time. For instance, if the teacher wishes to teach a new word, it should be a word that (a) is in the same semantic category as one the student already knows; (b) can be used for a communicative function the student already expresses; (c) is taught in a form the student already uses; and (d) is taught in a context in which the student already knows how to communicate.

An assessment of a student's communication skills will generally give the teacher a broad range of options for possible teaching objectives. Looking at the priorities that have been identified for the year will help in selecting a few of the many possible objectives to focus on in the student's program. We recommend that the teacher concentrate on no more than three or four objectives at any given time. As these objectives are achieved, the teacher and parents can discuss strategies for maintaining the student's use of recently acquired skills and then set new objectives that continually expand upon skills that the student has already acquired.

## Case Illustration

A brief illustration of these procedures will be given using Doug, the child for whom a partial communication sample was shown in Figure 1. Doug had a predominance of the "commenting" function in his communication, both at home and at school: on objects, on his own activities, and on other people. His parents and teacher felt that learning to make requests was a high priority for him. Doug had a number of words he used to comment on objects. For instance, when he was at the table with lunch on his plate in front of him, he would label what was on his plate by saying "sandwich," "cake," etc. Using some of these old words, such as "sandwich," "bubble," and "cake," one of the initial objectives for Doug was to learn to request objects, a "new" function. The initial context for teaching this function was in interaction with his teachers, because Doug was rarely observed to communicate spontaneously with his classmates.

Doug's teacher identified the expansion of Doug's category of action words as a high priority. The function chosen for initially teaching these new words was commenting on himself, which was a function Doug already used frequently. The teacher also expressed the desire to teach Doug the new semantic category of *actor*. Doug had a number of names of people, but they were not used to indicate a person was doing something. Rather, they were used to name people in the same way Doug named familiar objects around his environment. The teacher began working on this objective by eliciting the known names of classmates and teachers from Doug as responses to questions about the identity of a person carrying out a particular activity.

Another priority for both Doug's parents and his teacher was to improve his intelligibility, because his articulation was so poor that they frequently could not understand him. He was evaluated by the school's speech pathologist, who did not feel that articulation therapy could be successfully conducted at the time, given the limitations of his language and his behavior problems. The teacher suggested that Doug be taught to use total communication, and Doug's parents were willing to participate by learning some signs themselves. This new form of communication was first taught using Doug's old words and functions in familiar contexts.

Some further examples of objectives for students, along with activities used to teach the objectives, will be provided in the next section.

## Teaching Strategies and Activities

### Motivation

The task of making teaching activities motivating is accomplished to a large extent in the previous step, which was selecting teaching objectives. If teaching goals and objectives are chosen with the purpose of improving the student's everyday communication, this implies that they are chosen to help the student communicate what *he* or *she* wants or needs to communicate. The teaching activities should then be designed so that the student gets to engage in activities he or she wants or needs to engage in as a consequence of learning to communicate about these activities. In other words, there is a focus on "natural consequences." The student is not taught to identify a picture of the action "ride" and then given a piece of candy; he learns to say "ride" in order to gain access to a favored skateboard. More than other handicapped students, autistic students seem to lack an understanding of the power of communication—that is, that communicating can result in getting people to act and react in desired ways. Teaching objectives and activities must be designed to help students make this discovery.

### Shaping Responses

We wish to make it as easy as possible for a student to learn a communicative act. For many students, this will mean that teaching will begin in a structured situation in which what is expected of the student is repetitive and predictable. It will involve using a variety of prompts and cues, as described on the next page:

1. Guidance: Physical assistance is given to get a student to produce a certain sound, sign, motor act, or gesture (e.g., by molding the student's hand into the sign for "ball").
2. Models: A complete verbal or physical model is provided for the student to imitate.
3. Partial models: The initial sound of a target word is provided, or the initial word of a target phrase; or a partial physical model is given to get a student to begin a sign, etc.
4. Gestural cues: For instance, the teacher might point to an object or person, or to the relevant feature of an object or person, or might dramatize a relevant action, etc.
5. Question cues or direct instructions: The student is asked a question, such as "What do you want?" or "What is that?" or "Where is your math work?"; or given a direct instruction, such as "Tell John what that is" or "Tell Julie to come here."
6. Hints: Indirect cues are provided that indicate the student is expected to communicate something. Some examples are "time to play" (to get student to ask for toy); "Julie would like to see that" (to get student to show object); "Look!" (indicating a novel object of interest, to get student to comment on object); pregnant pause with expectant look; "Well?"; "I know where the toothpaste is" (to get student to ask for location of toothpaste).
7. Physical proximity and gaze directed at student: Often we observe that an autistic student will communicate when the listener is readily available, but will not seek out someone with whom to communicate. Getting another person's attention is a separate communicative skill, which, in our experience, usually requires explicit teaching itself.
8. No cues or prompts beyond those of the natural situation are given.

The initial intervention with a student might include all levels of cueing. For example, the teacher might say, "James, time to eat. What do you want?" and then hold up a cookie and say, "cookie." Gradually the prompts are faded, beginning with the most intrusive or direct ones and proceeding to the least direct ones.

## Making Communication an Everyday Event

Even though teaching will often begin in highly structured situations, the teacher should bear in mind the ultimate goal of communication in everyday life. Thus, the student should be getting experience with objects and activities that resemble situations that will be encountered in everyday life, even when the teaching situation is highly structured.

Teaching must move beyond the initial teaching context to provide the student with practice in as many different contexts as possible. The teacher will gradually decrease the use of ''unnatural'' cues with the aim of having the student eventually use the environment and ongoing events in the environment as cues for when to communicate and what to communicate about, rather than depending on cues from the teacher. A strategy that is useful at this point is to ''engineer'' the student's environment so that situations will arise with greater than normal frequency in which the student will need or want to use a new communication skill. For example, if a student has recently learned to request help to ''open,'' the teacher might send him to get playground equipment from a locked closet, put him in charge of making peanut butter crackers for a snack using a tightly sealed jar of peanut butter, or give him some materials for a prevocational task, which are in a child-proof container. It is not expected that the student will automatically use recently acquired skills for spontaneous communication in novel situations; the teacher must be alert to the teaching opportunities that occur in the everyday environment and be ready to provide cues and prompts if necessary when these situations arise.

## Aiding Comprehension

In contrast to most language and communication curricula, the TEACCH curriculum is not divided into receptive and expressive components. The intention is that receptive training will proceed concurrently with expressive training and will not be considered a prerequisite for beginning expressive training.

Language comprehension in the early stages of acquisition is based to a large extent on the child's general knowledge of the world, of the uses of objects, of typical actions of people, and of typical reactions of objects and people to the actions that affect them (Huttenlocher, 1974; Thompson & Chapman, 1977). The emphasis the TEACCH curriculum places on the use of functional activities during communication training is intended to counter the autistic student's deficits in knowledge of the world in general and comprehension of language in particular. Although it is important for the teacher to be aware of how heavily a student depends on contextual cues in an effort to understand language, we think that relevant contextual cues should be consciously employed to facilitate the student's comprehension and use of communication, rather than being deliberately eliminated, as is done when comprehension is trained in a multichoice discrimination paradigm. Autistic people, with the exception of a few, very high functioning individuals, will face lifelong difficulties in understanding what is said to them. The ability to use all available cues to figure out language meaning is therefore an important skill for them.

Another way to make teaching more understandable is for the teacher to simplify his or her own language and to cut down on the amount of language used. In most cases, students will understand communication at only a slightly more complex level than what they themselves produce. This means that many autistic students will have little or no understanding of verbal language. They may become confused when hearing a great deal of language, and their behavior may become disorganized and difficult to control. Cutting down on verbal language (or, in some cases, cutting it out altogether) and using more physical prompting and gestural cues may have a calming effect on such students by conveying the teacher's expectations more clearly with less "noise."

## Examples

### Teaching a New Word

Ned uses a few signs, including signs for the *actions* "eat" and "drink." The teachers wish to teach some new *words* for other actions. Most of Ned's communication is for the purpose of *requesting* (for instance, he asks to have his shoe laces tied by signing "shoe"). He communicates spontaneously only with his teachers while in the classroom.

The activity is set up to teach the new word *open* as a means for Ned to request a teacher to carry out the action. The initial activity involves having Ned put all his classmates' coats or swimsuits in their lockers. This is a motivating activity for Ned because he has a compulsion to put things in their proper places, but he cannot work combination locks. The teacher first hands Ned the clothing to be put away and lets Ned pull at the lock to discover that he needs help. Then the teacher prompts Ned to produce the sign for "open," subsequently opens the locker, and lets Ned put the clothing away. This is repeated at the locker of each classmate. The activity is conducted regularly on successive days until Ned produces the sign consistently without prompts.

Next, the contexts for using "open" are expanded. During his individual work session, Ned is given a variety of containers to put objects into or get objects out of. Some of these containers are extremely difficult to open (e.g., child-proof bottles). When Ned has difficulty with a container, the teacher uses prompts and cues as needed, and gradually fades them out.

The teacher now begins to concentrate on engineering Ned's everyday environment, as well as taking advantage of opportunities that arise naturally during the day. For instance, some of Ned's prevocational materials are placed at his work station in tightly closed containers. He is handed a new jar of peanut butter at snack time. He encounters a locked classroom door when he returns from lunch. The cabinet door in the kitchen area is latched. Again, cues are provided as needed to elicit the request "open" from Ned, and faded out when possible.

## Teaching a New Function

Phil needs a means of seeking information. He uses many location and object words and seems to understand simple *what* and *where* questions. His communication is through speech or total communication and is at a telegraphic and simple sentence level.

The teacher chooses to teach this new function initially by having Phil ask for information about the location of objects. The activities revolve around engineering Phil's environment in a variety of ways—removing his hall pass from its pocket or the pencils from his desk; not including his math or writing assignment in his work folder; asking him to get an object that is not in its usual location; failing to provide all the materials needed for a task; and so forth.

When the teacher sees that Phil has noticed that an object is needed, she initially prompts him by saying, "You ask, 'Where is (object)?' " (e.g., "Where is hall pass?"). The prompts are then faded to "You ask" (plus sign for "where"); then "You ask"; and then only by making eye contact with Phil and waiting.

## Teaching a New Semantic Category

At the point this program is begun, Phil has learned to get the attention of his teachers by approaching them and touching them on the shoulder. He knows their names and uses them in requesting actions and in giving information, but not to request their attention. The purpose of this activity is to teach Phil the new semantic category of "person called."

Phil's independent work time is set up so that he needs to make many requests of the teachers. For instance, as in teaching him to request information, he may find that pencils or work assignments are missing. He may be given a written work assignment to make labels for pictures or objects, some of which he does not recognize or cannot spell.

Phil knows that when he encounters difficulties with his independent work, he should go ask Robert, the teacher who sets up his work folder, for help. During Phil's independent work session, Robert is involved with conducting an individual instruction session with another student, so that Phil must get Robert's attention to ask for help.

The first few times when Phil approaches Robert for help, Jean, the other classroom teacher, accompanies him and models the desired behavior of saying Robert's name while touching his shoulder. After that, Jean simply reminds Phil to "Say Robert's name" if necessary when she observes Phil touching Robert's shoulder. Robert no longer responds to Phil if Phil only touches him—he waits until Phil says his name. When Phil has learned to request Robert's attention in this situation, other activities that require getting the attention of Jean and of his classmates are included in his day. For instance, Robert might ask him to go borrow a pencil from Jean at a time when Jean is busy. Or he might be sent to tell a classmate that it is time to go to the gym. He is given reminders when necessary to say the person's name.

## EVALUATION

The TEACCH curriculum received extensive evaluation in two classrooms (one primary and one adolescent) in the 1981–1982 school year and is being given the same evaluation in two additional classrooms during the 1982–1983 school year. In these classrooms we have collected data on the communication skills of the students over the course of the year, as well as soliciting feedback from the teacher and the assistant teacher in each classroom regarding the curriculum.

On an ongoing and long-range basis, we are also providing training on the curriculum to the teachers, assistant teachers, and TEACCH consultants in other classrooms. Although we are not collecting systematic data on the students in these additional classrooms, we are getting invaluable additional feedback from these teachers and consultants on the comprehensibility and usability of the curriculum.

This process of evaluation is incomplete; as we compile and assimilate the information we are getting, the curriculum is being revised to take into accout what we are learning from the students and teachers. No attempt will be made to give a full report on the evaluation in this chapter, but some of the findings will be described briefly.

## Students

We have evaluated changes in the student's behavior by taking a monthly sample of their spontaneous communication.

In the first year of evaluation, we did not have sufficient base-line data to determine whether global changes in the communication of individual students (e.g., number of different words, functions, or semantic categories used; mean length of an utterance; or rate of communication) were attributable to the implementation of the curriculum or to development that would have occurred anyway. For each student, there were at least some targeted communication skills which generalized to spontaneous communication. In our consideration of what had happened during the year, we were concerned that not all the communication objectives established for the students were consistent with the curriculum, and we were uncertain to what extent the curriculum had been implemented. Project staff reviewed the teachers' monthly classroom reports to determine the degree of consistency between objectives set and curriculum procedures. Table 3 shows the percentage of communication objectives which were consistent with the curriculum, the percentage not consistent, and the percentage questionable. As can be seen from Table 3, the curriculum was implemented to a large extent in the teachers' planning of their students' programs.

Next, the project staff analyzed these data to determine whether there were any differences in the generalization to spontaneous communication for those objectives that were consistent with the curriculum and those that were not. We found that 46% of the objectives that were consistent with the curriculum generalized to spontaneous communication, as opposed to only 26% of those that were not consistent with the curriculum. It appears, then, that the curriculum procedures do improve the chance of effecting changes in the students' everyday communication.

## Teachers

Overall, the teachers who have used the curriculum have been very positive in their reactions to it. Some of the major concerns have to do with whether the procedures for going from the assessment to the objectives to the teaching activities can be made more explicit and whether there are ways to decrease the time required by the process. There have also been problems with understanding the dimension of semantic categories.

The teachers who have used the curriculum have felt they have learned much about language and communication, in general, and the communication of their students, in particular. They have found that the curriculum addresses some issues that are crucial in the education of their students, but that have been ignored in other curricula they have used. The curriculum has helped them avoid some major pitfalls, such as spending extensive time training skills that are never used by the student except during training sessions. Although the curriculum is seen as requiring some extra work, the effort is considered to be worthwhile.

The feedback we have had from these teachers will be utilized as we revise the curriculum. We hope we can respond to the concerns in ways that will make the curriculum a more useful and effective guide to teaching communication to autistic students. The effort to achieve an individualized approach to improving multiple dimensions of a student's communication will inevitably result in a more complex approach than that taken in most language curricula. It is our hope that this increased complexity will be justified by increased returns in the student's everyday communication skills.

Table 3.  Consistency of Teachers' Monthly Objectives with Curriculum

| Class | Consistent | Not consistent | Questionable |
|-------|-----------|----------------|--------------|
| Primary | 83% | 13% | 4% |
| Adolescent | 73% | 21% | 6% |

# REFERENCES

American Psychiatric Association. (1980). *Diagnostic and statistical manual of mental disorders* (3rd ed.). Washington, DC: Author.

Bettelheim, B. (1967). *The empty fortress—infantile autism and the birth of the self.* New York: The Free Press.

Curcio, F. (1978). Sensorimotor functioning and communication in mute autistic children. *Journal of Autism and Childhood Schizophrenia, 8,* 281–292.

Donnellan-Walsh, A., Gossage, L. D., LaVigna, G. W., Schuler, A. L., & Traphagen, J. D. (1976). *Teaching makes a difference.* Sacramento, CA: State Department of Education.

Fay, W. H., & Schuler, A. L. (1980). *Emerging language in autistic children.* Baltimore, MD: University Park Press.

Ferster, C. B. (1961). Positive reinforcement and behavioral deficits of autistic children. *Child Development, 32,* 437–456.

Fish, B., Shapiro, T., & Campbell, M. (1966). Long-term prognosis and the response of schizophrenic children to drug therapy: A controlled study of trifluoperazine. *American Journal of Psychiatry, 123,* 32–39.

Frith, U. (1971). Spontaneous patterns produced by autistic, normal, and subnormal children. In M. Rutter (Ed.), *Infantile autism: Concepts, characteristics and treatment* (pp. 113–131). Edinburgh: Churchill Livingstone.

Hermelin, B., & O'Connor, N. (1970). *Psychological experiments with autistic children.* London: Pergamon Press.

Howlin, P. (1978). The assessment of social behavior. In M. Rutter & E. Schopler (Eds.), *Autism: A reappraisal of concepts and treatment* (pp. 63–69). New York: Plenum Press.

Huttenlocher, J. (1974). The origins of language comprehension. In R. L. Solso (Ed.), *Theories in cognitive psychology* (pp. 331–368). Hillsdale, NJ: Lawrence Erlbaum Associates.

Koegel, R. L., & Wilhelm, H. (1973). Selective responding to multiple visual cues by autistic children. *Journal of Experimental Child Psychology, 15,* 442–454.

Lotter, V. (1967). Epidemiology of autistic conditions in young children. II. Some characteristics of parents and children. *Social Psychiatry, 1,* 163–181.

Lovaas, O. I., Schreibman, J. P., Koegel, R. L., & Rehm, R. (1971). Selective responding by autistic children to multiple sensory input. *Journal of Abnormal Psychology, 71,* 211–222.

Martin, E. (1980). Implementing the right to education. *Proceedings, National Society for Children and Adults with Autism* (pp. 95–114). Washington, DC: The National Society for Children and Adults with Autism.

National Society for Autistic Children. (1978). National Society for Autistic Children definition of the syndrome of autism. *Journal of Autism and Developmental Disorders, 8,* 162–167.

O'Neill, P. J., & Lord, C. (1982, June). *A functional and semantic approach to language intervention for autistic children and adolescents.* Paper presented at the Symposium on Research in Child Language Disorders, Madison, WI.

Reichler, R. J., & Schopler, E. (1976). Developmental therapy: A program model for providing individual services in the community. In E. Schopler & R. J. Reichler (Eds.), *Psychopathology and child development: Research and treatment* (pp. 347–372). New York: Plenum Press.

Reynolds, B. S., Newsom, C. D., & Lovaas, O. I. (1974). Auditory overselectivity in autistic children. *Journal of Abnormal Child Psychology, 2,* 153–163.

Ricks, D. M., & Wing, L. (1975). Language, communication, and the use of symbols in normal and autistic children. *Journal of Autism and Childhood Schizophrenia, 5,* 191–221.

Rimland, B. (1964). *Infantile autism.* New York: Appleton-Century-Crofts.

Rutter, M. (1978). Language disorder and infantile autism. In M. Rutter & E. Schopler (Eds.), *Autism: A reappraisal of concepts and treatment* (pp. 85–104). New York: Plenum Press.

Schopler, E., & Reichler, R. J. (1979). *Individualized assessment and treatment for autistic and developmentally disabled children. I. Psycho-educational profile (PEP).* Baltimore, MD: University Park Press.

Schopler, E., Reichler, R. J., & Lansing, M. (1980). *Individualized assessment and treatment for autistic and developmentally disabled children. II. Teaching strategies for parents and professionals.* Baltimore, MD: University Park Press.

Schopler, E., Lansing, M., & Waters, L. (1983). *Individualized assessment and treatment for autistic and developmentally disabled children. III. Teaching activities for autistic children.* Baltimore, MD: University Park Press.

Tager-Flusberg, H. (1981). On the nature of linguistic functioning in early infantile autism. *Journal of Autism and Developmental Disorders, 11,* 45–56.

Thompson, J., & Chapman, R. S. (1977). Who is "Daddy" revisited: The status of two-year-olds' over-extended words in use and comprehension. *Journal of Child Language, 4,* 359–375.

Wing, L. (1978). Social, behavioral, and cognitive characteristics: An epidemiological approach. In M. Rutter & E. Schopler (Eds.), *Autism: A reappraisal of concepts and treatment* (pp. 27–45). New York: Plenum Press.

Wolff, S., & Chess, S. (1965). An analysis of the language of 14 schizophrenic children. *Journal of Child Psychology and Psychiatry, 6,* 29–41.

# 10

# Parents as Language Trainers of Children with Autism

SANDRA L. HARRIS and THOMAS D. BOYLE

We are all language trainers. Like the character in Molière's play who learns that "for more than forty years I have been speaking prose without knowing it," so too have all of us been teaching language all along, although it has taken us a while to find that out. Children acquire speech with such apparent ease and delight that we pay little attention to the role we play in tutoring them in language. The seeming simplicity of this acquisition makes all the more frustrating and puzzling the inability of autistic children and others with severe communication handicaps to learn to speak.

Although our role as "intuitive" teachers is quite sufficient for helping most children acquire an impressive range of communication skills, it is increasingly evident that if autistic children are to understand and use language we must use extraodinary means to help them. Much of the responsibility for this language facilitation typically rests upon parents, if only because they have many hours of daily contact with the child.

The notion that parents can serve as effective language trainers for their autistic children is not a new concept. Well over a decade ago, Schopler and Reichler (1971) described their treatment program for psychotic and autistic children as one in which parents were taught to serve as "primary developmental agents." Their innovative program demonstrated repeatedly the central function parents can play in the treatment of their handicapped child. The essential role of parent as teacher was further emphasized by Lovaas, Koegel,

SANDRA L. HARRIS and THOMAS D. BOYLE • Rutgers University, Piscataway, New Jersey 08854. Support for this research came in part from a grant from the National Institute of Mental Health (MH29897-04).

Simmons, and Long (1973) who provided follow-up data on 20 autistic children with whom they had worked on an intensive inpatient basis using the best behavioral technology available. Their findings showed that most children who were discharged from the treatment program to a state hospital evidenced marked regression, whereas those children who were returned home to parents who had been trained to help them were able to maintain their achievements. These parents were able to provide an environment that facilitated the child's growth.

Parents can teach language to their handicapped children in at least two domains—the formal and informal. The formal domain involves a highly structured setting like that developed by Lovaas, Berberich, Perloff, and Schaeffer (1966), which is widely used in schools, clinics, and other programs for autistic children. The informal domain involves all the language training that parents typically do (often without awareness) during their daily routine with their child. The present chapter explores how parents of autistic, mentally retarded, and other communication handicapped children differ from or resemble other parents in how they talk to their child and how the language environment might be modified to facilitate language acquisition by the handicapped child.

There have been a number of recent attempts to train parents in both formal and informal modes of facilitating speech, and the present chapter examines these reports to learn how effective parents actually are as speech teachers and what obstacles to parental efficacy have been identified. The chapter also looks at the kinds of skills parents need in order to function as teachers and the context in which these skills can be transmitted most readily to parents.

## SURROUNDED BY LANGUAGE: THE NATURAL ENVIRONMENT

From birth, children are talked to by their parents, other adults, and children. The ongoing existence of this language environment poses a variety of interesting questions. Of relevance for us here are two issues in particular: (a) How do parents of normally developing children modulate their speech when talking to their children? and (b) Do parents of language-delayed children talk to their children in a different fashion than parents of normally developing children? We will address each of these problems in turn.

### The Language Environment of the Normal Child

First, it is important to note that a child's language environment is not solely a product of the adults in that environment. The child plays an active role in shaping the speech of his or her parents and thus creates a mutual process of language transaction between adult and child. For example, a number of researchers have observed that parents of young normally developing children adjust their speech to match the complexity of the child's productions (e.g., Lederberg, 1980; Moerk, 1974, 1975, 1977; Phillips, 1973; Snow, 1972). Among the changes in adults' speech to young speakers is that it is slower (Broen, 1972), more repetitive, and drawn from a smaller semantic domain (Broen, 1972; Phillips, 1973) than is speech directed toward adults. This simplified speech, sometimes called "motherese," has, in fact, been shown to characterize the speech of both mothers and fathers (Fash & Madison, 1981; Kavanaugh & Jirkovsky, 1982).

Interestingly, mothers and fathers have somewhat different patterns of speech when they are both with their child together than when either one is alone with that child (Clarke-Stewart, 1978; Stoneman & Brody, 1981). Dunn, Wooding, and Herman (1977) also observed that a mother's speech to her child varies with the setting. Mothers have more child-oriented speech patterns when engaged in a joint task with the child, such as reading a book, and less facilitative when relaxing or busy with other tasks.

## The Language Environment of the Handicapped Child

Is the child who is speech delayed exposed to a different language environment than the child who has progressed at a normal rate in the acquisition of speech? The mothers of mentally retarded children have been examined more closely than any other group in an effort to answer that question. In an early study addressed to this problem, Buium, Rynders, and Turnure (1974) matched five normal 2-year-old children and their mothers with six 2-year-old Down's syndrome children and their mothers. According to their results, the speech of the mothers of the Down's syndrome children differed significantly from the normal children's mothers in that the Down's syndrome children heard more utterances of shorter length, more sentences of shorter length, and more incomplete sentences than the normal children (Buium et al., 1974). Interpretation of these data is made difficult because the children were matched for chronological age, not language age. The mothers of the Down's syndrome children, reflecting their reciprocal relationship with the child, may have used simpler speech because their children's language was less advanced than the children in the normal control group and not because they were providing poor language models.

Buckhalt, Rutherford, and Goldberg (1978) wondered whether these differences between mothers of Down's syndrome and normal children would exist when babies averaging just over one year of age were studied. They matched 10 Down's syndrome babies with 10 normal children of the same age and examined maternal speech during naturalistic observations and structured play. The Down's syndrome babies had significantly lower mental ages than the control babies. Buckhalt et al. (1978) found that the mothers of Down's syndrome babies spoke somewhat more quickly, and made more utterances, but were no more complex in their speech than the control mothers. In comparing their results in Buium et al. (1974), they note that the mothers of the older, normal children in that previous study had a longer mean length of utterance than the mothers of the younger normal subjects in their study, whereas the mean length of utterance for the mothers of the Down's syndrome babies remained constant across the two studies. Buckhalt et al. (1978) interpret their results to suggest that the mothers of the Down's syndrome children do not provide an abnormal learning environment, but rather adjust to the language level of their children.

In an effort to examine the impact of the child's language age, rather than chronological age, Rondal (1977; 1978) compared 21 Down's syndrome children and their mothers with 21 normal children and their mothers after matching the children for mean length utterance. There were no differences between the children on any of the eight speech dimensions assessed, except for a tendency for the Down's syndrome children to use a somewhat more diversified vocabulary. There were predictable differences between children grouped according to mean length of utterance, but these differences cut across diagnostic category. In addition, there were no differences between mothers of normal and mothers of Down's syndrome children on any of the 20 maternal speech variables tested, although mothers of children at different levels of language development did show different patterns of speech. These results point compellingly to the importance of matching children for language age rather than chronological age when studying maternal speech behavior.

When one looks at the speech of mothers of autistic children, one again finds few differences between these women and other mothers. Cantwell, Baker, and Rutter (1977) and Cantwell and Baker (1978) examined the speech of mothers of autistic and dysphasic children and failed to identify any differences between these two groups in terms of linguistic sophistication or grammaticality. Cantwell and his colleagues (1977) conclude from their research that the mothers of autistic children talk to their children in a fashion that is typical of mothers of language-impaired youngsters.

When parents of autistic children are compared to parents of normal children, a similar story emerges. Frank, Allen, Stein, and Meyers (1976) found that mothers of autistic and normal youngsters exhibited a similar pattern of good responses and nonresponses. It is interesting to note that the mothers of the autistic children showed a normal to superior level of performance on all the speech dimensions examined by Frank and his associates (1976).

Wolchik and Harris (1982) compared the language patterns of the mothers and fathers of four autistic boys with four normally developing boys who were matched for level of language development. They analyzed parental speech behavior during play sessions that were videotaped and later coded along a variety of dimensions. The only difference that emerged between the two groups was that the parents of the normal children spent a higher percentage of time talking to one another than did the parents of the autistic children. The mothers in both groups were more active speech teachers than the fathers.

Wolchik (1983) followed up this study with a more rigorous look at the speech behavior of the parents of 10 preschool autistic children who were matched with 10 normally developing children in terms of language age, sex, and parental education. The only difference she found between the groups were that during videotaped play sessions, the parents of the normal children talked to one another more, talked less overall, and used less speech directed at nonlanguage activities than did the parents of the autistic children. The mean length of utterance was the same for both groups. Wolchik (1983) also noted that the mothers of both groups of children were more active facilitators of speech (e.g., "say ball") than the fathers; the fathers devoted more of their effort to nonlanguage activities (e.g., "throw the ball").

Although parents of mentally retarded and autistic children appear to function as competent speech models for their children, this does not solve fully the problem of the long-term, potentially maladaptive impact of the child's slow rate of language acquisition upon the parent–child interaction. Mahoney (1975) took an ethological approach to the language problems of autistic and retarded children when he wrote "the potential non-verbal communication deficiency of autistic and mentally retarded children may not only impede language development by increasing the difficulty of the children's task of detecting the intention of the speaker, but may also interfere with the feedback system which provides language models with information necessary for regulating the complexity of their own language" (p. 144). There exists the possibility of a maladaptive pattern in which the child's reduced responsiveness gives less feedback to parents who, in their turn, are not stimulated to initiate increasingly more complex interaction with the child.

A couple of studies provide some support for the notion that there is a risk of developing a maladaptive pattern between parent and retarded child over time. Cunningham, Reuler, Blackwell, and Deck (1981) matched normal and retarded children in terms of their intelligence scores on the Peabody Picture Vocabulary Test. In a structured play situation, the retarded children initiated fewer social interactions, were less responsive to their mother's initiations, and engaged in more solitary play than the normal children. In addition, the mothers of the retarded children were more directive, initiated fewer interactions with their child, and were less responsive to their child's compliant behavior than were the mothers of the normal children. The mothers' mean length of utterance and complexity of speech did not differ for the two groups. Cunningham *et al.* (1981) express the concern that the more directive style of the mothers of the retarded children, although a response to the needs of the child, may have some long-term maladaptive consequences.

Eheart (1982) examined mother–child play interactions of eight retarded and eight nonretarded children who were matched for cognitive ability on the basis of play behavior. The study revealed that the mothers of the retarded children were more directive in the sessions and the retarded children were less responsive to their mothers than were the normal control subjects. Eheart (1982) notes that "many of the maternal skills that are important for fostering the development of social adaptability in children are less frequently demonstrated by mothers of retarded children than by mothers of nonretarded children" (p. 24). These studies by Cunningham *et al.* (1981) and Eheart (1982) both lend support to the concern that the retarded child's limited ability to respond may elicit greater directiveness by parents and that, over time, this pattern can become maladaptive if the parents do not modify their style to guide the child toward greater independence. At the present time, we lack the data to know to what extent parents change these controlling, directive behaviors as the child's skills increase.

If the apparently "normal" language environment parents typically provide the young mentally retarded or autistic speaker is not sufficient to stimulate these children, and if one speculates about the possibility of a decline in level of stimulation provided by parents as the child grows older, these problems point to the need to provide an enriched environment for these children and to produce in parents an awareness of their roles as language models. Cheseldine and McConkey (1979) suggest that "mentally handicapped children apparently need more than an adequate linguistic input" (p. 618). How shall we provide such stimulation?

## MODIFYING THE NATURAL LANGUAGE ENVIRONMENT

There is little evidence to suggest that deficient parental language causes the language delay of autistic or mentally retarded children. Nonetheless, a number of authors have argued that parents can create a linguistically enriched context for their children to learn language. Lord, Merrin, Vest, and Kelly (1983) found that simply telling preschool teachers that an autistic child was handicapped lead them to make greater modifications in their own speech and produced more on-task child behavior than the uninformed teachers. In our own program (Harris, 1983), we gave parents a list of specific behaviors that might be useful for facilitating the child's speech in everyday living. This advice focuses on such things as ensuring one has the child's attention before speaking, keeping speech simple, allowing the child time to reply, and rewarding all attempts to speak that are made by the child. Elsewhere (Sosne, Handleman, & Harris, 1979) we suggested that one structure the home environment to create more opportunities to demand speech from the child. For example, one might withhold access to desired items, such as juice or cookies, until the child asks for the item. Even though the child's communication might be primitive, perhaps no more than a grunt or gesture, such efforts are to be preferred to simply handling the child items without any effort to communicate. One does not want to frustrate a child to a point of sustained unhappiness, but modest demands can be helpful in shaping increasingly complex communication skills.

In a recent study of language-disordered children, Lasky and Klopp (1982) similarly note that they urge parents to (a) encourage and reinforce the child's efforts to communicate; (b) wait for responses from the child; (c) use expanded imitation of the child's vocalizations; (d) be aware of and responsive to the child's interests; and (e) encourage the child to imitate, ask questions, and describe the environment. Similarly, Rogers-Warren, Warren, and Baer (1983) suggest the following steps to facilitate speech in language-delayed children: (a) follow the child's lead by responding to events and activities of interest to the child; (b) build upon the utterances made by the child and shape these into gradually more effective communication; (c) reinforce the child for both verbal and nonverbal communication efforts; (d) emphasize the positive aspects of the child's efforts to communicate; and (e) talk with the child in an interactive not directive way.

It is evident that Rogers-Warren *et al.* (1984), Lasky and Klopp (1982), and Harris (1983) converge in many of their suggestions for facilitating children's speech development. It, of course, remains to be explored to what extent each of these suggestions is, in fact, effective and whether they are of differential value depending upon the child's level of language acquisition or clinical diagnosis. The guidelines do appear to contain a bit of "clinical wisdom" and good sense as well as at least peripheral empirical support.

## FORMAL LANGUAGE INSTRUCTION

Although informal language instruction in the natural environment is probably an important component of any comprehensive language program, many children require more structured, formal training as well. This may be particularly true of autistic children who sometimes have to be taught how to say words and be drilled repeatedly in the connection between sounds and their meaning.

Lovaas and his colleagues (1966) laid the groundwork for formal language training with their demonstration that previously nonverbal children could be taught the rudiments of speech using operant methods in a very intensive fashion over a relatively brief period of time. Since that original study, scores of other researchers have explored techniques for teaching specific components of the communication process, for increasing the efficiency of the training, and for enhancing the generalizability of the child's speech.

The process of formal language instruction may be divided conveniently into four components: (a) attending skills; (b) nonverbal imitation; (c) verbal imitation; and (d) functional speech. A research literature has grown up around each of these four areas and has shown that many autistic (Lovaas, 1977) and retarded (Buddenhagen, 1971) children can acquire at least a portion of these diverse skills.

The importance of *attending skills* is self-evident. Unless a child is capable of sitting quietly, and listening to and looking at his or her teacher or parent, it is not likely that the youngster will be able to attend to the instructional material. Although quiet sitting and eye contact do not ensure attending, they do set the scene for such behavior. Thus in the traditional model of language training, the child is taught to respond to the command "look at me" while sitting quietly (e.g., Lovaas *et al.*, 1966).

*Nonverbal imitation* is typically included as a building block in preparation for language training (e.g., Bricker & Bricker, 1970; Buddenhagen, 1971; Lovaas, 1977). Here the child learns to relate the movements of his or her body to those of the parent or teacher. In the later stages of training, this imitative training may focus upon the fine movements of the mouth and tongue in order to facilitate the verbal imitation training that is to follow. A child who is unable to learn basic nonverbal imitation is probably a poor candidate for speech training. Nonverbal imitation is also an integral component of instruction for the acquisition of a range of nonverbal behaviors from pulling on a shirt to spreading peanut butter with a knife or holding a screwdriver. One can view generalized imitative ability as a building block for instruction (Baer, Peterson, & Sherman, 1967).

Teaching the autistic child *verbal imitation* skills provides the first conspicuous step toward language production. Lovaas *et al.* (1966) followed a four-step model for verbal imitation that has been replicated many times in succeeding years. Using this model, one first reinforces any vocalizations made by the child and then gradually shapes these sounds until they resemble those made by the trainer. This complex teaching process demands considerable skill in shaping and prompting of verbal behavior on the part of the parent–teacher.

All of this preliminary training would be of minimal value if it did not lead to the end goal of *functional speech*. The sounds acquired during verbal imitation training can be combined into units that form words and the child taught the meaning of these words. This permits the child to begin to use speech to control events in the environment and thus to experience language as intrinsically reinforcing. Research has shown that some children are capable of acquiring the full range of language forms, including nouns, verbs, prepositions, adjectives, and asking questions, in both a receptive and expressive mode (Harris, 1975).

## PARENTS AS LANGUAGE TEACHERS: THE EMPIRICAL DATA

A modest, but very important literature that has emerged in recent years addresses the question of how effective parents can be as speech teachers and language facilitators for their language-delayed or nonverbal children. Much of this work has been done with mothers of Down's syndrome children or other mentally retarded children, but there also exists some specific data on the autistic child. Many of these studies have used a small number of subjects, sometimes one or two mother–child duos within a single subject design, whereas a few have used larger samples and analyzed their data using group statistics. Typically, the studies with mentally retarded children involve youngsters who already had a little speech; some of the work with autistic children included subjects who were mute initially. The studies have varied widely in terms of measures of change, assessment of change in parent, child, or both, duration of follow-up, home versus clinic setting for training and assessment, and other potentially critical variables.

### Early Case Reports

An early example of an informal case report of parents as speech teachers was Goldstein and Lanyon's (1971) description of their efforts to train the parents of a 10-year-old autistic boy to enhance their son's language. Whitehurst, Novak, and Zorn (1972) first assessed the speech patterns of a bright, language-delayed boy and his mother, then encouraged the mother to talk to the boy more often and to use speech prompts. These changes facilitated significant verbal growth for the boy. Similarly, Arnold, Sturgis, and Forehand (1977) showed the mother of a 15-year-old, mentally retarded girl how to stimulate her daughter's conversational skills. Kozloff (1973), in an early, important study of training parents as teachers, described his work with four families of autistic children, in which he trained the parents to deal with a full range of behavior problems and adaptive skills, including speech.

## Mentally Retarded Children

One of the early studies of parental facilitation of speech in Down's syndrome children was reported by MacDonald, Blott, Gordon, Spiegel, and Hartman (1974) who trained mothers to increase both the length of their child's utterances and the complexity of the child's speech. Three treated children showed significant changes posttreatment when compared to three control subjects. These gains were still present at a 3-month follow-up. The children apparently did not require training in precursor skills of attending, nonverbal imitation, and verbal imitation and were already engaged in single-word utterances when training began. The training for these children involved both formal sessions and an effort to encourage the child to use language skills in daily living. The study used a combination of professional trainers and parent trainers and thus does not allow one to disentangle the effects of these two groups, although the authors noted that the children continued to make progress in speech when responsibility for teaching was shifted exclusively to the mothers. Measures of parental skill were not reported.

Bidder, Bryant, and Gray (1975) used a group format to teach behavior modification skills and give parents of eight Down's syndrome children an opportunity to discuss their personal and family problems. Another group of eight families received no training. After twelve behavior modification training sessions and six group counseling sessions spread out over a year, the experimental group children showed improvement in their language and the mothers were more confident about their ability to handle their children. The idea of attending to the needs of the parents and the family as a whole may be an important component in parent training (Harris, 1983), although the study by Bider *et al.* (1975) has serious design problems, which limit the conclusions we can draw from it.

Becoming aware of one's role as a teacher may be facilitative for some parents. Cheseldine and McConkey (1979) asked the parents of seven Down's syndrome children to "introduce four action words" to their children, but did not give them instructions in how to do so. Three of the children showed an increase in their use of words over the course of the four play sessions that were observed. When Cheseldine and McConkey (1979) analyzed the speech of the parents who had been most effective in bringing about change in their children, they found that these parents had decreased their mean length of utterance, used fewer words, and increased their statements, while decreasing their questions. The authors argue that the parents of retarded children may have lower expectations for their children's speech productions and do not advance their language modeling as rapidly as the child requires (Cheseldine & McConkey, 1979).

Just as nonspecific instructions to increase a child's use of particular words can lead to change, so too can asking parents to record their child's speech output. Waters and Siegel (1982) used a multiple base-line design to examine the benefits of having parents who had been previously trained in speech facilitation write down the speech of their preschool Down's syndrome child. All four of the children showed an increase in speech when the parents recorded verbal output.

Salzberg and Villani (1983) employed a multiple base-line design with two mother–child duos to examine the acquisition and generalized use of vocal imitation skills by mothers of Down's syndrome preschoolers. The mothers were taught to use praise and prompts and to decrease their tangential statements in training sessions with their children. Changes in maternal behavior were related to improved vocal imitation by the children and a decrease in disruptive behavior. Skills taught in the clinic did not generalize to free play sessions at home until the mothers were told directly to use these skills at home and shown how to adapt them to the free play situation. Once this step was taken, there was a rapid increase in the use of the behaviors at home. Salzberg and Villani (1983) conclude that one cannot assume parents will generalize skills from one setting to another.

Although the bulk of studies examining the ability of parents to teach speech skills to their retarded children have shown some success in this mission, the literature is not without report of failure. Clements, Evans, Jones, Osborne, and Upton (1982) used a home-based language program to teach language skills to severely retarded preschool- and school-age children for a period of 16 to 18 months. Although both their treated and untreated subjects improved over time, their was no significant advantage for the treated subjects. These authors note that the parents were effectively able to teach the specific tasks assigned, but this had little generalized effect on speech acquisition (Clements et al., 1982). They point out that most of the studies on language acquisition by retarded children failed to provide appropriate long-term follow-up to determine how sustained the benefits of training were and to what extent the child's skills generalized beyond the specifics taught by the parents. Clements et al. (1982) suggest that it is important to begin to identify children who can benefit from this kind of language instruction and those who may require other forms of instruction. It may also be important to program systematically for generalized responding by the children.

## Autistic Children

Some of our own research has addressed the question of the language acquisition of autistic children who are trained by their parents (Harris, 1983). Over a period of four years, we trained more than 40 families of autistic preschool children in behavior modification skills and techniques of operant language training. These children were all quite delayed in language acquisition, with a mean communication age of 18.23 months of the Communication Scale of the Alpern and Boll (1972) *Developmental Profile* and an average chronological age of 46.2 months. Some of the children were mute, others had a few words or were echolalic. Of the children studied, 21% were girls and 79% boys, a distribution consistent with the report of DeMyer (1979). All of the children came from intact, middle-class families in which both the mother and the father were willing to participate in training and were fluent English speakers.

In one of our studies, we addressed the question of whether parents need specific training in facilitation of speech as compared to general training in behavior modification in order to be effective language trainers (Harris, Wolchik, & Milch, 1983). Using a multiple base-line design, we found no change in the parents' speech-oriented language (such as providing speech models, expanding the child's vocalizations, and reinforcing speech attempts) until they received specific training in these skills. Simply training parents to be skillful behavior modifiers who could teach their child to use a spoon, button a shirt, or come when called had little apparent impact on their use of speech training skills. We also noted that those children who had a little speech when training began made greater progress than those who were mute (Harris *et al.*, 1983). We speculated that a 2½-month training program may not have been long enough for these children to move from muteness to speech acquisition.

Weitz (1982) examined in detail the mastery of various behavior modification skills by the parents who participated in our treatment program. He found that parental teaching skills were quite stable during three pretraining assessment sessions and changed markedly after training. Both mothers and fathers were more skillful at providing discriminative stimuli, knowing when to use prompts, offering effective prompts, using reinforcements, shaping behavior, following a discrete-trial format, and recording data after training than they had been before.

In a second study examining the experiences of the children whose parents were the subjects of Weitz's (1982) project, we looked at changes in the children's speech before and after treatment and during one-year follow-up (Harris, Wolchik, & Weitz, 1981). The children's language skills were significantly improved after their parents completed training and the mute children, although not showing as much progress as the speaking children, did make some progress in the precursors to speech behavior. Interestingly, when the children were followed up at one year we observed that there had been little additional progress over that time period, although previously learned skills were retained.

These studies, taken as a package, suggest that parents can learn speech training skills during a 10-week course in behavior modification and operant speech techniques and can be significantly more competent in these skills after training than before. Their children show similar improvement in their prespeech and speech skills. It also appears that parents must be encouraged to continue to use these techniques after training is completed in order to promote more improvement in the child's language skills.

A very important contribution to the research on long-term benefits to autistic children of a home-based language training program was done by Howlin and her colleagues. These authors, in a series of reports, described their efforts to train parents of autistic children to provide a broad-based behavioral treatment package at home (Hemsley, Howlin, Berger, Hersov, Holbrook, Rutter, & Yule, 1978; Howlin, 1981a,b; Howlin, Marchant, Rutter, Berger, Hersov, & Yule, 1973). They studied 16 autistic boys between 3 and 11 years of age with nonverbal IQs of 60 or higher. There were two matched control groups, one group for a 6-month, short-term follow-up and one group for a longer follow-up. The parents of the experimental subjects were trained in their own homes to use language programs and other behavioral procedures. The treatment lasted for 18 months, with measures of change taken at 6-month intervals.

The treatment package employed by Howlin and her colleagues produced significant improvements in the children's functional speech (Howlin, 1981b). The frequency of their utterances was increased, speech was used more for communication purposes, and the incidence of echolalia and idiosyncratic utterances declined. It is important to note that language structure showed less change than the expanded use of existing structures. The children's behavior problems resolved more rapidly, with more improvement over time than did their speech.

Howlin (1981b) notes that those children who were at least echolalic made more changes than those children who had fewer speech skills or were mute when training began. This observation is consistent with the report of Harris *et al.* (1983). A very important aspect of Howlin's (1981b) research was her observation that on long-term follow-up the echolalic control subjects made the same kind of gains as the echolalic experimental subjects. Thus, although the program had a short-term impact upon the echolalic children, the passage of time appears to have had similar beneficial effects for the control subjects, with no apparent advantage for the earlier training.

Howlin (1981b) argues that the benefits of language training programs vary according to the ability level of the child and the level of language that is being trained. She regards those children who have the basic prerequisites of speech as most likely to benefit from training, whereas those who show little comprehension of speech, make no spontaneous vocalizations, and show severely retarded social and play skills are unlikely to show major gains. She indicates that the use of these speech programs for such children may lead to intense frustration on the part of both parents and child. Her data suggest that behavioral techniques are far more effective for motivating children to use the skills they already have than in creating new linguistic forms for the children. In addition, children who are already echolalic may not require this form of intervention, whereas mute children apparently derive little benefit. Perhaps the children most likely to make use of these intensive home-based programs for growth in language are those who are beginning to communicate by single words or approximations of single words (Howlin, 1981b). According to Howlin (1981b), the subjects in her study who were in this group made progress toward the use of phrases, whereas the control subjects did not.

Although Howlin's (1981b) data are compelling and important, they require replication and extension. She and her co-workers have clearly provided one of the most significant pieces of research in this area. It is now important to ensure that other studies of language acquisition with autistic children use the same long-term follow-up and systematic measures employed by Howlin and her co-workers. The outcome of such studies would have implications not only for parents as speech teachers, but also for our language curriculum in general. Although short-term studies examining one teaching technique or another have value in generating new methods of intervention, it is critically important that we determine to what extent we are, in fact, helping autistic children with our home-based treatment procedures. Sixteen children, even carefully studied, cannot provide all the answers to that problem. The data of Howlin and her co-workers have generated a series of very important hypotheses that must be followed up in the near future.

## METHODS OF TRAINING PARENTS TO TRAIN CHILDREN

Given the potential benefits of training parents as speech teachers, two important questions arise: First, what skills do parents need to learn in order to teach speech? And second, what methods are available for training parents to become effective speech teachers? For parents to be able to engage in formal and informal language instruction, they must first acquire a wide variety of skills, ranging from a working knowledge of basic behavioral techniques to more sophisticated skills, such as assessment and program planning.

### Skills That Parents Need to Learn

Formal language training is often conducted using a "discrete-trial procedure," as described by Koegel, Russo, and Rincover (1977). The ingredients of a discrete trial are the discriminative stimulus (SD), which is the instruction given to the child, the child's response, and the consequence. Effective discrete trial teaching requires that (a) the child be attending to the teacher; (b) the SD be presented only once, clearly and without superfluous words or gestures; (c) an appropriate target response be selected and operationally defined; and (d) an appropriate consequence must be delivered immediately, and be contingent upon the child's response. Parents must learn how to optimally pace the trials, choose appropriate target behaviors, and select and deliver effective positive and negative consequences. They must also become adept at implementing such techniques as behavior shaping or reinforcement of successive approximations, prompting, and prompt fading.

Technical competence is necessary, but not altogether sufficient for parents to become effective language trainers. Parents must also know how to conduct a functional analysis and modify a program that is not progressing as expected. Furthermore, ideally, they should be able to identify specific language or behavioral deficits and devise structured programs aimed at overcoming those deficits. It is also important that parents generalize the skills they have acquired for discrete-trial teaching and be able to implement them in informal settings, thereby creating a more facilitative language environment.

It is not unusual for developmentally disabled children to exhibit disruptive behaviors that interfere with learning. Such behaviors include tantrums, self-stimulation, aggression, and inappropriate attention-seeking activity. These behaviors typically occur across a variety of situations including, but certainly not limited to, formal language instruction. Parents should be able to assess the problem behaviors as they occur in specific situations, identify the factors maintaining those behaviors, and devise strategies aimed at controlling or eliminating them. They must therefore be capable of implementing behavior reduction procedures, such as time-out, extinction, and differential reinforcement of other behaviors, consistently, and without the use of threats or numerous warnings. Parents should also learn how to collect and analyze meaningful data on targeted behaviors. It is perhaps most important that parents develop the habit of reinforcing their child contingent upon appropriate behavior.

## Methods of Training Parents

Methods for teaching parents to train their children include the use of such media, as film, video tape, and written manuals (Flanagan, Adams, & Forehand, 1979; O'Dell, Mahoney, Horton, & Turner, 1979), and direct instructional methods, such as group training (e.g., Adesso & Lipson, 1981; Rinn, Vernon, & Wise, 1975) or in-home training (Howlin, 1981b).

Investigations of the relative efficacy of different methods of parent training are sometimes difficult to interpret. For example, Flanagan *et al.* (1979) found that the efficacy of training procedures varied depending on the particular outcome measure that was used. They compared four different instructional procedures for teaching time-out—written manual, lecture, video taped modeling presentation, and role-playing presentation—across three different outcome measures. The parent's knowledge of the time-out procedure was assessed by their responses on a questionnaire; all four groups performed approximately equally well, and they all performed better than a no-treatment control group. However, the role-playing group performed best on an audio-taped analog task, whereas the group that experienced the video taped modeling presentation performed best on the in-home assessment. Furthermore, the correlation between group scores on the audio tape analog measure and the in-home assessment was found to be negligible, which suggests that one must be cautious when comparing and generalizing the results of studies employing different outcome measures. As Flanagan *et al.* (1979) succinctly state, "it would appear that if research clinicians involved in parent training are primarily interested in changing behavior in the home, assessment of the effectiveness of their training should occur in the home" (p. 101).

Direct instruction need not take place on a single-family basis. Group training involving mothers, fathers, or couples is a viable alternative (Adesso & Lipson, 1981). Rinn *et al.* (1975) found that group training provided for parents by a community mental health center was effective in teaching parents to manage child behavior problems at home. Furthermore, 84% of the parents contacted at a 3-year follow-up reported that they had not sought any further treatment for their child, although some decrements in the initial treatment effects did occur. Rinn *et al.* (1975) concluded that the group training class incurred less cost to both the parents and the community mental health center than the "usual single-family clinical approach."

Do both mother and father need to participate in the parent program? Involvement of both parents is preferable, since it promotes generalization of child management skills and treatment effects (Kelley, Embry, & Baer, 1979), as well as maintenance over time (Adesso & Lipson, 1981). However, practical constraints, such as divorce or job commitments, sometimes prevent both parents from receiving direct professional training. In these cases, the parent who receives the professional training might train his or her spouse. Adubato, Adams, and Budd (1981) present evidence that some parents are capable of training their spouses in child management procedures; however, generalization of these results is limited since their study involved only one couple in which both parents were college-educated.

It is hard to draw any definitive conclusions from the research on parent training, especially when one is addressing the needs of parents of autistic or retarded children. Interpretation of the data is made difficult, since studies on parent training often differ on such variables as the training techniques employed, components of the training packages, outcome measures, parent demographics, and child populations. In addition, the efficacy of a given training technique may depend on the current skill level of the parent. For example, a parent who has already learned rudimentary behavioral principles and techniques may benefit more from a particular lecture presentation than a parent who is unfamiliar with behavioral principles and procedures. Furthermore, the majority of the research on parent training has focused on training parents of less seriously disordered children in behavior management skills and has not typically addressed the specifics of language training or other needs of the developmentally disabled.

In our experience training parents of developmentally disabled children in a number of settings, we have found a multifaceted approach to be effective. Incorporating different modes of instruction into a training program appears to facilitate learning, perhaps because the different methods often reinforce and supplement each other. Three componets appear useful for an effective parent training program: (a) information and instruction; (b) "hands-on" experience with direct feedback; and (c) posttraining ongoing consultation.

Information and instruction may be provided individually or in a group setting. Written material, films, and videotapes may be used to supplement a lecture-type presentation. Parents should be presented with an overview of the nature of their child's problem, instruction on how to implement behavioral techniques, and the rationale behind those techniques. Studies investigating whether or not educating parents in behavioral principles leads to stronger treatment effects have yielded equivocal findings (e.g., Hudson, 1982; McMahon, Forehand, & Griest, 1981). However, it is our impression that providing parents with a brief overview of the principles of operant theory can facilitate their learning of behavior management skills and promote generalization of those skills as they apply to other child problems.

"Hands-on" experience is perhaps the most important aspect of parent training. If possible, parents should work directly with their child and practice the newly learned techniques until they are mastered. This training should ideally take place at home in order to facilitate generalization. A trained professional should be present to provide constructive feedback and, if necessary, to model appropriate techniques. These "home visits" may initially occur on a weekly or monthly basis, but can be gradually faded and conducted on a less frequent schedule.

Parent training should not necessarily end when the formal instruction is over. Ongoing consultation by trained professionals, such as psychologists, speech therapists, and teachers, should be offered in order to assess the child's developmental progress, provide objective feedback, troubleshoot specific problems, assist in programming, monitor parents' goals and expectations, and ensure maintenance of child management skills over time. In some cases, family intervention may be required in order to facilitate maintenance of treatment gains (Harris, 1982, 1983; Kelley et al., 1979).

## SUMMARY

Teaching an autistic child to use language for effective communication is a complex process that demands intensive effort on the part of all the major members of the youngster's language community. There is little doubt but that parents can play a central role in the facilitation of speech for their child. Although we have little evidence to suggest that parents of autistic children talk to their children in a fashion that differs greatly from the style of other parents, nonetheless, it does appear that if these parents can learn to alter their speech patterns to be especially facilitative, they may enhance their child's language acquisition. In spite of this, it is important to recognize that the child's readiness for speech is a critical variable in terms of how well he or she will respond to parental instruction. Thus, teaching parents to be language trainers must be tempered by a realistic recognition that even with the best training and intent one is often limited in the degree of speech the autistic child will master. It is important to be open to teaching alternative modes of communication when speech does not appear to be a feasible goal.

ACKNOWLEDGMENTS

Our thanks to Linda Hoffman, who typed the manuscript.

## REFERENCES

Adesso, V. J., & Lipson, J. W. (1981). Group training of parents as therapists for their children. *Behavior Therapy, 12,* 625-633.

Adubato, S. A., Adams, M. K., & Budd, K. S. (1981). Teaching a parent to train a spouse in child management techniques. *Journal of Applied Behavior Analysis, 14,* 193-205.

Alpern, G., & Boll, T. (1972). *Developmental profile.* Aspen, CO: Psychological Developmental Publication.

Arnold, S., Sturgis, E., & Forehand, R. (1977). Training a parent to teach communication skills. *Behavior Modification, 1,* 259-276.

Baer, D. M., Peterson, R., & Sherman, J. (1967). The development of imitation by reinforcing behavioral similarity to the model. *Journal of Experimental Analysis of Behavior, 10,* 405-416.

Bidder, R. T., Bryant, G., & Gray, O. P. (1975). Benefits to Down's syndrome children through training their mothers. *Archives of Disease in Childhood, 50,* 383-386.

Bricker, W. A., & Bricker, D. D. (1970). A program of language training for the severely handicapped child. *Exceptional Children, 37,* 101-111.

Broen, P. (1972). The verbal environment of the language learning child. *American Speech and Hearing Association Monograph* (No. 17).

Buckhalt, J. A., Rutherford, R. B., & Goldberg, K. E. (1978). Verbal and nonverbal interaction of mothers with their Down's syndrome and nonretarded infants. *American Journal of Mental Deficiency, 82,* 337–343.

Buddenhagen, R. (1971). *Establishing vocalizations in mute mongoloid children.* Champaign, IL: Research Press.

Buium, N., Rynders, J., & Turnure, J. (1974). Early maternal linguistic environment of normal and Down's syndrome language-learning children. *American Journal of Mental Deficiency, 79,* 52–58.

Cantwell, D. P., & Baker, L. (1978). The language environment of autistic and dysphasic children. *Journal of the American Academy of Child Psychiatry, 17,* 604–613.

Cantwell, D. P., Baker, L., & Rutter, M. (1977). Families of autistic and dysphasic children. II. Mother's speech to the children. *Journal of Autism and Childhood Schizophrenia, 7,* 313–327.

Cheseldine, S., & McConkey, R. (1979). Parental speech to young Down's syndrome children: An intervention study. *American Journal of Mental Deficiency, 83,* 612–620.

Clarke-Stewart, K. A. (1978). And daddy makes three: The father's impact on mother and young child. *Child Development, 49,* 466–478.

Clements, J., Evans, C., Jones, C., Osborne, K., & Upton, G. (1982). Evaluation of a home-based language training programme with severely mentally handicapped children. *Behaviour Research and Therapy, 20,* 243–249.

Cunningham, C. E., Reuler, E., Blackwell, J., & Deck, J. (1981). Behavioral and linguistic developments in the interactions of normal and retarded children with their mothers. *Child Development, 52,* 62–70.

DeMyer, M. K. (1979). *Parents and children in autism.* New York: Wiley.

Dunn, J., Wooding, C., & Herman, J. (1977). Mothers' speech to young children: Variation in context. *Developmental Medicine and Neurology, 19,* 629–638.

Eheart, B. K. (1982). Mother–child interactions with nonretarded and mentally retarded preschoolers. *American Journal of Mental Deficiency, 87,* 20–25.

Fash, D. S., & Madison, C. L. (1981). Parents' language interaction with young children: A comparative study of mothers' and fathers'. *Child Study Journal, 11,* 137–152.

Flanagan, S., Adams, H. E., & Forehand, R. (1979). A comparison of four instructional techniques for teaching parents to use time-out. *Behavior Therapy, 10,* 94–102.

Frank, S. M., Allen, D. A., Stein, L., & Meyers, B. (1976). Linguistic performance in vulnerable and autistic children and their mothers. *American Journal of Psychiatry, 133,* 909–915.

Goldstein, S. B., & Lanyon, R. I. (1971). Parent-clinicians in the language training of an autistic child. *Journal of Speech and Hearing Disorders, 36,* 552–560.

Harris, S. L. (1975). Teaching language to nonverbal children—with emphasis on problems of generalization. *Psychological Bulletin, 82,* 565–580.

Harris, S. L. (1982). A family systems approach to behavioral training with parents of autistic children. *Child and Family Behavior Therapy, 4,* 21–35.

Harris, S. L. (1983). *Families of the developmentally disabled: A guide to behavioral intervention.* Elmsford, NY: Pergamon Press.

Harris, S. L., Wolchik, S. A., & Weitz, S. (1981). The acquisition of language skills by autistic children: Can parents do the job? *Journal of Autism and Developmental Disorders, 11,* 373–384.

Harris, S. L., Wolchik, S. A., & Milch, R. E. (1983). Changing the speech of autistic children and their parents. *Child and Family Behavior Therapy, 4,* 151–173.

Hemsley, R., Howlin, P., Berger, M., Hersov, L., Holbrook, D., Rutter, M., & Yule, W. (1978). Treating autistic children in a family context. In M. Rutter & E. Schopler (Eds.), *Autism. A reappraisal of concepts and treatment.* New York: Plenum Press.

Howlin, P. (1981a). The results of a home-based language training programme with autistic children. *British Journal of Disorders of Communication, 16,* 73–88.

Howlin, P. A. (1981b). The effectiveness of operant language training with autistic children. *Journal of Autism and Developmental Disorders, 11,* 89–105.

Howlin, P., Marchant, R., Rutter, M., Berger, M., Hersov, L., & Yule, W. (1973). A home-based approach to the treatment of autistic children. *Journal of Autism and Childhood Schizophrenia, 3,* 308–336.

Hudson, A. M. (1982). Training parents of developmentally handicapped children: A component analysis. *Behavior Therapy, 13,* 325–333.

Kavanaugh, R. D., & Jirkovsky, A. M. (1982). Parental speech to young children: A longitudinal analysis. *Merrill-Palmer Quarterly, 28,* 297–311.

Kelley, M. L., Embry, L. H., & Baer, D. M. (1979). Skills for child management and family support: Training parents for maintenance. *Behavior Modification, 3,* 373–396.

Koegel, R. L., Russo, D. C., & Rincover, A. (1977). Assessing and training teachers in the generalized use of behavior modification with autistic children. *Journal of Applied Behavior Analysis, 10,* 197–205.

Kozloff, M. (1973). *Reaching the autistic child. A parent training program.* Champaign, IL: Research Press.

Lasky, E. Z., & Klopp, K. (1982). Parent–child interactions in normal and language-disordered children. *Journal of Speech and Hearing Disorders, 47,* 7–18.

Lederberg, A. (1980). The language environment of children with language delays. *Journal of Pediatric Psychology, 5,* 141–160.

Lord, C., Merrin, D. J., Vest, L. O., & Kelly, T. (1983). Communicative behavior of adults with an autistic four-year-old boy and his nonhandicapped twin brother. *Journal of Autism and Developmental Disabilities, 13,* 1–17.

Lovaas, O. I. (1977). *The Autistic child.* New York: Irvington.

Lovaas, O. I., Berberich, J. P., Perloff, B. F., & Schaeffer, B. (1966). Acquisition of imitative speech by schizophrenic children. *Science, 151,* 705–707.

Lovaas, O. I., Koegel, R., Simmons, J. Q., & Long, J. S. (1973). Some generalization and follow-up measures on autistic children in behavior therapy. *Journal of Applied Behavior Analysis, 6,* 131–165.

MacDonald, J. D., Blott, J. P., Gordon, K., Spiegel, B., & Hartmann, M. (1974). An experimental parent-assisted treatment program for preschool language-delayed children. *Journal of Speech and Hearing Disorders, 39,* 395–415.

Mahoney, G. J. (1975). Ethological approach to delayed language acquisition. *American Journal of Mental Deficiency, 80,* 139–148.

McMahon, R. J., Forehand, R., & Griest, D. L. (1981). Effects of knowledge of social learning principles on enhancing treatment outcome and generalization in a parent training program. *Journal of Consulting and Clinical Psychology, 49,* 526–532.

Moerk, E. (1974). Changes in verbal child–mother interactions with increasing language skills of the child. *Journal of Psycholinguistic Research, 3,* 101–116.

Moerk, E. (1975). Verbal interactions between children and their mothers during the preschool years. *Developmental Psychology, 11,* 788–794.

Moerk, E. (1977). *Pragmatic and semantic aspects of early language development.* Baltimore, MD: University Park Press.

O'Dell, S. L., Mahoney, N. D., Horton, W. G., & Turner, P. E. (1979). Media-assisted parent training: Alternative models. *Behavior Therapy, 10,* 103–110.

Phillips, J. R. (1973). Syntax and vocabulary of mothers' speech to young children: Age and sex comparisons. *Child Development, 44,* 182–185.

Rinn, R. C., Vernon, J. C., & Wise, M. J. (1975). Training parents of behaviorally-disordered children in groups: A three years' program evaluation. *Behavior Therapy, 6,* 378–387.

Rogers-Warren, A., Warren, S. F., & Baer, D. M. (1983). Interactional bases of language learning. In K. Kernan, M. Begab, & R. Edgerton (Eds.), *Environments and behavior: The adaptation of mentally retarded persons*. Austin, TX: Pro-Ed.

Rondal, J. A. (1977). Maternal speech in normal and Down's syndrome children. In P. Mittler (Ed.), *Research to practice in mental retardation, education and training, Vol. II*. I.A.S.S.M.D.

Rondal, J. A. (1978). Maternal speech to normal and Down's syndrome children matched for mean length of utterance. In C. E. Meyers (Ed.), *Monograph of the American Association on Mental Deficiency*.

Salzberg, C. L., & Villani, T. V. (1983). Speech training by parents of Down syndrome toddlers: Generalization across settings and instructional contexts. *American Journal of Mental Deficiency, 4*, 403-413.

Schopler, E., & Reichler, R. (1971). Parents as co-therapists in the treatment of psychotic children. *Journal of Autism and Childhood Schizophrenia, 1*, 87-102.

Snow, C. (1972). Mother's speech to children learning language. *Child Development, 43*, 549-565.

Sosne, J. B., Handleman, J. S., & Harris, S. L. (1979). Teaching spontaneous-functional speech to autistic-type children. *Mental Retardation, 17*, 241-245.

Stoneman, Z., & Brody, G. H. (1981). Two's company, three makes a difference: An examination of mothers' and fathers' speech to their young children. *Child Development, 52*, 705-707.

Waters, J. M., & Siegel, L. V. (1982). Parent recording of speech production of developmentally delayed toddlers. *Education and Treatment of Children, 5*, 109-120.

Weitz, S. (1982). A code for assessing teaching skills of parents of developmentally disabled children. *Journal of Autism and Developmental Disabilities, 12*, 13-24.

Whitehurst, G. J., Novak, G., & Zorn, G. A. (1972). Delayed speech studied in the home. *Developmental Psychology, 7*, 169-177.

Wolchik, S. A. (1983). Language patterns of parents of young autistic and normal children. *Journal of Autism and Developmental Disabilities, 13*, 167-180.

Wolchik, S. A., & Harris, S. L. (1982). Language environments of autistic and normal children matched for language age: A preliminary investigation. *Journal of Autism and Developmental Disorders, 12*, 43-55.

# 11

# Sign Language and Autism

## RONNIE B. WILBUR

For over a decade, reports have documented the efficacy of sign language intervention techniques with autistic individuals who do not appear to benefit from traditional speech training. There has been much discussion and speculation as to the reasons for this apparent success in the various reviews that have surveyed the research literature (Bonvillian, Nelson, & Rhyne, 1981; Carr, 1979; Layton, Leslie, & Helmer, 1983; Wilbur, 1979). Concurrently, there has been an exciting revolution in our understanding of the structure of sign language and its function as a natural language. Although these recent linguistic insights do not solve the puzzles presented by sign language usage with autistic children and adults, they do provide fresh perspectives on the problems that may serve to stimulate innovative research and clinical creativity. This chapter then will take its title literally and allocate a substantial portion of its space to a description of sign language itself, even though in many cases only a portion of the language is being used for intervention purposes. Following this discussion, our attention will be turned to the problems posed by the need to develop communicative language in autistic individuals. We will suggest new directions for future intervention and research and reiterate several earlier suggestions for sign language usage with autistic children (Menyuk & Wilbur, 1981; Moores, 1981).

## LINGUISTIC DESCRIPTION OF SIGN LANGUAGE

### Fingerspelling, American Sign Language, and Signed English

The English language can be represented by many codes. Of these, the best known are speech and print. Other codes for English, such as Morse code

RONNIE B. WILBUR • Department of Audiology and Speech Sciences, Purdue University, West Lafayette, Indiana 47907.

and Braille, have been devised to serve special purposes. From this perspective, fingerspelling can be seen as a code for representing the English language on the fingers. The coding on the fingers is entirely arbitrary, and the English language may be represented by different fingerspelling alphabets depending on the country (England's fingerspelling alphabet is two-handed). To be a fluent user of a fingerspelling alphabet, one must not only be able to produce and comprehend the sequences of handshapes, but one must also be familiar with the structure of the spoken language and able to *spell* its vocabulary. On the other hand, sign language (in particular, American Sign Language, henceforth ASL) is not a code for a spoken language, but is instead a natural language itself.

Within the United States, ASL differs from region to region and from state to state. These differences are similar to those observed for spoken language, involving vocabulary items, pronunciation/formation, and syntactic structure. In the same way that one must learn when to use "soda," "pop," "soft drink," or "tonic," specific signs show considerable variation. Fluent users of a language normally have control over several communicative styles (formal/informal, addressing a person of superior or inferior social status, addressing strangers or children, etc.) and dialects. Thus within the normal language situation, there is no "correct" word or sign for a particular concept, but rather a regionally or socially "accepted" form.

Signing and fingerspelling differ from spoken languages in that the channel of transmission is manual/visual. Although it is not possible to simultaneously produce two spoken languages, the modality difference allows a unique situation to arise—the possibility of signing and speaking at the same time, often referred to as "simultaneous communication." Simultaneous communication should not be confused with total communication, this latter being used to refer to an educational philosophy that advocates use of signing, speaking, print, auditory training, and amplification, but not necessarily simultaneously. Another confusion occurs frequently in the literature: Authors refer to simultaneous production of speech and ASL (or Ameslan, as it is sometimes called). It is not, in fact, possible to produce spoken English and ASL at the same time; they have very different syntactic structures. Instead, one produces the *signs* from ASL along with the spoken English. In such a case, one is putting the signs from ASL into English word order.

The use of ASL signs in English word order also entails many "dialects." In some cases, only ASL signs are used, and therefore certain English words are spoken but not signed (because their translation into ASL does not involve a separate sign; see below). In many other cases, artificially created signs are used in addition to ASL signs in order to parallel those spoken English words that do not have separate ASL signs for translation, so that every spoken word may be signed. Both of these situations, and the many intermediate possibilities involving differing amounts of artificial signs and the use of fingerspelling, may be subsumed under the title "signed English," which is another code for the English language, not a language separate from English. Some of these have been published as systems, including Seeing Essential English (SEE I), Signing Exact English (SEE II), Linguistics of Visual English (LOVE), Manual English, and Signed English (for a review, see Wilbur, 1979, Chapter 7). Of these, the two most popular in the United States are SEE II and Signed English.

Bellugi and Fischer (1972) compared the amount of time and the number of words/signs needed to convey the same story in ASL, signed English (unspecified variety), and spoken English. They reported that the spoken version required 50% more words than the ASL signed version (because of the morphological and syntactic differences), but both were nonetheless produced in the same amount of time, because spoken words take considerably less time to produce than signs. This suggests that, at some level of processing, there is an optimum time or rate for transmission of information regardless of modality. They also found that the signed English version increased the time by almost 50%, although no additional information was transmitted.

The entire process of signed English acquisition remains to be investigated. One initial investigation (Maxwell, 1982) reported that because use of signed English with artificial signs for English words requires heavy linguistic stress on the morphological endings (for example, -ing), the students mistakenly perceive these endings as separate words (as would be appropriate within ASL), and when they use them, they may move them to an inappropriate place in the sentence. Thus, Maxwell reports that a sentence such as "John is eating the cake" might be signed by a young child as "John is eat the cake ing." The grammatical organization that seems so apparent to the adult user of English may not be obvious to the child, and the emphasis placed on the -ing sign to highlight its presence actually serves to reinforce its independence by giving it the linguistic stress usually reserved for an individual sign. This type of error has not been observed in deaf students' written English (see Wilbur, 1979, Chapter 8, for a review).

## Structure of the Sign

To further appreciate the differences between signed English and ASL and to lay the foundation for suggestions of new research and intervention techniques, a more thorough explanation of the structure of a single sign is needed, especially because, in certain circumstances, a single sign may translate an entire English sentence.

Components of Signs

When Stokoe (1960) first described the internal structure of a sign, he attributed three aspects to it: what acts, where it acts, and the action. As linguists began to apply phonological theory based on spoken languages to ASL, it became apparent that additional information was needed to fully describe a sign. For example, the difference in formation between the sign CHILDREN and the sign THING is that for CHILDREN, the palm faces down, whereas for THING, it faces up. Linguists identified several parameters or primes as components of a sign. These included the handshape, the place of articulation, the movement, the orientation of the palm and fingers, the point of contact, the facial expression, tension, the speed, and the direction of movement (see Wilbur, 1979, Chapter 2, for a review).

Syllable Structure of Signs in American Sign Language

More recent research has concentrated on the analogue of syllables in sign language. Liddell (1982) argued that a sign syllable contained at most three parts: an initial hold (no movement), the movement, and a final hold. Wilbur (1982a) modified this suggestion to take into account the different kinds of movement that may occur in ASL. For linguistic purposes, two main categories of movement are relevant: path movement (which may be linear or arcing and usually involves movement from the elbow) and local movement (movement at the wrist, knuckles, or fingers, such as finger wiggling, finger flicking, wrist rotation, or wrist nodding). A well-formed basic sign in ASL may contain only one path movement, only one local movement, or a combination of one path movement and one local movement. The majority of basic signs in ASL are monosyllabic; extra syllables may be added by some of the inflections to be discussed below. A change in direction of the path movement (accompanied by deceleration or acceleration) signals the end of one syllable and the beginning of another. Similarly, a change in the local movement (from one type to another) signals separate syllables. The smallest syllable contains only movement (path or local). The most common lexical syllable contains a movement and a final hold. Compounds and stressed signs (among others) utilize the initial hold, movement, and final hold pattern. There are some signs that contain an initial hold followed by movement, with no final hold, but these tend to be infrequent (e.g., BIG/LARGE). Additional details of syllable structure, such as the internal structure of syllables or the placement of stress, remain to be clarified by linguist.

Morphemic Structure of Signs in American Sign Language

Recent work (Bellugi, 1980; McDonald, 1982; Supalla, 1982; Wilbur, 1978) has demonstrated the validity of analyzing many signs into several morphemes (units of meaning), some of which may be simultaneously realized and others of which may be sequential.

Classifiers. Many verbal predicates in ASL are composed of a predicate portion, which is formationally represented by the movement, and a noun classification portion (classifier), which is formationally represented by the handshape. In order to have a "complete" sign, the predicate portion and the noun portion must be produced simultaneously. For example, the sign CHASE is composed of a movement portion (path movement forward and local movement wiggling of the wrist on the hand doing the chasing) and a handshape portion (the basic form is made with a fist with thumb extended, which is a classifier referring to unspecified objects) (see Fig. 1). This form of CHASE is not used in all situations. If one car is chasing another car, then the handshapes used must be the classifier for vehicles, which in ASL involves an extended thumb, index finger, and middle finger (the same handshape used for the number 3). If one person is chasing another, then the handshape used must be the classifier for persons, which is simply an extended index finger (the handshape used for the number 1). The classifiers in ASL include categories for people, animals, vehicles, an airplane, and a variety of object shapes (tall, cylindrical, hollow, flat, etc.) (Kegl & Wilbur, 1976; Wilbur, Bernstein, & Kantor, in press).

Classifiers are not found in English, but are common in other languages of the world (Allan, 1977). Classifiers have been recognized in ASL for a long time (Kegl & Wilbur, 1976; McDonald, 1982; Supalla, 1978, 1982) and have been shown to function in accordance with the constraints identified for classifiers in spoken languages (Wilbur, Bernstein, & Kantor, in press). Signs that are constructed of separate predicate portions and separate classifier portions belong to the *productive* lexicon of ASL; the substitution of different handshapes for different classifiers adds meaning to the basic predicate portion (in this case, chasing). To say that these forms are productive means that the actual form of the sign depends on the context in which it is being used (that is, talking about cars chasing, people chasing, animals chasing, etc.).

There are many other signs in ASL that cannot be analyzed into pieces, for example the sign IMPROVE. Although these signs, which form the *frozen* lexicon of ASL, may have been analyzable in the past, they are no longer and are treated linguistically as single morphemes. Signs from both the productive lexicon and the frozen lexicon can be morphologically modified by several derivational and inflectional processes.

Derivational and Inflectional Processes. What are some of these morphological distinctions? Supalla and Newport (1978) identified relationships that exist between pairs of nouns and verbs. The verb form may be made with a large continuous or hold manner (for example, FLY, SIT DOWN, COMPARE), while the noun is made with a small, restrained, and repeated movement (AIRPLANE, CHAIR, COMPARISON). Until their description was published, many people failed to realize that ASL made such distinctions.

Other inflectional processes add information about the actors (linguistic ar-

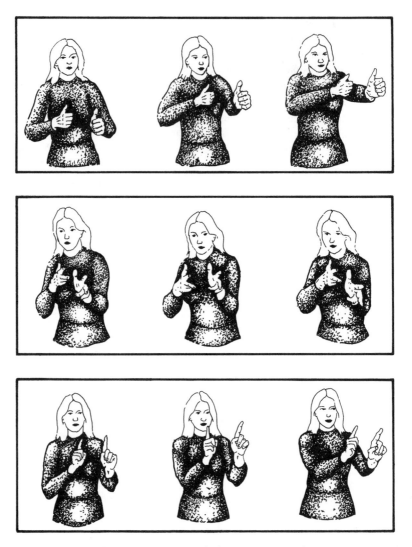

Figure 1. The signs CHASE (unmarked), CARS–CHASE, and PEOPLE–CHASE

guments such as subject and object) and the action (the predicate itself). The number and functions of these processes greatly exceed those that are present in English. Klima and Bellugi (1979) suggest at least eight categories of inflectional modifications (Table 1). There are two groups, separated by grammatical function and by how they are actually produced. The modifications that result from the first group affect the meaning of the predicate itself, providing

Table 1.   Inflections in ASL

I. Grammatical function: modifies predicate (action)
  A. Formational representation: affects rhythmic and dynamic qualities
    1. Changes in rate of signing (fast, slow)
    2. Differences in tension of muscles (tense, lax, normal)
    3. Changes in evenness of production
    4. Differences in size of production
    5. Differences in contouring of path (straight, circular, elliptical)
    6. Cyclicity (single, multiple repetitions)
  B. Types of inflection
    1. Temporal focus
      a. Inceptive: "starting to"
      b. Resultative: "resulting in"
      c. Augmentative: "increasingly"
    2. Temporal aspect
      a. Continuative: "for a long time"
      b. Durative: "continuously"
      c. Iterative: "again and again"
      d. Habitual: "regularly"
      e. Incessant: "incessantly"
    3. Manner
      a. Facilitative: "with ease"
    4. Degree
      a. Approximative: "approximately"
      b. Intensive: "very"
II. Grammatical function: modifies arguments (actors)
  A. Formational representation: affects spatial arrangements
    1. Planar locus (vertical, horizontal)
    2. Geometrical patterning (lines, arcs, circles, points/dots)
    3. Direction of movement
    4. Cyclicity (single, multiple repetitions)
    5. Doubling of the hands
  B. Types of inflection
    1. Referential indexing: Subject and/or object
    2. Reciprocal: "Each other"
    3. Grammatical number
      a. Dual: "two"
      b. Trial: "three"
      c. Multiple: "plural"
    4. Distributional aspect
      a. Exhaustive: "to each"
      b. Allocative: "to certain ones"
      c. Apportionative: "within or across groups"
      d. Seriated: "with respect to a series"

information that is often added by adverbs or prepositional phrases in English, whereas those which result from the second group affect the arguments (subject, object) of the predicate, adding information that is conveyed in English by pronouns, quantifiers, and prepositional phrases. (For further details, the reader is referred to Bellugi, 1980; Klima & Bellugi, 1979; Wilbur, 1979; Wilbur, Klima, & Bellugi, 1983.) Figure 2 illustrates several inflections with the sign ASK.

Implications of Morphemic Structure for Word Order in American Sign Language. The existence of numerous modifications on a single sign means that an enormous amount of information can be conveyed at once. Of particular interest is the fact that a single verb sign can potentially indicate the agent/subject and recipient/object of its action by means of Referential Indexing (see Fig. 2). A sign meaning "he gives her" would start at a specific point in space that had been established earlier in the conversation to refer to some male and would move to a specific ending point that had been earlier established to refer to some female. In ASL, each individual, whether male or female, is given a separate, unambiguous point in space. As a result of this type of verb inflection, the word order in ASL is not as fixed as it is in English because the endings mark the agent/action and object/recipient and therefore the word order is not as critical to understanding the meaning.

Another characteristic of ASL that affects word order is the previously discussed combination of predicates and classifiers. The classifiers represent a major argument (subject, object) of the predicate, and are produced simultaneously with the verb rather than sequentially as in English. It should be clear from this abridged discussion of ASL morphology and syntax why simultaneous production of spoken English and ASL is not possible. Actual simultaneous communication can only consist of spoken English and uninflected basic signs in English word order.

## SIGN LANGUAGE ACQUISITION BY DEAF CHILDREN

Considerably more is known about the acquisition of ASL by deaf children of deaf parents than is known about the acquisition of signed English. In many cases, the developmental progression displayed by young deaf children learning ASL reflects and confirms the theoretical complexities discussed above.

A comparison of the acquisition of ASL with that of spoken English reveals several interesting observations. It appears that a deaf child's first sign may emerge 2 to 3 months earlier than a hearing child's first spoken word (Wilbur & Jones, 1974). Similarly, in hearing children of deaf parents, the child's first sign may emerge several months before the same child's first spoken words (Wilbur & Jones, 1974). In addition, the child's spoken vocabulary does not initially overlap with the signed vocabulary, but instead complements it. After several months, the child begins to acquire spoken and signed names for the same objects or actions (Wilbur & Jones, 1974). Another comparison

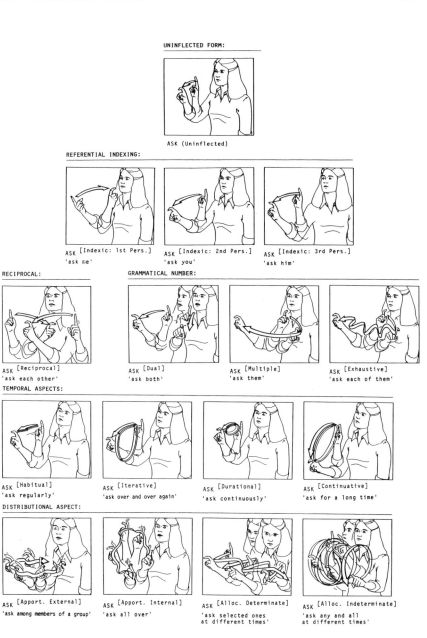

Figure 2. Inflectional operations on a single root: ASK (Copyright, Dr. Ursula Bellugi, The Salk Institute, La Jolla, CA 92037.)

made by McIntire (1977) indicates that a deaf child learning sign language may have a vocabulary of about 20 signs to age 10 months, the age at which a hearing child may be producing his or her first spoken word. McIntire also reports two-sign utterances at 10 months and three-sign utterances at 18 months, as compared to a hearing child beginning to produce two-word utterances at 18 months.

These comparisons must be viewed with caution. The number of children who have been studied is small. There is also considerable difficulty determining when a child has uttered his first word or signed his first sign. What may be intelligible to the parents may not be to an outside observer. Another factor that is often overlooked when interpreting these studies is that a deaf child learning to sign is given credit for many of his gestures as "baby signs" and for his pointing behavior, whereas a hearing child is only given credit for his spoken items. Thus, a hearing child who utters a word (even if it is only partially intelligible) and points is given credit for one word; the signing child who signs a name and points is given credit for two signs, even if he makes both signs at once. There is no doubt that pointing serves a multiplicity of functions in ASL and is linguistically and developmentally complex (Hoffmeister, 1977), but it is not clear that a young deaf child's early pointing can be separated from a young hearing child's early pointing. We will return to this issue below.

## Developmental Considerations

There is strong evidence that certain handshapes are harder to produce than others. McIntire (1977) reported developmental stages of handshape production that are affected by (a) opposition of the thumb; (b) extension of one or more fingers; and (c) contact of a finger with the thumb. In the first stage, only one of the handshapes requires a finger to make contact with the thumb. The remaining stages are progressively more complex, involving several of the above-mentioned factors. For example, the third stage includes extension of the weaker fingers (ring finger and pinkie), whereas the fourth stage included some handshapes that require crossing fingers.

Aspects of this developmental sequence were confirmed by Kantor (1980). Kantor's study of the acquisition of classifiers revealed that the development of classifiers reflects the linguistic complexity attributed to them (Kegl & Wilbur, 1976; Wilbur, Bernstein, & Kantor, in press). The classifiers were not acquired simply as basic lexical items, but rather as part of a syntactic process, as reflected by the fact that the same classifier might be used appropriately in one context but not in another. Of particular interest was the observation that children who could produce a particular handshape (e.g., the 3 handshape) when not part of a classifier (as when producing the number 3) substituted a simpler handshape (in terms of McIntire's stages above) when attempting a classifier (the vehicle classifier is made with the *3* handshape, but a child might substitute either the *5* handshape, all fingers extended and spread, or the *B* handshape, all fingers extended and together). The presence of this handshape substitution even at an early age implies that young deaf children learning sign language are sensitive to the distinction between the productive and the frozen lexicon. A developmental sequence was also observed in the noun categories associated with each classifier. The youngest children in Kantor's study (aged 3 years to 3 years 11 months) used the vehicle classifier for "car" and "motorcycle." An older group (aged 5 years 8 months to six years) expanded its use to include "train." Children aged six years to seven years expanded its use even further to a wider variety of syntactic contexts and to include "truck" and "parked car." The adult usage of the vehicle classifier centers primarily around transportation as the key notion, with the prototypical cases being water conveyances (boat, submarine) and long-distance land vehicles with wheels (i.e., cars, but not roller skates) (Wilbur, Bernstein, & Kantor, in press). Although classifiers begin to emerge in children as young as 3, full adult mastery is not seen until 8 or 9 years of age (Kantor, 1980).

There is evidence that young deaf children are also sensitive to the presence of the various inflections that may occur on verbs. Fischer (1973), Hoffmeister (1977), and Meier (1982) agree remarkably well that the beginning of verb inflection emerges before age 3. Meier (1982) compared three models that make predictions about how deaf children would acquire Referential Indexing. Two of the three models were in some part based on iconicity, whereas the third utilized notions of theoretical linguistic complexity. Meier's observations that deaf children of deaf parents produce uninflected verb forms that are counter-iconic and incorrect by adult standards confirmed previous observations by Fischer (1973), Hoffmeister (1977), Kantor (1982), and Newport and Ashbrook (1977). The literature on deaf children's early acquisition of sign language documents consistently that the extensive presence of iconicity in ASL contributes little if anything to the overall development of sign language as a communicative system (Bellugi & Klima, 1982; Bernstein, 1980; Fischer, 1973; Hoffmeister, 1977; Kantor, 1982; Launer, 1982; Meier, 1982; Newport & Ashbrook, 1977; Supalla, 1982; Wilbur, 1979).

As alluded to earlier, pointing performs several functions in ASL. Popular opinion views pointing as a fundamental gesture that is so basic that its use in ASL has often been overlooked or, when recognized, treated as evidence that ASL is concrete and context-bound. In fact, the full functions of pointing in ASL are so complex that even a summary would require more space than is available here. The reader is referred to Hoffmeister (1977) and Wilbur (1979, Chapters 4 and 5). Pointing forms the basis for part of the pronominal reference system as well as for part of the locative system (Hoffmeister, 1977).

While the hearing child's parents are busy teaching him that it is not nice to point at people, deaf children learning to sign are busy acquiring contraints on the use of pointing for person reference (*I/me, you, he/she, they*, etc.). If pointing is as basic, iconic, and concrete as is commonly thought, there should be no developmental progression in its acquisition by young deaf signers. Bellugi and Klima (1982) remarked that before beginning the study of the pronominal system, they "had fully expected that the learning of the equivalent of pronominal reference in ASL would be easy and early ('trivial' is the way we expressed it)." Working in their lab, Petitto (1983) reported that one deaf child as young as 10 months pointed to herself and others for pronominal reference as well as to objects and locations. Petitto observed that there followed a period of nearly a year during which the child ceased to use pointing for pronominal reference, substituting instead lexical items (primarily names), but continued use of pointing for other functions. At about 1 year 10 months, the child began using pointing for pronominal reference again, but much to everyone's surprise, the child made pronominal reversal errors of the type so familiar to those who work with mitigated echolalic autistic children. In this case, the child pointed to herself when she meant "you" and pointed to her mother when she meant "me." Over the next few months, the child continued to use these reversals and appeared to be unaffected by the mother's attempts to correct them. The errors essentially disappeared by 2 years 3 months. Bellugi and Klima (1982) noted that deaf children learning ASL appear to parallel hearing children learning English in terms of the emergence and disappearance of these reversal errors. Thus, although adults view pointing as a basic and trivial gesture, it is clear that, to the young learner who must master pointing as part of a linguistic system, the matter is far more complex.

## Parents' Signing to Children

In addition to the current explosion of research on deaf children's acquisition of sign language, there has also been considerable attention paid to the modifications that parents make when signing to their young children. Thus, in accordance with Hoffmeister's (1977) observation that many of the early two-sign and three-sign combinations produced by the deaf children he studied consisted in whole or in part of pointing, Kantor (1982) has reported that the deaf mothers she observed used extensive amounts of pointing with their young deaf children, even going so far as to replace the normal handshapes of signs such as MOTHER, EAT, and DRINK with the pointing handshape. This form of baby sign was later paired with the appropriate adult form of the sign, so that the child would see both together.

Launer (1982) reports extensive modifications made by the mothers she studied. She noted that mothers' signing to children contained the same features of simplicity and redundancy reported for spoken language motherese. Both Launer (1982) and Maestas y Moores (1980) reported that parents positioned their bodies and those of their children to maximize attention, interspersed nonvocal affective acts with language interactions, used alternate or simultaneous sensory modalities to communicate with the child, and repeated signs many times. Launer also observed that exaggerated size appears to be the signing counterpart of exaggerated intonation reported for spoken language motherese. She noted that mothers repeated the movement of a sign, occasionally as many as 12 times, even when the sign would not be repeated in the adult form. To this end, mothers were observed to exaggerate their productions of certain signs, so as to highlight the form for the child, while producing a counter-iconic form that would be unacceptable in adult signing. Launer (1982), Maestas y Moores (1980), and Petitto (1980, 1982) also observed several other important aspects of mothers' signing to deaf children: (a) the tendency to sign on the child's face and body rather than on the mother's; (b) the tendency to produce certain signs, in particular the names of objects, but also adjectives, on the object itself, highlighting the association between the object and the sign; and (c) the tendency of parents to move or mold the child's hand to form a particular sign.

    In summary, although there is extensive iconicity that is apparent to an adult viewing ASL, deaf children's early acquisition of ASL does not reflect this direct relationship. Instead, deaf children appear to be more affected by morphological and formational complexity of the forms to be acquired. Parents of signing children modify their input considerably, changing the place of articulation, the handshape, and the movement (not all at once) so as to heighten the child's awareness of particular qualities of a given sign. Parents are even willing to exaggerate their productions to the point of destroying both the iconicity and the morphological distinctions between related forms. In this latter case, Launer (1982) noted that mothers modified their movement of related noun and verb pairs, such as AIRPLANE and FLY, to the point that the actual form they produce was neither a noun nor a verb; in fact, it was not an ASL sign at all, but rather an unacceptable distortion. Apparently, parents do not concern themselves with complex morphological distinctions until they have evidence that the child is able to handle them. These observations parallel those regarding speaking mothers.

## SIGN LANGUAGE AND AUTISM

    The preceding information, although far from complete, raises many questions of relevance to sign language usage with autistic children and adults. The main issues that confront those who are involved in planning language intervention with the autistic population include whether to use sign language with a particular individual and how to proceed once the decision has been made.

## Alternative Communication Intervention

In fact, the first decision is usually not to use sign language *per se*, but rather to use any kind of alternate or augmentative communication intervention, of which sign language is but one form. The literature on alternative and augmentative communication devices and techniques contains several excellent and recent overviews of the available options. These include Carlson (1982), Cohen and Shane (1982), Lloyd and Karlan (1984), Rabush, Lloyd, and Gerdes (1982a,b,c), Schiefelbusch (1980), Vanderheiden and Grilley (1976), and Yoder and Kraat (1982). These reviews cover available unaided systems (signs) and aided systems (including equipment such as microcomputers or communication devices with synthetic voices as well as Blissymbolics, rebuses, and picture boards) for a wide range of nonspeaking populations (cerebral paysied, mentally retarded, and laryngectomy patients). To make a truly objective decision as to whether sign language or some other technique or device is appropriate for a given individual, familiarity with these different options is necessary. Two papers by Shane (1980a; Shane & Bashir, 1980) help in the planning stages by providing decision-making flowcharts and criteria for adopting different available systems.

## Indicators of Potential Success with Signing

The decision to use sign language with an autistic individual requires consideration of a number of characteristics of the individual and of the environment in which communication will take place. Potentially, any autistic individual whose communicative abilities are deficient or whose speech abilities are inadequate to the requirements of his communicative abilities is a candidate for sign language intervention. Bonvillian, Nelson, and Rhyne (1981) surveyed the literature on sign language usage with autistic children and reported that nearly all of the 100 children learned receptive and expressive signs, with many learning to produce combinations of signs. They also noted that several investigators indicated informally that individuals who could signify their desires through pointing prior to initiation of the sign intervention program seemed to do well when presented with signs, although there is no formal data to support this observation. Howlin (1981), in her review, found that neither age nor IQ were good indicators of potential language learning for autistic individuals and that prior language abilities and social skills were important predictors.

Helmer, Layton, and Wolfe (1982) attempted to determine subgroups of autistic children (aged 3 to 9) on the basis of language skills and to indicate which of them would be good candidates for sign language programs. They identified five groups on the basis of the Sequenced Inventory of Communication Development (Hedrick, Prather, & Tobin, 1975). The first group of children had better expressive skills than receptive skills, tended to use the few spoken words they had spontaneously, but had poor imitation skills and did not speak when requested. These children used gestures and vocalizations in their attempts to communicate, and the authors suggested that this group may include the children most likely to benefit from a simultaneous communication approach, with the probability of their eventually developing usable speech from it. Helmer *et al.*'s second group was identifed by overall better receptive skills than expressive skills, a better response to words alone as compared to words and gestures combined, and infrequent attempts at initiating communication. This group actually contained two subgroups, one with nearly normal nonverbal IQs and echolalic tendencies and the other with the lowest IQs in their survey (below 30) and muteness. The authors suggested that, for both subgroups, significant amounts of prelingual training in general communication skills would be necessary before language training and that some alternative mode of communication would probably be required, given the poor speech capabilities of these children. The children in the third group had good receptive skills and poor expressive skills, responded well to gestured directions, appeared to understand speech well without additional cues, but had poor vocal imitation skills and no functional speech. Helmer *et al.* (1982) suggested that this group would profit from a sign language training program. Group four included children who were echolalic, had good vocal and verbal imitation skills, and were highly interactive. They differed from the echolalic children in group two in that they had low IQs (around 50) and that they scored higher on the expressive scale because of their interaction with others. Helmer *et al.* predicted that children in group four would need special training on speech comprehension because they were already communicatively active, whereas group two would need training in communication *per se*. They suggested that sign language intervention appeared to be detrimental to the children in group four, but did not provide further details. Finally, the fifth group that Helmer *et al.* identified contained children who had generally low receptive skills and expressive skills, were aided in comprehension by the presence of gestures in addition to spoken words, had poor vocal and verbal imitation skills, and were relatively noncommunicative. They suggested that this group also would benefit from training on prelingual communication skills before the initiation of language intervention and that sign language or other alternative communication would be appropriate.

Further investigations along the lines of Helmer *et al.* are needed to clarify the situation. Similar studies comparing responsiveness to spoken words only with words combined with different types of symbol systems (Blissymbolics, rebuses, pictures) would contribute to early decision-making, especially in those cases in which sign language intervention appeared to be detrimental. Because the upper age limit on these children was 9, it is difficult to extend these findings to older autistic children or even adults. Studies to confirm Helmer *et al.*'s predictions are also needed. An important additional concern is that language is not only used for communicative purposes, but also for helping self-direction, maintaining a line of thought, and aiding memory. Bonvillian *et al.* (1981), in their review, noted that for many children who developed speech after sign language training, the signs were retained and used as an aid to communication, the signs were used to maintain a train of thought even when actual communication was conducted in speech (Schaeffer, Kollinzas, Musil, & McDowell, 1977), and the signs may have functioned as a mediator to speech (Baron & Isensee, 1976). Thus, even if Helmer *et al.* are correct in their predictions about the communicative outcomes of sign language intervention with the different groups of children, there may still be additional benefits to be achieved by including sign language at some point in the intervention and education process.

## When to Begin Intervention

Helmer *et al.* (1982) also raise the question of when (sign) language intervention should begin. For two of their groups, they suggested prelingual communication training prior to the initiation of language training. This issue has been of concern to speech/language pathologists for many different populations (Chapman, 1982; Kemp, 1982; Rees, 1982; Snyder, 1982) as well as for autistic children (Seibert & Oller, 1981; Yoder & Calculator, 1981). Menyuk and Wilbur (1981) argued that, although a clear distinction must be made between merely communicative behavior and truly linguistic behavior, there is no strong evidence that early gestural or facial communication must precede early linguistic communication. One thing is clear, namely, the emphasis on establishing eye contact as a prerequisite to initiating language training should no longer be a major concern and may, in fact, be counterproductive (Shane, 1980b; Yoder, 1980; Yoder & Calculator, 1981; Yoder & Kraat, 1982).

In one particularly instructive instance, W. Reagan (personal communication, 1975) taught the sign SOAP to an autistic child as the very first sign. He accomplished this despite the fact that eye contact was not established and that SOAP is not considered to be among the first signs that would be included in an initial lexicon (Fristoe & Lloyd, 1980; Riechle, Williams, & Ryan, 1981). Instead, Reagan took advantage of the child's propensity for self-stimulation by rubbing his palms together, a gesture that resembles the sign for SOAP. Using shavings from a soap bar, he dropped them onto the child's hands whenever the child rubbed his palms together. Eventually, an association between rubbing and soap shavings was established. The child then began to rub his hands together and stop and wait for the shavings. Reagan increased the delay time between the child's hand-rubbing and the deposit of the soap shavings, resulting in the child's beginning to look around for the expected soap. This interaction led to requesting behavior (that is, requests for soap shavings), which although obviously a game, was also the beginning of communicative interaction. If there is a moral to this story, it is undoubtedly that, in spite of the best guidelines that can be provided on who will benefit from signs, when to begin sign training, which signs to begin sign training with, and how to procede training signs, there is also considerable room for innovation, creativity, and flouting of the guidelines. There is no recipe waiting to be discovered or made up that, when followed exactly, will produce a successful result every time.

## Considerations in Choosing a Sign System

One major question faced by many programs is what sign system to use. As a general rule, programs that use ASL signs are preferable to those that create their own. This is partly a sociolinguistic preference, but more importantly, there are many artificially created signs that violate sign structure constraints that are presumed to be perceptually and motorically based (Wilbur, 1979, Chapters 2, 7, and 9). Another general observation is that a system that requires use of fingerspelling requires the ability to spell, fine motor control for production, and excellent perception of dynamically presented handshapes. A child who is deficient in any of these areas will have considerable difficulty communicating through fingerspelling.

Of concern to many is the presentation of English syntax, an often-cited reason for choosing a signed English system over ASL or its dialect variants. For normal deaf children, the decision usually involves two considerations. One is the desire to expose deaf children to English syntax with the expectation that this will result in the development of reading and writing skills when the child gets older. Thus, a form of signed English is chosen so that simultaneous communication may take place. The research clearly shows that deaf students experience considerable difficulty in the acquisition of English syntax, even after many years of formal schooling (Quigley, Wilbur, Power, Montanelli, & Steinkamp, 1976; Wilbur, 1977, 1979). The research also clearly shows that deaf students' problems with English are not the result of interference from

ASL syntax (Wilbur, 1977, 1979). Educators who introduce signed English as an early communication form tend to overlook the fact that signed English is still English, and that to be fluent users of it, the deaf students must still learn the syntactic structures of English. These syntactic rules must be developed over time, primarily through communicative interaction with other fluent users, regardless of the modality of interaction.

The same situation holds for autistic children. Grammatically well-formed sentences are a luxury that the early communicator, autistic or not, can ill afford (Menyuk & Wilbur, 1981; Moores, 1981; Yoder & Kraat, 1982). Little communication between hearing mother and normal child takes place in grammatical sentences. The evidence from deaf mothers' exaggerations and substitutions with their young deaf children shows that they are not concerned about the "well-formedness" of the signs they present, much less the structure of the sentences they use. Robbins (1976) argued that the goal of choosing an intervention system should be "*not* to select *a* system, *not* to determine which system is the 'best,' *nor* which system represents English the least imperfectly," but rather "for a preferred method for a particular child at a particular stage." Robbins expressed her personal preference for "language goals relating to functional use and development of meaning and of concepts which would enable the student to relate more completely to the world of objects, events, and persons as he learns, than goals focusing on production of correctly formed English kernel sentences with perfect morphological components." If, and when, there is reason to believe that the individual is ready for syntactic structure (presumably beyond the three-sign stage), English word order can be introduced. Even then, however, it is not clear that extensive morphological markings, such as the artificial signs for -*ing*, and -*ed*, are necessary.

## Functional Communication in Intervention

The focus on functional communication, rather than sentence structure, is emphasized in Bonvillian *et al.*'s (1981) discussion of teaching and training strategies, including discourse therapy. They are concerned that communicative interaction with autistic children follow "more closely the normal child's pattern of language development" (p. 132). They offer several suggestions, which include contingent language training in any context as the events and topics arise, especially if the child selects the topics by indicating attention, more than one language trainer in more than one training setting, the explicit inclusion of discourse routines, and exposing the child to conversations between two or more fluent communicators using the sign language system being taught (this means that adults in the communication environment should possess considerably better sign language skills than the individuals they are trying to teach; see, in this regard, Kopchick & Lloyd, 1976).

Bonvillian *et al.* (1981) also noted that sign language programs for autistic children have been inhibited by the misperception of institutional staff members and parents that it is difficult to learn to communicate manually. A contradictory perception is held by hundreds of college students who shun foreign language courses (e.g., French, German), but flock to sign language courses and enjoy themselves while they learn, primarily because they do not expect it to be difficult. As indicated earlier in this chapter, there is a considerable amount of linguistic complexity that must be mastered by these beginning sign language students, but they have no preconceived anxieties about sign language and they master it quite well. Bonvillian *et al.* point out that, given the slow rate of acquisition and production of signs by most autistic children, the parents and staff probably need only spend a few minutes a week learning to sign and that the optimal effectiveness of sign language training with autistic children will likely not be reached until teachers and parents become fluent signers with each other and the children. An excellent beginning text is *A Basic Course in American Sign Language* (Humphries, Padden, & O'Rourke, 1980; note—this is not the *older* ABC book, but rather a completely new one with a similar name).

One final concern expressed by Bonvillian *et al.* with respect to functional communication is that when a child is attempting to communicate a message, especially an urgent one, and the adult is not able to understand, the strategy should be one of "patient, imaginative attempts to help the child get his meaning across" (p. 134). Yoder and Kraat (1982) concerned themselves almost entirely with communication problems between adults and users of augmentative or alternative communication systems (whether the users are children or adults, hearing-impaired or normally hearing, cerebral palsied, mentally retarded, or autistic). They feel that not only does the user of the augmentative or alternate system need communication training, but also those who will communicate with them (parents, teachers, non-educational staff). They emphasize the flexibility that is needed, both in terms of training not only linguistic information, but also paralinguistic communicative behaviors, and that the successful user of these systems must occasionally break down conventional linguistic rule usage. They illustrated their concern with the following two samples of interaction (*V* vocal user, *A* augmentative/alternate systems user):

V: "Halloween. What are you going to be?"
A: B. Man (*Bliss/board user.*)
V: "Yeah, I could have guessed. . . . Hey, you know they took Batman off the air?"
A: (*Vocalizes, bangs fist, points in the direction of the bulletin board.*)
V: (*Reads letter on the board from Joey and a friend, protesting Batman off the air.*) "That's beautiful, Joe!"

(Kates, McNaughton, & Silvermann, 1977)

V: "What do you want?"
A: (*Points to ball.*)
V: "No, tell me with your board."
A: (*Points to ball again.*)
V: "How can you tell me with your board?"
A: (*Puts head down on laptray. No response.*)

(Harris, 1978)

In linguistic terms, this second interaction would not be considered a conversation. It illustrates a typical interaction that focuses heavily on desired future communicative skills, in this case, the ability to label objects. What it ignores is the fact that it is pragmatically odd to label an object that is present in the communicative environment when no additional information about it is provided. Thus, the child who is pointing to the ball is using an appropriate communication strategy that is not being accepted by the adult who is focusing on linguistic form. This interaction fails to provide the child with a reason to label the object with a linguistic term (functional communication) and fails, as well, to interest the child in continued communicative interaction.

## Future Research Needs

Several themes have pervaded this discussion. They include (a) the need for careful consideration of when introduction of English syntax and morphology is necessary and appropriate; (b) the recognition of a major distinction between communicative behavior and linguistic ability; (c) a concern for pragmatic development as well as phonological, syntactic, and semantic; and (d) the need for flexibility and creativity in intervention techniques, including starting points, initial signs, settings for interaction, and continual determination of the appropriateness of each decision for the individual child. The review of ASL structure in the first part of this chapter suggests several new directions for both intervention and research. Current investigations of factors that contribute to the ease of sign acquisition in populations other than the hearing-impaired indicate that there is some memory advantage to signs that are perceived as more iconic over those that are not (Daniloff, Lloyd, & Fristoe, 1983; Griffith & Robinson, 1980; Karlan & Lloyd, 1982; Karlan, Lloyd, & Fristoe, 1984; Luftig & Lloyd, 1981) and to signs that include contact with the body or between the hands over those without contact (Lloyd & Doherty, 1983), but these remain to be replicated with autistic individuals. If there is an iconicity effect, does it contribute to communicative behavior? What are the effects on perception and production difficulty of the different types of movement (local, path, combination of both) that may occur in basic ASL signs? Does syllable structure contribute to ease of learning? Are autistic children sensitive to differences between the frozen lexicon and the productive lexicon? If so, what differences are they aware of, how did they develop this awareness, and what are the implications for proceding with sign intervention? Are there developmental sequences of handshape acquisition, and if so, should the practice of molding the child's hands be eliminated on the assumption that the child will eventually develop the correct handshape or should molding be increased to try and speed the developmental sequence? Do signing autistic children make the same type of pronoun reversals as young deaf children and, if so, do they finally correct them? Are echolalic autistic children poor risks for sign language intervention (Helmer *et al.*, 1982; Bonvillian *et al.*, 1981) and is pronominal reversal a clue to the reason why they have excessive difficulty with signs? Can the inflectional capabilities of ASL that utilize three-dimensional space and rhythmic dynamic qualities be used for autistic children in a linguistically productive way? (Moores, 1981, also raised this question). What types of semantic analysis are autistic children capable of in their learning of language, and can this semantic processing be used to suggest the types of signs that can be taught fruitfully (for example, signs from the productive lexicon containing classifiers)? What pragmatic functions are autistic children capable of displaying with their acquired signs (Oxman & Blake, 1980) and what can be done to increase them? Finally, what are the implications of the modifications the deaf mothers make for their deaf children? Is there any benefit to using baby sign with beginning signers? Such modifications as replacing the lexical handshape with the pointing handshape, exaggerating the size and shape of the sign, repeating the sign inordinately many times, and signing on the object when appropriate appear to be strategies that would not be too difficult to implement, but remain to be documented as beneficial. Other strategies, such as reducing the complexity and increasing the redundancy of the message, maximizing the child's attention by guiding his face (but not to establish eye contact), and signing on the child's body as well as on the adult's, are also candidates for further investigation, but should be easy to test clinically.

In a discussion of the overall problems of language intervention with children, Rees (1982, p. 310) summed up the main point that many other researchers and clinicians have been trying to make: "Things started getting rough for the language professional when it became apparent that morphology plus syntax plus semantics does not equal language." To these she added "perception, neurolinguistics, cognitive development, social development, reading, pragmatics, and learning (p. 311)," as well as phonology. Some recent linguistic theories support Rees' view. For example, Givón (1979) argued that pragmatic factors in discourse are the source of syntax, both historically in the evolution of languages and developmentally in the acquisition of language by children. Wilbur (1982b) argued that in order to address the questions of who should receive language intervention, what kind of intervention it should be, when this intervention should start, how it should proceed, and where it should take place, a better understanding of the *what*, the nature of the language being taught or trained, is required. By providing the description of ASL at the beginning of this chapter and only loosely suggesting ways in which it may be utilized, this author hopes to stimulate creativity in research and clinical applications.

## REFERENCES

Allan, K. (1977). Classifiers. *Language, 53,* 285-311.
Baron, N., & Isensee, L. (1976). *Effectiveness of manual versus spoken language with an autistic child.* Unpublished manuscript, Brown University, Providence, RI.
Bellugi, U. (1980). The structuring of language: Clues from the similarities between signed and spoken language. In U. Bellugi & M. Studdert-Kennedy (Eds.), *Signed and spoken language: Biological constraints on linguistic form* (pp. 115-140). Dahlem Konferenzen. Weinheim/Deerfield Beach, FL: Verlag Chemie.
Bellugi, U., & Fischer, S. (1972). A comparison of sign language and spoken language: Rate and grammatical mechanisms. *Cognition, 1,* 173-200.
Bellugi, U., & Klima, E. (1982). The acquisition of three morphological systems in American Sign Language. *Papers and Reports on Child Language Development, 21,* K1-35.
Bernstein, M. E. (1980). *Acquisition of locative expressions by deaf children learning American Sign Language.* Unpublished doctoral dissertation, Boston University, Boston, MA.
Bonvillian, J. D., Nelson, K. E., & Rhyne, J. M. (1981). Sign language and autism. *Journal of Autism and Developmental Disorders, 11,* 125-137.
Carlson, F. (1982). *Alternate methods of communication.* Danville, IL: Interstate Printers.
Carr, E. G. (1979). Teaching autistic children to use sign language: Some research issues. *Journal of Autism and Developmental Disorders, 9,* 345-359.
Chapman, R. (1982). Deciding when to intervene. In J. Miller, D. Yoder, & R. Schiefelbusch (Eds.), *Contemporary issues in language intervention* (pp. 221-225) (ASHA Reports 12). Rockville, MD: The American Speech-Language-Hearing Association.
Cohen, C., & Shane, H. (1982). An overview of augmentative communication. In N. Lass, L. McReynolds, J. Northern, & D. Yoder (Eds.), *Speech, language, and hearing.* Philadelphia, PA: Saunders.
Daniloff, J., Lloyd, L., & Fristoe, M. (1983). Amer-ind transparency. *Journal of Speech and hearing Disorders, 48,* 103-110.
Fischer, S. (1973, December). *The deaf children's acquisition of verb inflections in ASL.* Paper presented at the Linguistic Society of America Annual Meeting, San Diego, CA.
Fristoe, M., & Lloyd, L. (1980). Planning an initial expressive sign lexicon for persons with severe communication impairment. *Journal of Speech and Hearing Disorders, 45,* 170-180.
Givón, T. (1979). From discourse to syntax: Grammar as a processing strategy. In T. Givón (Ed.), *Syntax and semantics: Vol. 12: Discourse and syntax.* New York: Academic Press.
Griffith, P., & Robinson, J. (1980). Influence of iconicity and phonological similarity on sign learning by mentally retarded children. *American Journal of Mental Deficiency, 85,* 291-298.
Harris, D. (1978). *Descriptive analysis of communicative interaction processes involving non-vocal severely physically handicapped children.* Unpublished doctoral dissertation, University of Wisconsin-Madison, Madison, WI.

Hedrick, D., Prather, E., & Tobin, A. (1975). *Sequenced Inventory of Communication Development.* Seattle, WA: University of Washington Press.

Helmer, S., Layton, T., & Wolfe, A. (1982, November). *Patterns of language behavior in autistic children.* Paper presented at the American Speech-Language-Hearing Association Annual Convention, Toronto, Canada.

Hoffmeister, R. (1977). *The acquisition of American Sign Language by deaf children of deaf parents: The development of demonstrative pronouns, locatives, and personal pronouns.* Unpublished doctoral dissertation, University of Minnesota, Minneapolis, MN.

Howlin, P. (1981). The effectiveness of operant language training with autistic children. *Journal of Autism and Developmental Disorders, 11,* 86–106.

Humphries, T., Padden, C., & O'Rourke, T. J. (1980). *A basic course in American Sign Language.* Silver Spring, MD: T. J. Publisher.

Kantor, R. (1980). The acquisition of classifiers in American Sign Language. *Sign Language Studies, 28,* 193–208.

Kantor, R. (1982). Communicative interaction: Mother modification and child acquisition of American Sign Language. *Sign Language Studies, 36,* 233–278.

Karlan, G., & Lloyd, L. (1982). *Considerations in the planning of communication intervention: II. Manual and gestural sign systems for representing the lexicon.* Unpublished manuscript, Purdue University, Lafayette, IN.

Karlan, G., Lloyd, L., & Fristoe, M. (1983). The effects of presentation modality upon learning in a comprehension task using oral, manual, and dual mode stimulus cues. *Journal of Speech and Hearing Research, 26,* 436–443.

Kates, B., McNaughton, S., & Silvermann, H. (1977). *Handbook for instructors, users, parents, and administrators.* Toronto, Ontario, Canada: Blissymbolic Communication Foundation.

Kegl, J., & Wilbur, R. (1976). When does structure stop and style begin? Syntax, morphology, and phonology vs. stylistic variation in American Sign Language. In S. Mufwene, C. Walker, & S. Steever (Eds.), *Papers from the Twelfth Regional Meeting, Chicago Linguistic Society.* Chicago: The University of Chicago Press.

Kemp, J. (1982). The timing of language intervention for the pediatric population. In J. Miller, D. Yoder, & R. Schiefelbusch (Eds.), *Contemporary issues in language intervention* (pp. 183–195) (ASHA Reports 12). Rockville, MD: The American Speech-Language-Hearing Association.

Klima, E., & Bellugi, U. (1979). *The signs of language.* Cambridge, MA: Harvard University Press.

Kopchick, G., & Lloyd, L. (1976). Total communication for the severely language impaired: A 24 hour approach. In L. Lloyd (Ed.), *Communication assessment and intervention strategies.* Baltimore, MD: University Park Press.

Launer, P. (1982). *"A plane" is not "to fly": Acquiring the distinction between related nouns and verbs in American Sign Language.* Unpublished doctoral dissertation, The City University of New York, New York.

Layton, T., Leslie, C., & Helmer, S. (1983). *A critical review pertaining to sign language acquisition in autistic children.* Unpublished manuscript, University of North Carolina, Chapel Hill.

Liddell, S. (1982, July). *Sequentiality in American Sign Language signs.* Paper presented at the Linguistic Society of America Summer Meeting, University of Maryland, College Park, MD.

Lloyd, L., & Karlan, G. (1984). Nonspeech communication symbols and systems: Where have we been and where are we going? *Journal of Mental Deficiency Research, 28,* 3–20.

Lloyd, L., & Doherty, J. (1983). The influence of production mode on recall of signs in normal adult subjects. *Journal of Speech and Hearing Research, 26,* 595–600.

Luftig, R., & Lloyd, L. (1981). Manual sign translucency and referential concreteness in the learning of signs. *Sign Language Studies, 30,* 49–60.

Maestas y Moores, J. (1980). Early linguistic environment: Interactions of deaf parents with their infants. *Sign Language Studies, 26,* 1–13.

Maxwell, M. (1982, December). *The acquisition of signed English by deaf children.* Paper presented at the Linguistic Society of America Annual Meeting, San Diego, CA.

McDonald, B. (1982). *Aspects of the American Sign Language predicate system.* Unpublished doctoral dissertation, The State University of New York, Buffalo.

McIntire, M. (1977). The acquisition of American Sign Language hand configurations. *Sign Language Studies, 16,* 247-266.

Meier, R. (1982). *Icons, analogues, and morphemes: The acquisition of verb agreement in ASL.* Unpublished doctoral dissertation, University of California, San Diego, CA.

Menyuk, P., & Wilbur, R. (1981). Preface to special issue on language disorders. *Journal of Autism and Developmental Disorders, 11,* 1-13.

Moores, D. (1981). Issues in the modification of American Sign Language for instructional purposes. *Journal of Autism and Developmental Disorders, 11,* 153-162.

Newport, E., & Ashbrook, E. (1977). The emergence of semantic relations in American Sign Language. *Papers and Reports on Child Language Development, 13,* 16-21.

Oxman, J., & Blake, J. (1980, September). *Sign language use by autistic children: A pragmatic analysis.* Paper presented at the American Psychological Association Convention, Montreal, Quebec, Canada.

Petitto, L. (1980). *On the acquisition of anaphoric reference in American Sign Language.* Unpublished manuscript. The Salk Institute for Biological Studies, La Jolla, CA.

Petitto, L. (1982). *From gesture to symbol: The acquisition of pronominal reference in American Sign Language.* Unpublished manuscript, Harvard University, Boston, MA.

Petitto, L. (1983). *From gesture to symbol: The acquisition of pronominal reference in American Sign Language.* Unpublished doctoral dissertation, Harvard University, Boston, MA.

Quigley, S., Wilbur, R., Power, D., Montanelli, D., & Steinkamp, M. (1976). *Syntactic structures in the language of deaf children.* Urbana-Champaign, IL: Institute for Child Behavior and Development, University of Illinois.

Rabush, D., Lloyd, L., & Gerdes, M. (1982a). Communication enhancement bibliography: Part I. *Communication Outlook, 3,* No. 1, 4-10.

Rabush, D., Lloyd, L., & Gerdes, M. (1982b). Communication enhancement bibliography: Part II. *Communication Outlook, 4,* No. 1, 4-12.

Rabush, D., Lloyd, L., & Gerdes, M. (1982c). Communication enhancement bibliography: Part III. *Communication Outlook, 4,* No. 2, 4-12.

Rees, N. (1982). Language intervention with children. In J. Miller, D. Yoder, & R. Schiefelbusch (Eds.), *Contemporary issues in language intervention* (pp. 309-316) (ASHA Reports 12). Rockville, MD: The American Speech-Language-Hearing Association.

Riechle, J., Williams, W., & Ryan, S. (1981). Selecting signs for the formulation of an augmentative communication modality. *Journal of the Association for the Severely Handicapped, 6,* 48-56.

Robbins, N. (1976, November). *Selecting sign systems for multi-handicapped students.* Paper presented at the American Speech and Hearing Association Convention, Houston, TX.

Schaeffer, B., Kollinzas, G., Musil, A., & McDowell, P. (1977). Spontaneous verbal language for autistic children through signed speech. *Sign Language Studies, 17,* 287-328.

Schiefelbusch, R. (1980). *Nonspeech Language Intervention.* Baltimore, MD: University Park Press.

Shane, H. (1980a). Non-speech communication: A position paper, Ad Hoc Committee on Communicative Processes for Non-speaking Persons. *ASHA, 22,* 262-272.

Shane, H. (1980b). Early decision-making in augmentative communication system use. In R. Schiefelbusch & D. Bricker (Eds.), *Early language: Acquisition and intervention.* Baltimore, MD: University Park Press.

Shane, H., & Bashir, A. (1980). Election criteria for the adoption of an augmentative communication system: Preliminary considerations. *Journal of Speech and Hearing Disorders, 45,* 408-414.

Seibert, J., & Oller, D. K. (1981). Linguistic pragmatics and language intervention strategies. *Journal of Autism and Developmental Disorders, 11,* 75-88.

Snyder, L. (1982). From assessment to intervention: Problems and solutions. In J. Miller, D. Yoder, & R. Schiefelbusch (Eds.), *Contemporary issues in language intervention* (pp. 147-164) (ASHA Reports 12). Rockville, MD: The American Speech-Language-Hearing Association.

Stokoe, W. (1960). Sign language structure: An outline of the visual communication system of the American deaf. *Studies in Linguistics occasional papers,* No. 8. Buffalo: University of Buffalo Press.

Supalla, T. (1978). Morphology of verbs of motion and location in American Sign Language. In F. Caccamise (Ed.), *National symposium on sign language research and teaching.* Silver Spring, MD: National Association of the Deaf.

Supalla, T. (1982). *Structure and acquisition of verbs of motion and location in American Sign Language.* Unpublished doctoral dissertation, University of California, San Diego, CA.

Supalla, T., & Newport, E. (1978). How many seats in a chair? The derivation of nouns and verbs in American Sign Language. In P. Siple, (Ed.), *Understanding language through sign language research* (pp. 91-132). New York: Academic Press.

Vanderheiden, G., & Grilley, K. (1976). *Nonvocal communication techniques and aids for the severely physically handicapped.* Baltimore, MD: University Park Press.

Wilbur, R. (1977). An explanation of deaf children's difficulty with several syntactic structures of English. *The Volta Review, 79,* 85-92.

Wilbur, R. (1978). On the notion of derived segments in American Sign Language. *Communication and Cognition, 11,* 79-104.

Wilbur, R. (1979). *American Sign Language and sign systems.* Baltimore, MD: University Park Press.

Wilbur, R. (1982a, December). *A multi-tiered syllable structure for American Sign Language.* Paper presented at the Linguistic Society of America Annual Meeting, San Diego, CA.

Wilbur, R. (1982b). Where do we go from here? Speculations of the future of language intervention research. In J. Miller, D. Yoder, & R. Schiefelbusch (Eds.), *Contemporary Issues in Language Intervention* (pp. 137-143) (ASHA Reports 12). Rockville, MD: The American Speech-Language-Hearing Association.

Wilbur, R., & Jones, M. (1974). Some aspects of the bilingual/bimodal acquisition of sign language and English by three hearing children of deaf parents. In M. LaGaly, R. Fox, & A. Bruck (Eds.), *Papers from the Tenth Regional Meeting, Chicago Linguistic Society.* Chicago: Chicago Linguistic Society.

Wilbur, R., Klima, E., & Bellugi, U. (1983). Roots: The search for the origins of signs in ASL. *Chicago Linguistic Society, 19,* 314-336.

Wilbur, R., Bernstein, M., & Kantor, R. (in press). *The semantic domain of classifiers in American Sign Language. Sign Language Studies.*

Yoder, D. (1980). Communication systems for nonspeech children. *New directions for the exceptional child, 2.*

Yoder, D., & Calculator, S. (1981). Some perspectives on intervention strategies for persons with developmental disorders. *Journal of Autism and Developmental Disorders, 11,* 107-124.

Yoder, D., & Kraat, A. (1982). Intervention issues in nonspeech communication. In J. Miller, D. Yoder, & R. Schiefelbusch (Eds.), *Contemporary issues in language intervention* (pp. 27-51) (ASHA Reports 12). Rockville, MD: The American Speech-Language-Hearing Association.

V

# General Issues

# 12

# Autism and the Comprehension of Language

## CATHERINE LORD

## INTRODUCTION

### What is the Comprehension of Language?

The comprehension of language is one of the most difficult constellations of skills for children and adults with autism to acquire and to use. Yet our knowledge of what we can do about these difficulties is at an extraordinarily rudimentary level. Part of the problem is that the meaning of the term *comprehension* has varied from highly specific and idiosyncratic descriptions (e.g., reaction time to negative, passive sentences read silently by psychology undergraduates) to characterizations that are too broad to be scientifically tractable (e.g., comprehension as the "full understanding of world events"). To have some idea what we can do to facilitate language comprehension in persons with autism, we need to first ask "What is the comprehension of language anyway?"

Formally, comprehension has been defined as the "complete process of understanding a sentence" (Chapman, 1978). A child who truly comprehends a sentence should therefore understand all aspects of the sentence when the structures (i.e,. specific linguistic rules such as those for combining words or sounds) are presented in isolation as well as in context. A child who comprehends "those skates were thrown in the garbage by your father because you left them out there again" should theoretically understand each word in the ut-

---

CATHERINE LORD • Department of Pediatrics, University of Alberta, Glenrose Hospital, Edmonton, Alberta T5G 0B7, Canada.

terance; grammatical markings such as those for plural *s*, irregular past tense, and possession; syntactic constructions using active and passive voices; deictic references to person (i.e., "you") and place (i.e., "there"); and logical connections between leaving skates out and having them thrown away. Yet, it is the relationship between *the sentence and the situation* that, in reality, we are most often called on to comprehend in everyday life. Sentences seldom appear typed out in mid-air or proclaimed by bodiless voices. Children need to understand the relationship between what has been said, who has said it, what they see when they look around them, and what they know about the situation in general.

The situation often provides as much, if not more, information for the listener as the sentence. Given redundancies in information and knowledge provided by immediate contexts or past experience, understanding the individual terms in a sentence or the relations of these terms to each other is often unnecessary in order to respond appropriately. Thus for the sentence above, we can imagine a girl peering into an empty closet looking for skates, facing an angry mother who abruptly points at the skates placed in the garbage can across the garage. As a repeat offender, the child may need to understand little more than her mother's facial expression or tone of voice, and possibly the word *father*, to know what has happened.

One of the difficulties in studying language comprehension is that there are many different possible relationships between sentence and situation. The situation often helps or eliminates the need for the child's understanding of specific linguistic aspects of the sentence, as occurred in the preceding example, where the child could use her experience to determine what was said. However, the situation can also place additional demands on the listener for understanding more than is stated in the sentence. Even a statement as simple as "Where's your blanket?" made by a parent to an irritable 2-year-old may carry numerous situational implications from "Do you want me to help you find your blanket?," "Go get your blanket," "Cheer yourself up, grumpy," to "It's time for your nap." Normally developing children can work back and forth from sentence to situation using what they know about the specific context as well as the general likelihood of events to determine which of these meanings is intended.

## What is Language Comprehension for the Child with Autism

It is in these ways that children with autism are doubly handicapped. Not only are many autistic children slow in developing the linguistic concepts necessary for communication, but they also may not have the knowledge about particular meanings or predictable relationships, social or otherwise, to be able to interpret situations in the same way as other children. If, as some psycholinguists feel, the origins of comprehension lie in the child's use of knowledge he or she already has about the world in order to make sense out of initially meaningless words and sentence forms (Macnamara, 1972), the child with autism may be left without a way even to begin the process of comprehending.

The purpose of this chapter is to discuss the implications for children with autism of what is currently known and proposed about the development of language comprehension. Working hypotheses about the nature of comprehension deficits associated with autism are proposed, although at this point there are few data available to support or refute these speculations. Two major deficits associated with autism will be considered as they related to language comprehension. The first of these deficits involves social skills. The second deficit involves a cognitive disorder in the extraction of rules and redundancies from verbal information. Thus, the chapter begins with a discussion of the relations between language comprehension and social behavior, which is followed by a description of language comprehension as a function of cognitive skills. Next, on the basis of the hypotheses relating each area to the comprehension difficulties experienced by autistic persons, suggestions are made for the assessment of comprehension in children with autism. Finally, intervention strategies to improve functional communication are proposed.

## LANGUAGE COMPREHENSION AND SOCIAL DEVELOPMENT

Rutter (1983) has proposed that autism is characterized by a cognitive disability in processing social meanings. Persons with autism have difficulty making sense out of and responding appropriately to information from and about other people. In particular, Wing (1981) has suggested that people with autism have difficulty understanding and responding to *species-specific* social and communicative behaviors. The significance of the term *species-specific* is that these behaviors, like language, are not usually taught in any systematic fashion, but rather are acquired in similar ways very early on in development by normally developing human beings across cultures. These behaviors include facial expressions, tone of voice, direction of gaze, gestures, imaginary play, and structural aspects of speech and language. Failure to develop spontaneous play or creative, imaginary use of objects forms the third factor in what Wing sees as a *triad* of deficits, including language comprehension, social relatedness, and play (Wing & Gould, 1979).

In recent years, Wing (1978) has used the diagnostic category of autism (which she defines narrowly using Kanner's 1943 criteria of extreme aloofness and use of elaborate, obsessive routines) to describe a small subgroup of children with the triad. Here, the term autism will be used more broadly to describe children whose difficulties conform to *DSM III* (American Psychiatric Association, 1980) and Rutter's (1978) definition of autism (i.e., onset before 30 months, uneven development including delayed or deviant use of language, extremely deficient social skills, abnormal insistence on sameness, or unusual responses to the environment). However, many of the points covered here are relevant as well for nonautistic children with multiple social and language deficits, such as those described by Wing (Wing, 1978; Wing & Gould, 1979).

## Socially Determined Comprehension Strategies

When looking at studies of normal development or observing a normally developing child, it is easy to become quickly overwhelmed by how rapidly and well most children learn to respond to social cues and to language. In a recent study, babies under 15 months were all found to respond discriminately to the name of one person (e.g., Mommy) and one-half responded discriminately to the name of an object (e.g., blanket) *without* contextual cues or gestures (Miller, Chapman, Branston, & Reichle, 1980). Equally impressive is work showing that infants under 3 months of age look at faces differently when they hear someone speaking to them. Infants discriminate the voices of familiar people and even process the rhythms of speech and gestures at some level (see Stern, 1974).

For the infant, many of whose interactions are with an adult, social and communicative meanings are constantly intertwined. For adults speaking to each other, relationships between specific social behaviors and language still exist, but these relations become more flexible (i.e., as adults, we can read factual reports of nonsocial phenomena and understand them; we can acknowledge the fine verbal skills of an articulate politician, but doubt his intentions and information). In the last 10 years, interest has been generated in the social behaviors associated with language comprehension in young children. In fact, more and more frequently, structural aspects of language are seen as only gradually entering the equation of comprehension, long after the child has begun to respond appropriately to sentences in social contexts. The child-as-listener is seen first as a communicative social being, only gradually becoming a linguistic one (Curtiss, 1981). The child's early responses to language are appropriate, not because of "language" comprehension, but rather because of early developed abilities to use social and world knowledge in context and early established attention to speech and speakers. Table 1 presents a summary of young children's strategies in responding to language.

## Social Behaviors as First Determiners of Attention and Response

For the clinician or teacher of autistic children, one is struck by how easily the strategies observed in normally developing 8- to 12-month-olds could be confused with a list of the deficits in social behaviors associated with autism. As shown in Table 1, following a gaze and imitating ongoing actions are identified as two of the three major ways infants respond to language in context. For an autistic child whose attention is captured by unusual aspects and uses of objects, even the third response, acting on an object noticed, may not be very

Table 1.   Summary of Nonlinguistic Response Strategies
and Comprehension Strategies[a]

| Approximate age range | Comprehension strategy |
| --- | --- |
| I. Context-determined responses | |
| (Child uses immediate environment to determine how to act) | |
| 8–12 months | 1. Look at objects that adult looks at |
| | 2. Imitate ongoing action |
| | 3. Act on objects that you notice |
| II. Lexical guides to context-determined responses | |
| (Child uses one word at a time to direct attention to relevant objects or to suggest actions appropriate to the immediate environment) | |
| 12–18 months | 1. Attend to object mentioned and . . . |
| | 2. Give evidence of notice |
| | 3. Take objects offered |
| | 4. Do what you usually do in the situation |
| | (a) Put objects into containers |
| | (b) Use in conventional way |
| III. Lexical comprehension with context-determined sentence meaning | |
| (Child uses words to determine elements referred to by speaker, but depends on immediate environment to know how these elements go together) | |
| 18–24 months | 1. Locate the objects mentioned and |
| | 2. Give evidence of notice or |
| | 3. Do what you usually do |
| | (a) Put objects into containers |
| | (b) Perform conventional use or |
| | 4. Act on the objects in the way mentioned |
| | (a) Child-as-agent |
| | (b) Choose handier object as instrument |
| IV. Lexical comprehension with context or knowledge-determined sentence meaning | |
| (Same as III with addition of the ability to use knowledge from past experience) | |
| 2–4 years | 1. Do what is usually done |
| | (a) Probable location strategy (in, on, under) |
| | (b) Probable event strategy for simple reversible actives |
| | 2. Supply missing information to questions not understood (2-year-olds) |
| | 3. Supply explanation to questions not understood (3-year-olds) |
| | 4. Infer most probable speech act in context |

*(Continued)*

Table 1. (*Continued*)

| Approximate age range | Comprehension strategy |
|---|---|

V. Lexical and syntactic comprehension for simple structures; context, knowledge, and overgeneralized syntactic strategies determine complex sentence meaning
(Child can use words and syntax independent of context and past experience when sentences are simple; as sentences become more complex, previous social and knowledge-based strategies reappear, as well as incorrect use of simple syntactic rules)

4-11 years
1. Word order strategy for agent–object relations
2. Order of mention strategy for clauses
3. Probable relation of events for causal conjunctions
4. Understanding of contrastive conjunctions *but* and *although* as though they mean *and then* when probable relations not obvious

*a*Modified from R. S. Chapman (1978). Comprehension strategies in children. In Kavanagh, J. E., & Strange, W. (Eds.), *Implications of basic speech and language research for the school and clinic* (pp. 308–327). Cambridge, MA: M.I.T. Press.

helpful, since the objects noticed may differ from those in which most people are interested. Children who are more interested in lint or vacuum cleaner nozzles than in a doll or car or blanket may be less likely to respond clearly when their attention is directed to these objects than children whose interest in objects is more social or more comprehensible to the people who care for them.

One of the most important characteristics of parental language to children during this period (8 to 12 months) is that it generally attempts to control or modify only one aspect of behavior at a time (Chapman, Klee, & Miller, 1980). Many of the commands that infants are given by parents actually describe behaviors in which the children are already engaged (e.g., such as a parent saying "give me the spoon" as the infant hands it to him). Parents also frequently call for their child's attention (e.g., saying "look!" and "see") when they in fact already have it (see Snow & Ferguson, 1977). Only when adults are assured that the child understands *what* they are talking about *and* is attending to them, is the linguisitic component—the name of the object or action— added. Almost every label is accompanied by a gesture or physical manipulation of the object. Thus, to take in the information being given him fully, the child must not only listen to, but also watch the speaker. Recent research has verified subjective impressions of the overwhelming importance of visual attention in early communicative interaction. For example, it was found that when an infant was watching his mother as she began to speak and gesture, 70% of the time he successfully looked at the object she indicated (Chapman *et al.*, 1980). When the child was not watching the mother, the rate of correct response was only about 10%.

It is interesting to note that the usual inference drawn by adults about a child who imitates, attends to, and acts on objects in typical ways is that he understands the accompanying language (Patterson, Cosgrove, & O'Brien, 1980). However, for a child who does not attend to, imitate, or reproduce familiar actions, the inference is more often that he is not *interested* in the situation, rather than that he does not understand what is being said (Lord, Merrin, Vest, & Kelly, 1983). One question is what effect an infant's tendency to respond (or not to respond) in this way has on parental behavior. If, with normally developing children, obtaining overt visual attention is so often a prerequisite to providing initial verbal labels and comments, what happens with the child whose parents find it difficult to even catch his gaze? Since autism is rarely diagnosed during infancy, we are dependent on retrospective data in most cases to know what interactions are like between parents and babies who are later diagnosed with autism.

As part of a large twin study conducted for entirely different purposes, Kubicek (1980) identified some interesting records of mother–infant interactions with two 16-week-old fraternal twins, one of whom was later diagnosed as autistic. She found, in a very brief observation, that the child later considered to be autistic had far fewer different behaviors than his brother (e.g., his facial expression did not vary from "neutral") and showed no variation in the intensity of these behaviors (e.g., how rapidly or forcefully he moved his arms). He never, during this admittedly brief observation, looked directly at his mother. The interactions between the mother and the normally developing twin typically contained a sequence of behaviors beginning with eye contact, followed by a "game" initiated by the mother—a response of smiling, attending to, or withdrawing by the infant and then a response by the mother, depending on the child's preceding behavior. For the baby with autism, the sequence of behavior involved an approach without eye contact by the mother and then an arm or torso movement by the child that terminated the sequence. How the mother and child behaved did not depend on the behavior of each other.

If initial language comprehension involves the overlay of language onto already meaningful social behaviors of looking, acting, and imitating, the child with autism may make it very difficult for the parent to even "set up the stage." Some parents of children with autism, or with other pervasive developmental delays and social deficits, have described what "good" babies their children were as they lay in their cribs entertaining themselves for hours without demanding attention. On the other hand, infants later judged to have autism have sometimes been described as upset by human interaction and impossible to soothe. Neither of these patterns would provide a strong basis for building language comprehension.

## Single Words as Guides to Attention Behavior

As shown in Table 1, the first intrusion of language into the development of comprehension in exchanges between normally developing children and their parents involves the parent offering the child a specific word as a target or guide to determine the object to which the child should attend. Thus, the child can no longer use *only* social or situational cues to determine his or her response. Some abstract association between word and referent has been formed. Before this time, the adult could have said any word or made any sound and, as long as relevant intonation, gesture, and gazing occurred, the child would have responded appropriately. Thus, a distinction is made between responses that are determined by the context (but that do not require attention to even a single word) and this next stage of comprehension, in which words serve as *guides* to the targets for communicative interaction. For an autistic child, a *word* might even provide a welcome addition to what may be meaningless social demands. Yet, for a child who does not attend to the usual aspects of social information, the difficulties in even acquiring first words cannot be underestimated.

However, although language at the single word level begins to make its own contribution in terms of directing the child's attention, typical *responses* by the child at this time continue to be primarily imitative actions or socially determined behaviors. Again, these are the same behaviors that are usually seen as difficult for children with autism (e.g., giving clear evidence of notice, playing such social games as taking objects offered, using objects in a conventional way). For example, the behaviors typically expected from a child in response to language at this stage would often be highly social or conventionalized games involving facial expressions or gestures (e.g., "How big are you?"; "Where's Susie?" "There she is!"). Many autistic children have difficulty producing these behaviors even during much later stages of development. It is interesting that, at this stage, parents of normally developing children have been reported as noting a marked increase in how often their children comply with their requests (Chapman *et al.,* 1980). Relevant for autistic children is the question of the extent to which this compliance indicates beginning comprehension of particular words or the acquisition of more explicit ways of responding to language or, in all likelihood, both.

## Beyond One Word at a Time

In the next stage of language comprehension, the normally developing child begins to use more than one word at a time to determine his behavior, although physical and social contexts still determine how the child conceives of the relationship between words in a sentence. A child may respond differentially to various word combinations indicating possession and action–object and agent–action relationships. Word order is not yet expected to be a significant factor. Nonlinguistic strategies continue to be important. A child assumes that *she* is the actor of most sentences (e.g., that "Where is the cup?" means that *she* should find the cup). The effect of nonlinguistic knowledge is also seen in the child's response to utterances referring to instruments (e.g., spoons are to stir with, pencils to write with) on the basis of familiarity and appropriateness of the objects themselves, rather than the linguistic information.

An important cognitive shift proposed to occur at about this time is the ability to locate objects that are not immediately observable. For some children with autism, this step in the acquisition of comprehension may be less difficult than were the more socially dependent behaviors required in the preceding stages (Sigman & Ungerer, 1981). However, if children with autism do not attend to social cues and if they have few behaviors that would clearly indicate to others that they "comprehend" what has been said, even such children who can form representations of objects that are not present are still left without much language behavior. Interestingly, in a recent intervention study using incidental teaching to increase the spontaneous language of seven school-age children with autism (O'Neill & Lord, 1982), the semantic relation of *location* was found to be used less often than expected by the children, given the earliness with which it appears in the language of normally developing children (Brown, 1977). However, location was one of the semantic relations most easily taught. Even more important, it was the relation that most quickly and consistently generalized to new contexts, in contrast to such relations as *possession and state* (O'Neill & Lord, 1982). One could speculate that such rapid learning and generalization occurred because the autistic children had the cognitive skills to maintain an interest and memory of an object and its location (Shah & Frith, 1983). Since they did not have the prerequistite social skills to communicate their knowledge, the autistic children had not conveyed their information to others very often. When they had, no one may have recognized it.

Conventional uses of objects have been identified as important for language comprehension at all levels of development because they give the child a predictable way of responding to what other people say and do. In many cases, comprehension of an utterance will make little difference if it is not apparent to the speaker that he or she is being understood. For a child who has little interest in doing what others do with the same object, there is not a great deal of inherent joy in "stirring" a spoon around an empty bowl or "wearing a hat" (i.e., placing a knitted cover over his or her head). Further, one cannot help but be struck by how limited in behavior a child is who cannot easily imitate others' behaviors, but must depend on his or her own ideas of interesting actions. In this light, such behaviors as placing objects in lines, dropping things, and unusual visual inspection may be seen as not altogether unreasonable alternative ways to interact with objects. The child's responses to objects are primarily determined by properties of the objects themselves rather than by their social–behavioral possibilities.

## Transition from Social- and Strategy-Based Responses to Linguistic Comprehension

One theme that remained constant across the first three levels of comprehension has been a gradual decrease in dependence on the specific, immediate contexts of an utterance. Thus, during the first level of comprehension, the child's responses were described as primarily imitative or attentional and so totally dependent on the immediate actions of others. During the second level, the child was seen as beginning to move one step further toward abstraction by responding by "doing what he usually does" *in that situation.* By the third level, the child used objects in conventional ways that no longer had to be specific to the situation (e.g., he no longer had to be sitting in his highchair in the kitchen with his own cereal bowl in order to stir). In addition, he could search for objects that were not immediately visible (Ungerer & Sigman, 1981). In order to move beyond being dependent on information supplied completely by the present situation, the child must begin to extract some predictable rules that allow identification of important features of objects or events occurring in varied environments. For example, in order to comprehend the word "stir," the child needs to learn that it applies to a certain intention and a certain kind of movement through a real or imagined substance regardless of the kind of container holding the substance or the kind of expression on his mother's face during his action. In the comprehension of language, formal relationships between linguistic concepts occur on many levels, from rules that determine when to use specific words (such as what constitutes "stirring" versus "mixing" or "banging") to rules that describe multiple interrelated privileges of occurrence or syntax (such as which words go where in constructing a passive sentence). One could argue that linguistic rules are not really very different from rules governing the social behaviors discussed earlier. However, for the purposes of this chapter, linguistic rules will be treated separately because they are typically described more formally than social conventions, and because linguistic rules involve more independence from immediate context than the particular social behaviors (i.e., imitating, directing gaze) discussed here.

## LANGUAGE COMPREHENSION AND COGNITIVE DEVELOPMENT

The ability to form or use linguistic or similar rules has been described as a second major deficit for autistic children, in addition to difficulties in social cognition. Hermelin and O'Connor (1970) have suggested that the cognitive pathology associated with autism is the inability to reduce information through the appropriate extraction of such crucial features as rules and redundancies.

Linguistic deficits are seen as one aspect of a general cognitive disability in encoding and higher order processing. For a child faced with the task of mastering the arbitrary nature of English syntax, for example, the extraction of the critical rules for combining and ordering words into sentences is paramount. It is not known whether autistic children are able to come up with the rules, but not able to use them meaningfully and reliably, or whether they fail to recognize or create the necessary rules in the first place, but when taught these rules, are able to use them adequately.

## Comprehension and the Extraction of Meaningful Rules

One hypothesis about a deficit in rule-learning in autism is based on a series of experiments by Hermelin and O'Connor (1970) and Frith (1970). In a study of the recognition of sound patterns, Frith found that, when presented with random series of sounds, both autistic and normally developing children reproduced the sounds by creating their own patterns. However, when presented with predetermined patterns of sounds, the normally developing children produced sounds in the same pattern that they had heard, often in exaggerated form, whereas the autistic children continued to create their own patterns. Studies of verbal memory tasks with autistic children have also indicated that, although the recall of retarded, nonautistic children was dramatically improved when words were presented in sentences or were semantically clusterable, the performance of autistic children was much less affected by the expected relationships among words. In general, the autistic children used the meaning of (and rules for combining) words and sentences to remember them, but they did so to a lesser extent than nonautistic children of equivalent cognitive levels. It seems unlikely that these difficulties were due to memory problems *per se*, since in general, autistic children remember as many or more terms than nonautistic controls when meaning is not a major variable. Memory span may be more closely related to nonverbal intelligence than to autism and so, through that relationship, memory may affect the acquistion of language in both autistic and nonautistic retarded populations. However, simple deficits in verbal memory do not seem to be necessary or specific to autism.

In a recent experiment, we looked at comprehension strategies in autistic, normally developing, and sociable-retarded children's responses to a series of instructions (Lord & Allen, 1979). These instructions consisted of requests to move familiar objects from one location to another within two dollhouses. How the objects were specified (by their location or by an attribute such as size) and the number of different relations were varied across sentences. Pretesting had indicated that all of the children were able to identify receptively each of the individual words included in the sentences. The experiment was deliberately designed so that a child could use everyday comprehension strategies related to the physical properties of the objects (in addition to more formal linguistic structures) to determine the correct response. Thus, objects were always moved from the dollhouse on the right to the one on the left and objects that filled the same semantic role all had visible properties in common (e.g., objects of actions were all of a single color, under 1½ inches in diameter and "rollable"; recipients were all multicolored representations of animate beings with a head, eyes, and a mouth). In response to a sentence such as "roll the big pencil to the clown," children had to select the pencil from among three other rollable objects in a dollhouse and roll it to a clown, who was one of three other dolls sitting in different rooms in another dollhouse. In one condition, the alternatives for the object included a small pencil, something large, and something that was neither large nor a pencil. In the "redundant" condition, the only visible pencil was conspicuously larger than all other objects, so that a child who responded to either "big" or "pencil" would make the correct response.

The autistic children, who were matched on nonverbal IQ and chronological age to a group of sociable retarded children (mean chronological ages equal to 10.9 and 11.4 years, respectively; mean nonverbal mental ages equal to 4.8 years for both groups) were consistently the least competent group compared to the retarded children and to normal 2- and 3-year-olds. The autistic children made errors more frequently than did any other group on both the easier and the more difficult sentences. They used fewer rules for determining the relationships between the words and their behavior. However, the pattern of sentence difficulty across diagnostic groups was identical. When asked to imitate the same sentences, the autistic children did as well or better than any of the other children (Svornos, 1979).

The difficulty of various utterances was generally associated with the number of terms to which the children actually had to attend, rather than the number of terms expressed in the instruction. Thus, when presented in the redundant condition, a four-term utterance, such as "roll the big pencil to the clown," was only slightly more difficult than a straightforward three-term instruction (i.e., "roll the pencil to the clown") because both utterances required comprehension of only three terms. For the straighforward utterance, the terms were *roll, clown,* and *pencil.* For the redundant utterance, the child had to respond to *roll, clown,* and either *big* or *pencil,* since the only large object in sight was a pencil. The exception to this finding was not the children with autism, but rather the sociable retarded children whose performance deteriorated significantly when four terms were presented in a sentence, even if all the terms were not needed for a correct response. The autistic children had more difficulty than the sociable retarded children in using three or more rules, but were no more confused by redundant information than the normally developing children. Thus, the autistic children did not have difficulty using *known* or familiar rules when embedded in complex input, but were less able to extract the rules. They were less able to use both physical contexts and syntactic information (e.g., word order, prepositions) to determine the relations of words, even when they knew the meanings of the words in isolation.

This study did not give a clear answer to the question of whether rule knowledge or use is at fault, but it does suggest that one needs to be certain that autistic children have perceived rules or meanings before deciding that the problem lies in their failure to use them. One cannot necessarily conclude that autistic children are failing to use meanings unless it is certain these meanings are available for them to use.

## Linguistically Determined Behaviors in Comprehension

### Using Knowledge from Past Experience

The distinction between having and using meanings or rules is critical when considering the fourth level of comprehension (Table 1). At this level, linguistic comprehension is still seen as primarily occurring for individual words with contexts determining the overall sentence meaning. However, Chapman (1978) proposes that at this stage children begin to use their past experience not only to select among a limited number of responses, but also to identify probable events within specific contexts. In fact, in a study comparing autistic children to normally developing children, Tager-Flusberg (1981) found that the autistic children, in contrast to other children, failed to use knowledge about probable relationships in acting out sentences. Yet, how we define "probable event" has implications for our description of the autistic child's disability. An event that may be probable for researchers (e.g., "the mouse dropped her mittens") may seem no less improbable to an autistic child who does not understand the rules for temporary suspension of disbelief typically assumed by experimental psychologists, than its reverse (e.g., "the mittens dropped the mouse"). Years ago, Bever (1970) found that normally developing 3-year-olds used a probable event strategy in responding to sentences, but 2-year-olds were not sufficiently familiar with the events to use this information. One therefore has to ask what events 2-year-olds and autistic children consider to be probable and then ask if they use this knowledge to determine their responses to language. Otherwise, we cannot tell if the children are simply unfamiliar with the situations or are failing to use the knowledge that they do have.

Task-specific strategies also become important at this stage, not only in research, but also in everyday contexts. In a pilot study, we were surprised when a 3-year-old girl perfectly identified pictures associated with negatively biased passives (e.g., the cereal is eating the boy), an ability usually not seen in children at this age. However, at one point during the experiment, the child asked how she was supposed to answer when there were no eyes. In rendering pictures of improbable relationships between objects and people, the artist had personified each object that served as actor with a pair of Mickey Mouse eyes and hands. The child's strategy was simply to find the eyes and label the object with the eyes as the actor.

Huttenlocher (1974) has identified variables in physical relationships between objects (e.g., mobility) that affect reaction time and comprehension of sentences describing these objects. Other strategies, such as supplying missing information to questions not understood or answering all positively stressed questions with "yes," also begin to occur at this time. The role of active experience cannot be underestimated. The child who has not attended to a relationship between certain objects or people cannot be expected to have established normal expectations for language describing it.

## The Appearance of Linguistic Strategies

By age 4 years or so, children begin to use purely linguistic strategies to comprehend sentences. Word order and syntactic markers become more important. Several studies have indicated that, like identification of locations of objects, this skill may be an area of strength within communication for autistic children. Tager-Flusberg (1981) found that the high-functioning autistic children she studied were as able to use word order as were normally developing children. In fact, Bishop (1982) has suggested that language-handicapped children in general may overuse this strategy under circumstances in which normally developing children would be more flexible. The excessive reliance on a word order strategy could be due to the paucity of alternatives for language-handicapped children, if immediate contexts and probable events contain fewer meanings for them than for other children.

Certainly, comprehension of connected discourse remains a problem for many people with autism throughout their lifetime, but there are also autistic adolescents and adults whose comprehension of syntax and relational semantics is quite good (Cantwell, Baker, & Rutter, 1978). A delay in the *acquisition* of most aspects of comprehension, as compared to nonverbal skills, appears to be a necessary and relatively specific criterion for autism (at least as compared to general retardation or childhood emotional problems). However, difficulties with *all* areas of comprehension may not continue for some autistic children and adolescents. For high-functioning children, syntactic comprehension and receptive vocabulary may become quite adequate; there, the problem may be one of *learning* the rules, not of lacking the capacity or capability to understand them. Thus, if the child can overcome social and learning-related deficits to acquire basic units, he or she could be capable of employing them. Difficulties may still remain, however, with the child's use of social aspects of language and comprehension of more social or contextual cues.

Alternatively, there are many children and adolescents with autism whose language comprehension remains severely impaired throughout their lives. Wing and Gould (1979), using a cutoff on the Reynell Scale of 20 months, found almost 60% of a geographically defined, epidemiological sample of autistic children and adolescents aged 2 to 15 years so impaired. Some of these children may gradually overcome much of their social deficit, but their difficulties in extracting rules or in other, perhaps more language-specific areas, remain so strong that the basic aspects of language are never acquired. This pattern is frequently associated, although not always, with severe mental retardation in nonverbal areas as well (Wing, 1981). One important point is that in neither of these patterns of development would autism be considered a language-specific disorder. This is not to deny that language is a critical factor in both the diagnosis and treatment of autism. Deficits in language development have major implications for other aspects of development as well. However, according to the assumptions made in this chapter, difficulties in language are seen primarily as part of even more pervasive social and cognitive deficits for *most* children with autism. The specific deficits in speech production and the production of meaningful sounds seen in *some* children with autism may be an exception to this statement, but are not within the scope of this chapter.

In summary, prior to age 4 years, the comprehension of sentences is not *primarily* a task requiring language skills, except for the pairing of specific referents and words. In fact, prior to 18 months, it is suggested that what appears as language comprehension in a normally developing infant is a combination of social behaviors and cognitive strategies for acting on the world. The normally developing child begins to show "linguistic" knowledge after having produced numerous responses to language that, well-buttressed by social and physical contexts, look like comprehension. For the child who cannot or does not use these contexts, questions emerge: (a) How can one help him acquire the linguistic rules that typically arise out of these more general strategies? (b) Once the child has *some* linguistic rules, how can the probability be increased that these rules will be used in the social and intellectual situations in which they are needed?

## SUGGESTIONS FOR ASSESSMENT OF COMPREHENSION

Specific suggestions for the assessment of functional language comprehension of children with autism or other social deficits arise out of this information. Some of these suggestions are listed in Table 2. First, because the knowl-

Table 2.  Suggestions for Assessment of Functional Comprehension

1. Assess child's nonverbal cognitive level and adaptive functioning
2. Observe child's nonverbal, even noncommunicative, use of nonverbal concepts likely to be taught (e.g., size, color, open/closed, number). This can often be done during a standard assessment, but might include such methods as:
   (a) Hiding things (e.g., hiding a favorite toy under a series of objects of a certain color)
   (b) Matching
   (c) Sorting
   (d) Establishing contingencies (e.g., requiring a child to turn a knob to activate a toy, waiting for him to indicate he wants "more")
   (e) "Engineering" the environment (e.g., giving a child a wrapper or package with nothing in it or a container that will not open)
   (f) Observing child's behavior in familiar contexts with common objects (e.g., put a brush, cup, pencil in front of the child and see what the child does)
3. Assess child's receptive vocabulary and ability to use syntactic rules in comprehension using standardized measures (e.g., Sequenced Inventory of Communicative Development, Peabody Picture Vocabulary Test—Revised Version (PPVT—R), Northwestern Syntax Screening Test, Preschool Language Scale, Preschool Language Assessment Inventory, Reynell)
4. Observe the behavior of people familiar with the child when they are trying to communicate with him or her
5. Observe child's response to specific words and instructions that child is reported to comprehend. Experiment with the contexts in which this comprehension occurs (e.g., Do the objects referred to have to be present?)
6. Observe child's social and information-getting strategies for comprehension while the child is with several different people (see Table 1).
7. Observe child's *response* strategies (e.g., position preference, preference for size, preference for order) across several familiar situations (start from Table 1). Try to encourage the child to make overt errors. Such situations might include:
   (a) Teaching tasks
   (b) Familiar instructions from parents
   (c) Behavior with other children
8. Experiment with factors that may enhance or decrease comprehension:
   (a) Focus of child's attention (e.g., is child looking at speaker?)
   (b) Speed of speech
   (c) Intonation
   (d) Length of utterance
   (e) Total amount of speech
   (f) Gesture

edge and behaviors required for comprehension go beyond "language" behavior, there is a need for an estimate of the child's nonverbal cognitive skills. A child with very good nonverbal cognitive skills is in a much better position to use world knowledge or to use more complex linguistic strategies than is a child whose cognitive skills are very limited. This assessment should include use of formal nonverbal intelligence tests (e.g., Merrill–Palmer, PEP, Leiter, Raven's; see Gould, 1976 for review) and adaptive measures (e.g., Handicaps, Behaviour, Skills Schedule; Vineland Social Maturity Scale; see

Wing & Gould, 1978). In addition, a child's familiarity with specific concepts that one might wish to teach (e.g., visible or functional characteristics of objects or events such as *open/closed, empty/full, to eat/to wear*) must be informally observed. Does the child know which actions are associated with common objects? Can he or she show you somehow that he or she associates certain objects and/or actions together (e.g., by sorting or matching them, by using them in context)? These observations appear as individual items on a number of formal language (e.g., Sequenced Inventory of Communicative Development, Preschool Language Assessment Inventory; see Stremel-Campbell, 1977) and psychological tests (see Schopler & Reichler, 1979, for examples). The need for additional assessment is often less than the need to re-group, for the purpose of specifically considering comprehension, observations, and results already obtained. In a sense, these observations are the first step of an intervention strategy similar to that described by Watson (Chapter 9) in this volume. The goal is to find evidence of meanings that the child already possesses to which language can be overlaid.

Language-specific aspects of comprehension that need to be assessed would include receptive vocabulary; comprehension of specific syntactic rules, such as word order and grammatical morphemes; and the number of different elements per utterance that the child can differentially process. These measures would typically form part of a standard speech and language assessment. It is important to remember that this assessment is really evaluating two different sets of skills: What the child's *functional level* of response to "normal" language input is, in which case numerous, redundant cues are usually provided (Does a child get his shoes when asked "Where are your boots?" as he heads out the door barefoot?). The other ability involves using linguistic information in isolation, such as selecting the picture that depicts "the deer sleep" versus "the deer sleeps."

One technique, drawn from research by Chapman *et al.* (1980), provides an interface between the two questions above. Situations are created in which the child has to select between some minimal contrasts, but in which these contrasts are created to resemble those typically seen in everyday contexts. An example at the single word level, for a child who is reported by his parents to "understand" the word "daddy," would be to place the child in a room with his father, mother, an unfamiliar man, and several familiar toys all in his sight. One could then ask "Where's daddy?" and observe how the child behaves. As a further contrast, one could also ask, in the same tone of voice, "Where's ball?" and "Where's Miss Piggy?" to see if the child continues to look at his father. Alternatives to "Where?" such as "Go get..." or just "Daddy?" could be used, depending on the routines familiar to the child. Testing somewhat higher level comprehension, one could also have the child watch the father leave his line of sight and then repeat the sequence. Such an informal assessment, starting from skills identified by parents, may be especially useful for children for whom standardized tests of language are generally too advanced.

Along with cognitive level of language-specific skills, the assessment of comprehension also requires deliberate observation of the child's strategies for determining what response is made when the child knows a response is expected. Since many of these strategies would be associated with specific contexts, the strategies need to be observed in the contexts in which they occur as much as possible. A child may show a definite position preference in discrete-trial tasks at school, but follow a different strategy at home (e.g., when in doubt, at home he may go to the bathroom; at school he may stare at finger movements or say "No!"). Common task-specific strategies of which to be conscious would be position preferences (i.e., for left or right), response to order of presentation (e.g., choosing the first one) or acting on preferences (e.g., choosing the object or action liked best), familiarity, size, or ease of handling. These strategies can be quite useful to children; as part of their communicative repertoire, they are not necessarily something to eliminate. However, it becomes confusing if we mislabel them or fail to identify the more idiosyncratic cues to which the child may be responding (e.g., we do not want to conclude that a child understands "apple" when he or she is actually attending to the erased pencil marks on the picture of "apple" used every day in speech therapy).

More general strategies, such as looking where someone else is looking or doing whatever one did last time, are also important to observe systematically. These strategies could be divided, somewhat arbitrarily, into social strategies that involve observation or interaction with other people and experience-based strategies that involve the use of knowledge about probable events. Since it is not feasible to observe all possible strategies in all situations, one may first want to identify situations in which the child's comprehension of language is seen as an important goal by parents or teachers. Then, observations can be made of possibly helpful or confusing strategies used by the child in these circumstances (see Watson, Chapter 9, for a discussion of this decision sequence as used in an intervention program to increase communicative language production). One could also contrast situations in which the child is described as being particularly confused and those in which he or she seems most comfortable.

Another strategy to help the teacher or clinician understand what, and, more important, *how* the child understands language is to create an environment that encourages the child to produce as many *overt* errors in comprehension as possible (as opposed to failing to respond at all). This can be done in the context of highly structured situations, such as using forced choice procedures, or it can be done in a more relaxed fashion in everyday environments, if children think they should act when a statement is directed to them. The more mistakes that children make that can be observed, the more certain one can be about the strategies they are using. Using a forced choice, discrete-trial procedure, one could begin by providing the child with a great deal of redundant information (e.g., instructions to throw the big ball, when there is a choice of a ball and a cup, and the examiner holds out her hands in order to catch the ball) and then gradually eliminating the gesture and the helpful association between "ball" and "throw" and increasing the number of objects from which to choose.

Watching how parents and teachers who are familiar with the child attempt to communicate can also provide insight as well. Asking the child's mother to repeat the same instruction in another context or to use different words or a different tone of voice, or without gestures, can be helpful. Observation of the child in familiar contexts is also of critical importance so that judgments about comprehension are made in situations when the child has the opportunity to relate what is heard to what is already known. Otherwise, it is difficult to tell if the child cannot respond because of lack of experience or lack of comprehension.

For older, higher functioning children with autism, one particular note of warning is needed. For some of these children, comprehension of linguistic aspects of sentences becomes quite good, especially in structured, familiar settings. However, these abilities can be quite variable in confusing, anxiety-provoking, overstimulating environments, such as in large groups of people, emotionally laden situations, or demanding academic activities. Being aware that this variation may occur is important so that a performance problem is not treated as lack of competence. A child needs to be observed both in maximally facilitative and in typical environments.

## TREATMENT STRATEGIES

The overriding principle for interventions aimed at increasing language comprehension of children with autism is to make language meaningful for the individual child. Thus, meanings must be valid for him or her at an individual level. Since autistic children are different from normally developing children and from each other, to meet this goal requires taking into account each child's nonverbal developmental levels, experience, social skills, motivation, and current language skills. Meaningful language is language that the child spontaneously associates with events or relationships in his or her world. The child should be able to identify the context in which the language occurs as an event that corresponds to or differs from what is anticipated and that provides new information or that supports or disputes his or her expectations.

Within this framework, the lexicon, or words to be taught, should first be selected for functionality and interest to the child (see Table 3). For the child with limited comprehension, words should describe objects and events with which the child is already familiar. Presenting a child who has very limited understanding of language with a new word (e.g., "lion") and a new concept (e.g., a picture of a lion in a zoo) is counterproductive, unless there is another goal besides comprehension (e.g., to facilitate social interaction in a particular context such as if the child were going to visit a zoo with his or her daycare group). The use of language to introduce new ideas becomes almost impossible to avoid when a child must acquire new abstract concepts, especially in school, but with younger children or those with comprehension skills less than that of normally developing 4-year-olds, new concepts can be presented in nonverbal as well as verbal ways, before specific responses to language can be expected.

At the same time as words are being provided to go along with concepts that are familiar in nonverbal ways, for young children with autism, it is equally important to provide new nonverbal experiences to which language will ultimately be added. Children cannot use the strategy "Do what you usually do in this situation," if the situation *or the expectation that they will do something in it* is entirely new to them. Using interactions between parents and normally developing young children as a model, the autistic child needs to be engaged in active experiences, onto which language is gradually imposed (e.g., as in the study where the mothers were observed telling their children to do what they were, in fact, already doing). Activities such as these have been discussed extensively elsewhere (Schopler, Lansing, & Waters, 1983), but it may be helpful to deliberately fit them into a comprehension-oriented intervention program, as well as to consider them as primarily play skills.

In addition, more general comprehension strategies, both for getting contextual information and for determining a reasonable response, can be taught. In addition to simple imitation with objects (which certainly has a long history of training), taking what is offered, following the direction of a gaze, and picking up the nearest object are also strategies (see Table 1) that can be taught.

Table 3.  Suggestions for Intervention to Improve Language Comprehension

1. Overriding principle: make language meaningful to *this* child
2. Assess child's nonverbal developmental level and familiarity with concepts, social skills, motivation and current language skills (receptive and expressive). Select a starting point
3. Choose lexicon for current functionality and potential generalization. Teach formally and informally
4. Provide nonverbal experiences related to target concepts accompanied by "verbal" narrative
5. Provide guided practice by placing child repeatedly in a similar contexts for comprehension. Allow him to develop his own strategies for comprehension
6. Explicitly teach general comprehension strategies
7. Explicitly teach behavioral responses to language
8. Modify input

Verbal or gestural or facial cues that bring about these behaviors can be systematically generalized. Although these are *not* language-specific strategies, they provide a way for the child to participate in communicative interactions (which may provide stronger motivation for others to include the children in these interactions) and they provide the child with both social and cognitive experiences to underlie later language acquisition.

Another approach is to put the child repeatedly in the same situation, in which he or she must comprehend the same language and, by preventing incorrect responses, encourage the child to come up with his or her own strategies for responding. This guided practice/errorless learning paradigm is used every day in many classrooms, but, again, may not be construed as comprehension training. It might be used, for example, in the context of having an older child choose appropriate clothes for the weather and to help in answering the question "What is the weather today?" or "What is it like outside?" The child might be discouraged from answering the question immediately (since it might already be known that he or she typically answers "What" questions by giving locations), but be encouraged to repeat "The weather" or "Like outside?" Any number of behaviors, such as looking at unshod feet and bare arms, looking out the window or turning on the news might be reinforced as a first step to help the child get the needed information from the environment. Once the child appears to have arrived at a behavioral strategy by which to get the needed information, various ways of communicating the information could be shaped, depending on the child's skills and interests. For example, having somehow established what the weather was, the child could be prompted to first state a type of weather (e.g., "raining") and then go get a raincoat, or if it seemed easier in the reverse order, to go get the raincoat and then either label the weather on the basis of the clothes needed (e.g., "raincoat") or by its most salient characteristic (e.g., "wet"). Sentence frames, such as "the forecast says" or "today it's [hot]," could also be taught, depending on what the child seems to use most easily and the situations in which it might be helpful for him or her to respond to inquiries about the weather.

A final strategy for intervention may have the quickest results. This strategy, that of modifying the input to the child, has the least direct long-term value because it places the responsibility for change on the speaker. On the other hand, if we believe that comprehension is learned through experience and communication, modified linguistic environments should allow for more learning than environments that require responses in isolation and that provide little contextual support. Although there are still not very good data to show which modifications make the greatest differences, assumptions are often made that shortening sentences, using gestures, limiting vocabulary, and exaggerating intonation and facial expressions increase understanding (Lord & Baker, 1977; Lord *et al.*, 1983). The social cues a child is given before language is presented also are as integral a part of comprehension-oriented modifications as are the lexicon and word order. Thus, requiring the child to do only one new thing at a time (including attend to the speaker, attend to the object, observe a way to use the object, listen to its name, or use the name) may result in much better "comprehension" and much more effective communication, as it did for mothers of normally developing infants, than multiple, simultaneous demands. Potential modifications of comprehension could come from two approaches. First, rather than waiting for the child to respond to a highly predictable instruction with a conventionalized response (e.g., "make the car go" by running a toy car on the ground), the mother can adjust her behavior and language to accompany the actions the child is already doing. For example, if the child is spinning the wheels on the toy car the mother can talk about *spinning* (and also spin the wheels herself). Another approach, more common and certainly not mutually exclusive, would be for the mother to first teach the child conventional uses of objects through demonstration and repeated example, and then introduce the appropriate language. An important distinction between this notion and typical "compliance training" would be that no requirement is made for the child to respond to language until he or she clearly possesses the behavior in question, although language could be used to accompany nonlinguistic teaching.

In addition, how much language is expected from the child seems very important. For some children, if they are made to feel that their role in the situation is *always* to say something, energy that could be devoted to listening may be spent looking for cues for what to say rather than trying to figure out what is meant. Alternatively, the child needs to have an active role in the interaction for the situation to have any meaning.

Thus, we have come full circle to the initial notion that comprehension is the understanding of relations between situations and sentences. This concept requires some introspection, on the part of those of us who work with or live with autistic children, concerning the kinds of situations with which we provide them. If what we are after is a response to be marked on a data sheet or compliance to our not-very-interesting instructions, what kind of situations are we giving children to which to tie their understanding of our sentences? In a paper about language and mental retardation, Ryan (1977) wrote about what she called the silence of stupidity. Her argument was that although professionals may try to teach linguistic structures to mentally retarded children, often we do not want to hear the content of what the children have to say, anyway, so that the teaching of language becomes an empty intellectual exercise.

One could make the same point for teaching comprehension skills. It is easy to lose sight of the fact that language comprehension is but a step toward more important roles of participating in social encounters and acquiring knowledge about the world. If we forget those goals and concentrate on the language itself, the social and cognitive environment we provide becomes highly restricted and "stupid." We fail to provide the necessary experiences during which everyday comprehension of language is acquired. Language is a social skill. We need to keep it so in the classroom, in the clinic, and at home for the autistic child. By working from hypotheses about the underlying deficits in autism, we can make a stab at designing interventions that improve functional communication. By modifying input by teaching specific social skills and rules about how the world operates, and by providing varied social and cognitive experiences, we can increase the ability of autistic children to process social meanings and to recognize the rules and redundancies in the world that help others feel that life is comprehensible. Looking at *how* normally developing children and autistic children attempt to understand language is as important as looking at *what* they comprehend. As soon as we think we understand comprehension as a simple process, we should know we are wrong.

# REFERENCES

American Psychiatric Association (1980). *Diagnostic and Statistical Manual of Mental Disorders* (3rd ed.). Washington, DC: American Psychiatric Association.

Bishop, D. (1982). Comprehension of spoken, written and signed sentences in childhood language disorders. *Journal of Child Psychology and Psychiatry, 23,* 1–20.

Bever, T. G. (1970). The cognitive basis for linguistic structures. In J. R. Hayes (Ed.), *Cognition and the development of language* (pp. 279–352). New York: Wiley.

Brown, R. (1977). Introduction. In C. E. Snow & C. A. Ferguson (Eds.), *Talking to children* (pp. 1–12). Cambridge, England: Cambridge University Press.

Cantwell, D., Baker, L., & Rutter, M. (1978). A comparative study of infantile autism and specific developmental receptive language disorder, IV. Analysis of syntax and language function. *Journal of Child Psychology and Psychiatry, 19,* 351–362.

Chapman, R. S. (1978). Comprehension strategies in children. IN J. F. Kavanagh & W. Strange (Eds.), *Speech and language in the laboratory, school and clinic* (pp. 308–327). Cambridge, MA: M.I.T. Press.

Chapman, R. S., Klee, T., & Miller, J. F. (1980, November). *Pragmatic comprehension skills: How mothers get some action.* Paper presented at the American Speech and Hearing Association, Detroit, MI.

Curtiss, S. (1981). Dissociations between language and cognition: Cases and implications. *Journal of Autism and Developmental Disorders, 11,* 15–31.

Frith, U. (1970). Studies in pattern detection in normal and autistic children: I. Immediate recall of auditory sequences. *Journal of Abnormal Psychology, 76,* 413–420.

Gould, J. (1976). Assessment: The role of the psychologist. In M. P. Everard (Ed.), *An approach to teaching autistic children* (pp. 31–52). Oxford: Pergamon Press.

Hermelin, B., & O'Connor, N. (1970). *Psychological experiments with autistic children.* New York: Pergamon Press.

Huttenlocher, J. (1974). The origins of language comprehension. In R. L. Solso (Ed.), *Theories in cognitive psychology* (pp. 331–368). Hillsdale, NJ: Lawrence Erlbaum Associates.

Kanner, L. (1943). Autistic disturbances of affective contact. *Nervous Child, 2,* 217–250.

Kubicek, L. F. (1980). Organization in two mother–infant interactions involving a normal infant and his fraternal twin who was later diagnosed as autistic. In T. M. Field, S. Goldberg, D. Stern, & A. M. Sostek (Eds.), *High risk infants in children: Adult and peer interactions* (pp. 99–112). New York: Academic Press.

Lord, C., & Allen, J. A. (1979, May). *Comprehension of simple sentences in autistic children*. Paper presented at the Midwest Psychological Association, Chicago, IL.

Lord, C., & Baker, A. (1977). Communicating with autistic children. *Journal of Pediatric Psychology, 2,* 181–186.

Lord, C., Merrin, D. J., Vest, L. O., & Kelly, K. M. (1983). Communicative behavior of adults with an autistic four-year-old boy and his nonhandicapped twin brother. *Journal of Autism and Developmental Disorders, 13,* 1–17.

Macnamara, J. (1972). Cognitive basis of language learning in infants. *Psychological Review, 79,* 1–13.

Miller, J. F., Chapman, R. S., Branston, M. B., & Reichle, J. (1980). Language comprehension in sensorimotor stages V and VI. *Journal of Speech and Hearing Research, 23,* 284–311.

O'Neill, P. J., & Lord, C. (1982). Functional and semantic characteristics of child-directed speech of autistic children. In D. Park (Ed.), *Proceedings from the International Meetings for the National Society for Autistic Children* (pp. 79–82). Washington, DC: National Society for Autistic Children.

Patterson, C. J., Cosgrove, J. M., & O'Brien, R. G. (1980). Nonverbal indicants of comprehension and noncomprehension in children. *Developmental Psychology, 16,* 38–48.

Rutter, M. (1978). Diagnosis and definition of childhood autism. *Journal of Autism and Developmental Disorders, 8,* 139–161.

Rutter, M. (1983). Cognitive deficits in the pathogenesis of autism. *Journal of Child Psychology and Psychiatry, 24,* 513–532.

Ryan, J. (1977). The silence of stupidity. In J. Morton & J. M. Marshall (Eds.), *Psycholinguistics: Developmental and pathological* (pp. 99–124). Ithaca, NY: Cornell University Press.

Schopler, E., & Reichler, R. (1979). *Psychoeducational profile*, Vol. 1: *Individualized assessment and treatment for autistic and developmentally delayed children.* Baltimore, MD: University Park Press.

Schopler, E., Lansing, M., & Waters, L. (1983). *Individualized assessment and treatment for autistic and developmentally delayed children,* Vol. 3: *Teaching activities for autistic children.* Baltimore, MD: University Park Press.

Sigman, M., & Ungerer, J. (1981). Sensorimotor skills and language comprehension in autistic children. *Journal of Abnormal Child Psychology, 9,* 149–166.

Shah, A., & Frith, U. (1983). An islet of ability in autistic children: A research note. *Journal of Child Psychology and Psychiatry, 24,* 613–620.

Snow, C., & Ferguson, C. (1977). *Talking to children.* New York: Cambridge University Press.

Stern, D. (1974). The goal and structure of mother–infant play. *Journal of American Academy of Child Psychiatry, 13,* 402–421.

Stremel-Campbell, K. (1977). Communication skills. In N. Haring (Ed.), *Developing effective IEP's* (pp. 58–71). Bethesda, MD: U. S. Department of Health, Education and Welfare.

Svornos, F. M. (1979). *Imitation and comprehension in autistic children.* Unpublished senior honors thesis, University of Minnesota, Minneapolis.

Tager-Flusberg, H. (1981). Sentence comprehension in autistic children. *Applied Psycholinguistics, 2,* 5–24.

Ungerer, J. A. & Sigman, M. (1981). Symbolic play and language comprehension in autistic children. *Journal of American Academy of Child Psychiatry, 20,* 318–337.

Wing, L. (1978). Social, behavioral and cognitive characteristics: An epidemiological approach. In

M. Rutter & E. Schopler (Eds.), *Autism: A reappraisal of concepts and treatment* (pp. 27–45). New York: Plenum Press.

Wing, L. (1981). Language, social and cognitive impairments in autism and severe mental retardation. *Journal of Autism and Developmental Disorders, 11,* 31–44.

Wing, L., & Gould, J. (1978). Systematic recording of behaviors and skills of retarded and psychotic children. *Journal of Autism and Childhood Schizophrenia, 8,* 79–97.

Wing, L., & Gould, J. (1979). Severe impairments of social interaction and associated abnormalities in children: Epidemiology and classification. *Journal of Autism and Developmental Disorders, 9,* 11–29.

# 13

# Logico-Affective States and Nonverbal Language

## B. HERMELIN and N. O'CONNOR

## INTRODUCTION

### The Dual Functions of Verbal Language

*Between the idea/And the reality/Between the motion/And the act/Falls the shadow.* These lines from T. S. Eliot's poem, "The Hollow Men," are presented as an introduction to this chapter because they raise in one's mind the question "What intervenes?" In what follows it will be argued that the shadow between motion and act is frequently "affect." Affect, it will be suggested, interacts with reason, producing a cognitive–emotional or logico-affective mental state or system. It will be argued that what gives autism its distinctive quality is a distortion in this logico-affective system, a disturbance that is particularly evident in language, whether spoken, written, or signed, partly because language serves both a cognitive and a communicative purpose. Language as a medium of communication, rather than as a vehicle for thought, involves not only cognitive, but also affective elements, although these are also often conveyed through nonverbal expressions. In this chapter, evidence will be presented that indicates not only abnormalities in the verbal, but also in the nonverbal language functions of autistic children.

It is not only in the syntactic or semantic properties of language, but particularly also in pragmatics, that is, in language in its interactive role between speaker and listener, that we find distortions of form and content in psycholog-

---

B. HERMELIN and N. O'CONNOR • Medical Research Council, Institute of Education, 2 Taviton Street, London, WC1 England.

ical maldevelopment (Baltaxe, 1977). However, for reasons that are probably accidentally as well as historically determined, the psychological study of language functions during abnormal development has, until recently, been concentrated on the effects that an inadequately developed verbal language system may have on the level and on the quality of cognitive processing. The main impetus for research in this area was, in recent times, provided by the work of Luria (1961) and his colleagues from the Soviet Union (Tikhomirova, 1956; Nepomnyashchaya, 1956) who derived their ideas primarily from the brilliant insights and observations of Vigotsky (1939). In a series of influential studies, these Soviet psychologists demonstrated that a dysfunction in what Pavlov (1927) had termed "the second signaling system," that is, verbal language, led to inadequate manipulation of mental concepts and general systems of classification and even to an inability to act consistently under implicit verbal self-instructions. Even in studies in which Luria (1959) made language serve an apparently communicative purpose, words were primarily regarded as reflecting cognitive processes. In the relevant experiment, he asked retarded children to describe the workings of a simple piece of machinery to another child, and found that, although the children could work the machine, they could not give an adequate verbal description of its working. But the reason for this failure was clearly that the children were unable to structure and formulate the situation to themselves, and the presence of a listener was incidental.

Work with autistic children has shown that they suffer from a cognitively based language disorder (Hermelin & O'Connor, 1970; Rutter, Bartak, & Newman, 1971; Rutter, 1978). However this disorder does not affect verbal development alone, but is also evident in other rule-governed behavior. The more complex and flexible such rules are, the less autistic children are able to generate or extract them (Hermelin & O'Connor, 1970). Frith (1970a,b) has shown that in such situations autistic children tend to impose their own repetitive and rigid rules, with the result that the behavioral repertoire becomes increasingly limited, stereotyped, and inappropriate.

Recently, there have been reports in the literature that focus on pragmatic deficits in the language of autistic children. Thus for instance, Baltaxe (1977) concluded that they showed impairments that could not be attributed to phonological, syntactical, or semantic aspects of language. Deficits were additionally evident in the assignment of speaker–listener roles, in the rules of conduct governing normal dialogue, and in the relative stress given to foreground and background information.

## Nonverbal Language

It should not be forgotten that in spite of the primary importance that the emergence of a verbal language system has had for human development, there is another, phylogenetically older communication system, which mankind shares with other organisms and which, in humans, finds expression mainly through gestures, facial expressions, and nonverbal vocalizations.

Neurological and neurochemical mechanisms that might add affective tone to the function of thought or memory are speculative at present. The influence of the right cortical hemisphere, and also the "coloring" or affective tone given to encoded thought by the nucleus basalis, the hippocampus, and the amygdala must be considered. Additionally, such neurotransmitters as nroephinephrine and vasopressin or the variety of emotional triggers that are currently called encephalins undoubtedly contribute to the quality and perhaps the direction of thought.

Ploog (1979) points out that, in contrast to monkeys and apes, nonverbal vocalizations in humans can be elicited from stimulation of cortical areas. In other nonhuman primates, the ponto-mesencephalic as well as the limbic systems play a role in phonetics and, according to Ploog (1979), the human infant's babbling is also governed from subcortical areas.

Human facial expressions and gestures have also been linked phylogenetically with those of other primate species (Chevalier-Skolnikov, 1973; Andrew, 1972). Spontaneous facial expressions and automatic movements are controlled by motor systems in the precentral gyrus, and in humans, damage to these structures causes deficits in these behaviors (Geschwind, 1975). It seems thus highly probable that some nonverbal signaling for communicative purposes has developed long before verbal language and is based on phylogenetically old neural structures.

Verbal language functions as an internalized system that serves cognition, as well as being made explicit for communicative purposes. Nonverbal language, however, consists of cognitively controlled, learned, propositional and symbolic communication, as well as biologically determined, spontaneous, universal, and unlearned signs that signal emotional states.

## Thoughts and Feelings

Of course, propositions and feelings can be expressed and understood through both verbal and nonverbal means. However, it could be argued that in the course of evolution, if not a total distinction, yet a differentiation in emphasis and efficiency, has occurred between the two communication systems. Words seem to be particularly well suited to express observations, experience, ideas, and intentions, more than emotions. This remains true in spite of the achievement of poets and other gifted individuals who are skilled in verbal descriptions of the precise quality of pain, joy, love, fear, or hate. But such people are rather rare exceptions. For most of us, the verbal expressions of emotional states remain sadly inadequate and by themselves often convey little of our true feelings to the listener. Simply using the words "I am very sad today," without the accompanying and corresponding intonation, posture, and facial expression, will elicit scant sympathetic response from the listener. This is quite a different state of affairs from a response to statements such as "the aim of socialism is equality" or "I just saw three cats outside." The listener can adequately respond to the verbal information conveyed in these statements with agreement, disagreement, boredom, or astonishment. However, coming amongst our friends and showing in gestures, expressions, and vocalizations an emotional state of mirth or distress needs no accompanying words to evoke concern and empathy. Thus, it is argued here that although the verbal system is particularly well equipped for those communications that refer to knowledge of ideas, facts, or events, the nonverbal system can most efficiently communicate emotions and feeling states. What should be stressed is that this distinction does not refer to a dichotomy of function, but rather to a bias in emphasis inherent in the development of verbal and nonverbal language systems.

## Cortical Organization

For both verbal and nonverbal language, a distinction between propositional and expressive functions seems to be partly reflected in cortical organization. Thus, there is general agreement now that most verbal language functions are, in right-handed people, localized in the left cerebral hemisphere. However, in dichotic listening tasks, the left ear (i.e., the right hemisphere) better identifies the emotional tone of speech (Haggard & Parkinson, 1971; Safer & Leventhal, 1977). Heilman, Scholes, and Watson (1975) and Tucker, Roth, Arneson, and Buckinham (1977) found that patients with damage in the right hemisphere had impairments in the recognition and expression of affective, but not propositional speech. Correspondingly, people with left hemisphere lesions have not only difficulty with speech, but also with such nonverbal propositional communication systems as Morse code and sign language (Kimura, 1979). Many studies have also demonstrated impairment of propositional, nonemotional nonverbal communication, such as in the use of enactive gestures and pantomime, which occur in patients with left hemisphere damage (Goodglass & Kaplan, 1963; Pickett, 1974; Varney, 1978; Duffi & Duffi, 1981). In contrast, Buck and Duffi (1980) found that spontaneous, emotional nonverbal expressiveness showed no association with left hemisphere impairment. Buck's (1982) conclusion is that propositional communication that uses symbols, whether verbal or nonverbal, is associated with left hemisphere processing, whereas expressive verbal and nonverbal language that communicates feeling states is associated with processing in the right cerebral hemisphere.

## The Origin of Nonverbal Language

Verbal and nonverbal communication systems share features that are self-generated, universal, and spontaneously emerging, as well as aspects that are developed through learning, environmental modeling, and cognitive progress. The evidence for these contributing factors is well attested in verbal language and will not be reviewed here. In regard to nonverbal communication, Darwin (1872, p. 187) stated that "one must regard certain behaviours which we regard as expressive of certain states of the soul, as the direct result of the constitution of the nervous system, and thus being from the beginning independent of the will and to a large extent also of habit." Many subsequent studies, notably the work of Ekman (1972, 1977), show that many expressive signs are universal and therefore not culturally determined. Ekman's published photographs of members of a remote New Guinea tribe will allow unmistakable identification of the feelings their faces and postures communicate. Ekman reports no difficulty in the recognition of not only feelings of disgust or surprise, but also in the identification of such relatively complex and sophisticated emotions as embarrassment, friendly interest, and shy uncertainty.

While thus acknowledging the biologically determined spontaneous emergence of signs that communicate feeling states, one must yet remember that just as Chinese children learn to speak Chinese rather than Hungarian, and just as the kind of English used by the Public School boy is markedly different from that of a working-class child, so the extensive gesturing and voluble laughing and crying of the southern Italian can be perceived to differ from the subtle raising of eyebrows and telling silences that are the Anglo-Saxon expression of profound emotions. Such differences, as much as those found in the actual nature of gestures to convey propositions in different cultures, are environmentally determined and due to learning.

Nevertheless, that much of nonverbal language behavior is unlearned can be demonstrated through studies of those who are deprived from birth of an opportunity to perceive and learn from other people's situation-appropriate expressions. A number of investigators (Goodenough, 1932; Thompson, 1941; Freedman, 1964; Charlesworth, 1970; Eibl-Eibesfeldt, 1973) have all observed that, in most respects, the facial expressions of congenitally blind and sighted children are essentially the same. Similar conclusions have been reached for the congenitally deaf, who show the same early intonation, vocalization, and babbling patterns as the hearing, although that similarity disappears with the onset of language proper (Goodenough, 1932; Eibl-Eibesfeldt, 1973). Research shows that development brings an increase in the capacity for controlling and simulating emotional expressions in face, gesture, and voice, which allows the individual to conform to social expectations and permits some voluntary control of spontaneous expression. Cognitive development also leads to an increased use of propositional, nonverbal language (Riseborough, 1982).

## Outline of Areas of Experimentation

In what follows, we will be concerned with nonverbal language and with experimental investigations of the autistic child's perception of faces, both for the purpose of person identification and emotional expression. The autistic child's ability to produce facial expressions voluntarily is also tested. Further studies investigate the ability of autistic children to use and recognize symbolic gestures in relation to objects and people. They also test the spontaneous use of these and other gestures by such children. Finally, a series of experiments reports on the autistic child's ability to integrate different sources and modalities of stimulation concerned with cognitive or emotional indicators in people and things. All the studies have been carried out while the investigators were associated with the authors. As most of this work is as yet unpublished, we gratefully acknowledge our colleagues' permission to quote their data. In particular, we would like to give credit to Dr. Peter Hobson, Research Fellow of the Medical Research Council, Institute of Psychiatry. During joint discussions, he has contributed a number of the ideas put forward here and has also developed them further in his own investigations. However, prior to our review of this recent research, we will also reconsider some of our earlier experiments (Hermelin & O'Connor, 1970), which were not so much concerned with nonverbal communication as with the autistic child's orientation toward, attention to, and interest in other people as compared with nonpersonal objects.

We will suggest a possible mechanism that may give rise to the peculiar quality of the autistic child's attempts to orientate and communicate. We will propose that these qualities are a function of abnormal cognitive, as well as emotional processes, which interact with each other. This interaction, we will argue, results in the production of a psychological system we have termed a logico-affective state. We suggest that it may be the particular characteristics of this state that give the communications of autistic children their particular quality.

## FREQUENCY OF ORIENTING RESPONSES

The autistic child is frequently described as not paying any attention to the presence of other people. Kanner (1943) noted that not only did autistic children fail to establish affective contacts with other people, they also treated them as objects, and did not seem to register a fundamental difference between people and things. In order to test how far such clinical observations could be verified experimentally, we compared the attention and behavioral orientation of autistic and retarded children (Hermelin & O'Connor, 1963). Orientations toward things as well as toward a person were recorded. Twelve children were tested in each group covering a wide range of age between 5 and 16 years, with a mean age of 9 years. All children functioned on a severely retarded cognitive level. Each child was introduced into a room in which an adult was present. The adult at first remained silent and passive, then initiated physical contact by stroking the child's hair, taking his hand, or cuddling him and finally attempted a verbal interchange and tried to obtain compliance to simple verbal commands. These conditions were compared with others in which pictures or recorded music or toys were presented to the subject. The frequency and duration of orientation responses by the child to each of these conditions was noted and recorded. Orientations were defined as turning toward, looking at, or approaching the stimulus, remaining in close proximity to and establishing physical contact with, or responding to, such contact or speech.

An analysis of the data demonstrated that both groups of children showed the same amount of orientation to pictures and music. The subnormal controls handled the toys significantly more often and for longer periods than did the autistic children. When the stimulus was a person, significantly more responses were obtained from the retarded than from the autistic children, particularly when the measures included a period of verbal interchange. However, a further analysis of the data showed that when the person sat passively, only one child from each group failed to make at least one approach to her. Ten autistic children retreated at times from the adult, compared with only five of the controls. Such retreating behavior occurred most frequently in the period during which the experimenter spoke to the child. But it must also be noted that although in this study the autistic children oriented toward a person less frequently than did the controls, nevertheless in both groups children made many more responses to the person than to any of the other stimuli. For both autistic and retarded children, this increase in responsiveness to an adult from that to other nonpersonal stimuli was highly significant.

## Distance and Mobility

In a further experiment (O'Connor & Hermelin, 1963), we measured the relative distance autistic and retarded children kept from various stimuli. We also recorded how often a child vacillated between approach and retreat. The aspects we selected as simulating characteristics of human contact were warmth and potential protection, represented by a blanket, and activity, represented by a rocking platform, which simulated comforting rocking movements. A human voice and a life-sized doll represented auditory and visual aspects of persons. In a further condition a person was seated in the room. The subject's position, in any part of the room, and mobility were continually monitored.

The autistic children stayed further away from the blanket, the rocking platform, and the voice; however, both groups of children kept equal distance from the life-sized doll and from the person. Both groups approached most closely to the person. When the autistic children spent time close to a stimulus, including a person, they did this for shorter durations than did the retarded children. As in the previous study, their behavior toward all stimuli alternated frequently and repeatedly between approach and retreat.

That such qualitative differences between groups cannot be primarily due to cognitive factors is indicated by the difference found between the autistic and the retarded children on many of the measures used here, although the two groups were matched for intelligence level. Similarly, the dual characteristic of the autistic children's attentions to people, that is, orienting toward persons more than toward nonpersonal things, yet making such orientation responses significantly more rarely and briefly than the intelligence-matched controls, also cannot be explained by either cognitive or emotional impairments alone. Instead, we suggest that the particular quality of this attentional process is due to an interaction of cognitive with emotional abnormalities and deficits, which produces a logico-affective state typical of the autistic syndrome.

Next we examine how the autistic child perceives and interprets interpersonal nonverbal signals, and we relate these to expressive as well as receptive capacities. We will also examine how such signals from different sources and modalities are integrated and understood.


## EXPERIMENTS WITH FACES

### The "Eyes" Have It

The role of facial expressions in nonverbal communication has been outlined in the introduction to this chapter. Many investigators have concluded that neonates exhibit little particular preferential fixation on faces when compared with other complex stimuli (Herschenson, 1964; Fantz, 1963; Koopman & Ames, 1968). The findings point instead to a visual preference of newborns for a certain intermediate level of complexity in a stimulus, with very simple or very complex visual displays being looked at less often. In the infant's face perception, the eyes seem to elicit most smiling and fixating responses (Gibson, 1969; Wolff, 1963 Greenman, 1963; Haith, Bergman, and Moore (1977) reported that infants between 5 and 11 weeks spend most of their time, when looking at the face, in fixating the eyes, and this eye fixation tends to increase when the baby is spoken to. Even then there is no reorientation toward the mouth. Caron, Caron, Caldwell, and Weiss (1973) found that the eyes are the most salient feature for 4-month-olds and that babies are more sensitive to distorting their position in a schematic face than they are to the spatial distortion of other features.

"Gaze avoidance" or lack of eye-to-eye contact has been a frequently reported characteristic of autistic children (Hutt & Ounsted, 1966). However, Churchill and Bryson (1972) failed to find support for active gaze avoidance and we had previously found no differential visual fixations by autistic children on a face with open eyes when compared with one with closed eyes (O'Connor & Hermelin, 1967). More recent studies (Langdell, 1978, 1981) presented children with photographs of the faces of classmates in which only certain features were visible while others were masked. Comparing the relative effectiveness of the masks, the results showed that there was a tendency for normal and retarded children to recognize photographed faces of their classmates by their upper facial features better than by the lower. In contrast the gaze of the younger autistic children was concentrated on the lower half of faces during their visual inspection for recognition, although older autistic children tended to give about equal attention to the upper and lower halves of faces. This change in emphasis may reflect a cognitive development in the autistic children. Findings by Field (1982) that neonates concentrate their gaze on the mouth of faces expressing emotion, will be discussed presently. The points we would like to stress here are that autistic children were as efficient as others in identifying partially masked faces, but that the hierarchical structure of the salience of features was qualitatively different for them than for other children.

Autistic children might have been efficient in using the lower facial features for identification because they tend to concentrate in general on the lower part of visual displays. Thus in the next study, they were asked to sort pictures of houses into two groups. The houses had flat or pointed roofs, straight or arched doors, and two storys of windows, either round or square. Children were free to select any one of these features for sorting, and were simply asked to put houses that "went together" or "looked similar" into one of two groups. Nine autistic and nine age- and IQ-matched retarded children were tested. All nine retarded and eight autistic children sorted according to the shape of the roofs or the upper windows. There was thus no tendency for dominant salience of the lower part of these displays. One other study was carried out in this series. In this, five congenitally deaf children were first presented with the masked faces task. A comparison with scores obtained from the previous study showed that these children, like the autistic, were significantly better in recognizing faces in which only the mouth was was visible than were normal or retarded children. It was thus thought possible that, like the deaf, autistic children might attempt to obtain speech cues by watching lip movements. Such a hypothesis seemed plausible because of the autistic children's specific difficulty in attending to and processing information via the auditory channel (Hermelin & O'Connor, 1970). Consequently, the autistic children were compared with the retarded for their ability to identify the names of their classmates, when these names were "mouthed" silently by the experimenter. Autistic and retarded children were equally good at this, obtaining, respectively,

73% and 79% correct identifications. This finding is in line with that of Dodd (1977), who found that for normal children, lip movements and speech sounds contributed equally to speech perception. There was, however, no evidence that the autistic children relied more on lip reading than did the retarded controls, and it seems therefore unlikely that the salience of the mouth area in the perception of faces could be accounted for in this way.

## Salience of Features for Facial Expression

It has already been mentioned that the discrimination of different facial expressions seems to be present soon after birth (Field, 1982) and that many expressions, particularly those signaling emotions, seem to be universal (Ekman, 1972). There is little evidence regarding the ability of autistic children to identify emotions in the facial expressions of others. In the present series of studies (Langdell, 1981), the children were given photographs of different faces and were asked to sort them according to the emotions expressed. Though the performance of the 10-year-old autistic children was worse than that of any of the other groups, they too performed significantly above chance level. Then the faces were partially masked, so that only the lower or only the upper portion of the face remained exposed. No deterioration in comparison with the complete faces was found when the mouth area remained visible, and this was again true for all groups. However, the ability to sort according to emotion dropped significantly when the autistic children could only see the upper half of the face. In contrast, retarded children could use the eyes effectively for the identification of emotional expression. Also, the autistic children were not affected by inversion of the upper facial features. For the retarded, however, inversion of the eyes led to a significant decrease of correct responses from 72% in the right orientation to 48% with the inverted eyes, a chance score. This last result confirms those obtained from infants, that distortion in the position of the eyes has a considerable effect (Caron et al., 1973).

These results thus indicate that the retarded children performed significantly better than the autistic when sad eyes had to be distinguished from glad eyes, and that they were also more affected by distorted eye positions. However, all children found it easier to identify the expression from the mouth of a face with a sad or happy expression than from the eyes. Thus, it seems that not only for infants, but also for older normal children and for those who are retarded or autistic, the mouth provided most information regarding the sad or happy expression of a face. On the one hand, infants are reported to concentrate their gaze on the eyes (Haith et al., 1977), as did older normal and retarded children in the present study when they had to identify not an emotional expression, but rather a particular person. One might conclude from this that information about an individual's identity is most clearly obtained from looking at his eyes. On the other hand, feelings might be conveyed best by the mouth. It is of interest that the autistic children could thus identify expressions, relying mainly on the mouth area, as well as could others. However, although salience shifted to the eyes for the normal and retarded children for the identification of individuals, the autistic children did not make this shift, but persisted in relying mainly or equally on the lower facial features. It must, of course, be stressed that such reliance on different facial features represented a differential emphasis only, and all children used both the eyes and the mouth to identify both people and feelings. Nevertheless, different strategies for identifying people and emotions seemed to be employed by autistic children compared with controls.

## Producing Controlled Facial Expressions

The last series of experiments in this section on faces is concerned with the ability of autistic children to produce or mime facial expressions themselves (Langdell, 1981). Adults have learned to control their facial expression of emotions (Ekman & Friesen, 1975). With children, Saarni (1982) found that 6-year-olds could conceal their feelings and Shennun and Bugenthal (1982) report that 6- to 12-year-olds could assume neutral or pleased expressions when they in fact disliked something. Younger children exaggerated such play acting more than older ones, and 6- as well as 12-year-olds were less able in acting dislike or indifference when in fact they felt pleased. De Paulo and Jordan (1982) reported that girls between 5 and 12 years became increasingly better in masking facial expressions of their true feelings, although gestures were less effectively inhibited. The reverse trend was found in boys.

In an early study, Dumas (1932) asked congenitally blind 12-year-olds to act afraid, sad, angry, and happy. Although the blind children were absolutely normal in their spontaneous expressive behavior, they were not easily able to produce these expressions at will. Similar results were obtained by Charlesworth (1970). However, Fulcher (1942) reported that when asked to produce facial expressions there were marked similarities between sighted and congenitally blind children. Blind children showed the same range of feelings in their faces as the sighted in a study by Fraiberg (1968). Only a few studies report on spontaneous facial impression in abnormal development. Sorce and Emde (1982) found that the faces of children with Down's syndrome expressed feelings less intensely than did those of normal children. In contrast, Ricks and Wing (1976) observed that autistic children show signs of pleasure, distress, fear, and anger only in their extreme forms. In the present experiments (Langdell, 1981), autistic children were asked either to produce or to imitate a happy or sad facial expression.

In the first study, the children were asked simply to look happy or sad. Photographs of these attempts were taken and were given to three independent judges for rating on a 7-point scale for appropriateness. Agreement between judges was high and resulted in a mean score of 2.8 for the autistic and 6.0 for the retarded children in attempts to look happy. Both groups were relatively poor in assuming sad expressions, with a mean rating of 3.0 for the autistic and 3.5 for the retarded children. There were, however, qualitative differences between the groups. Although the retarded children frequently received low ratings because they failed to register any emotion in their faces, the autistic children produced inappropriate grimaces and at times even expressed the opposite emotion to that required. Indeed, some of these children's faces were misclassified by the raters, something that never happened with the facial expressions produced by the retarded.

In a second experiment, the children were asked to imitate the sad or happy expression modeled by an adult. In one condition, the child sat opposite the model, and in another, both were facing a mirror. The most interesting result in this study was that though children from both groups achieved only moderate success when opposite the model, the retarded children improved markedly when they received feedback from the mirror, but the autistic children did not.

## Contact and Information

One could perhaps hypothesize that in ordinary circumstances normal children might seek frequent eye contact with others because there is no reciprocal contact with the mouth of a nonspeaking person, and therefore the mouth need not be looked at often. As the mouth does not observe one, but the eyes do, normal and retarded children may look at people's eyes to ensure that those people look at and make contact with them. The autistic child may not be primarily interested in this, but may base his distribution of attention on an information analysis, for which, these studies show, the mouth is the main source of information. But there was, in fact, a tendency for the retarded children to be less able than the other groups in identifying people by looking only at the lower facial features; they tended to be more able than the rest to use the eyes. The reverse trend was found in the autistic groups. One could thus assume that retarded children are primarily interested in establishing contact, whereas autistic children attempt to obtain information.

In this series of studies, different groups of children had been matched for age and for their level of cognitive ability. Nevertheless, differences in face perception emerged, indicating the use of qualitatively different strategies by autistic children when seeking information from faces. Such strategy differences may be attributable to different "cognitive styles," which in turn may be influenced not only by cognitive, but also by noncognitive factors. These factors may include those responsible for much social and affective behavior, and they may interact with cognitive ability to produce the specific and characteristic approaches of autistic children when they try to obtain information from other people's faces.

## THE PRODUCTION AND COMPREHENSION OF GESTURES

### Gestural Development and Classification

Gestures are expressed through movement of either the whole or part of the body, usually the arms and hands. Although facial expressions primarily communicate emotions, gestures can, in addition, express intentions or commands and can also be used to enact through mime the characteristics and use of objects. They are also used to underline and emphasize verbal language by a speaker or express the reactions of a listener. Barton (1979) has developed a system to classify gestures into five categories. The first refers to "deictic" that is, indicating and pointing gestures, which develop early, and are probably an extension of the infant's reaching behavior. Second, "instrumental gestures" are those that are intended to regulate the behavior of others, such as requests to "come here" or "stop." The third category are "expressive gestures," which communicate feelings, such as placing an arm around a person to show affection or clenching a fist in anger. The turning away of the head in rejection or disgust, which can be observed in the young infant, also belongs to this category, as do clapping hands or jumping for joy. "Enactive gestures" are performed to represent the use of objects and can be frequently observed at the age of 5 or 6 according to Riseborough (1983). Finally, "depictive" gestures represent properties and aspects of objects and events, such as the opening and closing of the thumb and index fingers to represent the opening and closing of a bird's beak, or the use of the hands and fingers to illustrate the size of an object. Piaget (1952) thinks that such gestures emerge at the same time as verbal language. Barton's (1979) terms are the ones used here.

The gestural system is supposed to have been developed prior to verbal language (Hewes, 1973). Apes have a large and natural repertoire of gestural communication (Argyle, 1975) and nonhuman primates use this to manipulate their social environment from soon after birth. In contrast, the human infant is comparatively immobile for the first few months of life, although some gestures, such as head turning, occur very early, and pointing as well as stretching out the arms as a request to be picked up are observed at 4 months (Bates, Benigni, Bretherton, Camaioni, & Volterra, 1979). Pointing at this stage usually expresses the desire to obtain an object, but later it also serves to direct an adult's attention to an object or event (Lobato, Barrera, & Feldman, 1981; Clark, 1978). The infant will also respond by placing an object into an upturned hand.

Instrumental gestures such as signing "go away" or "stop" are first noticed at around 2 years (Carver, 1975) and are well established at age 4 (Michael & Willis, 1968). Expressive gestures toward other children signaling affection or aggression are fully established at age 4 (Lewis, 1978), although gestural responses of affection in response to cuddling or movements to express frustration appear much earlier.

## Gesturing in Abnormal Children

The use and comprehension of gestures by children who do not follow a normal developmental course has not been investigated frequently. Curcio and Piserchia (1978) replicated with autistic children the study by Overton and Jackson (1977). Most of these children used body parts to represent objects, whether the gestures were self-directed or not. Snyder (1978) and Greenwald and Leonard (1979) reported that the appearance of pointing was delayed in mentally retarded children. Volkmar and Cohen (1982) found that verbal requests for nonverbal responses were more effective in eliciting gestures from autistic children than were nonverbal requests. Whereas Kirk and Kirk (1971) and Evans (1977) found that children with Down's syndrome were better at demonstrating the use of objects than verbally describing them, Tubbs (1966) obtained results that showed this not to be the case for autistic children. Bartak, Rutter, and Cox (1975) investigated communicative ability in 7- to 8-year-old autistic and aphasic children of near normal intelligence. They included the use of mime by the experimenter appropriate for one of several objects placed before the child. For example, the experimenter mimed throwing the ball and catching it, and the child had to select the appropriate object or had himself to enact its function and use. The results showed that the autistic children were less able to comprehend and execute gestures, than were the aphasic subjects. In the series of experiments that follow, comprehension and production of gestures in relation to objects and people will be investigated, and the spontaneously produced gestural repertoire of autistic children will also be described.

## Enactive Gestures

In this study, Attwood (1984) tested the ability of autistic children to select a pictured object appropriate to a mime performed by the experimenter.*

The autistic children were significantly less successful than either the normal or the retarded in pointing to the appropriate pictured object. Thus these results confirmed those obtained by Bartak, *et al.* (1975). When the errors were analyzed it appeared that although the autistic children had made more errors, a large proportion of these was due to a plausible object confusion. Apparently, there had been a tendency by the autistic chldren to base their analysis of the experimenter's gesture on only one feature of the mime, rather than on the whole gestural sequence.

Attwood (1984) also tested the competence of autistic children to enact the use of objects. The autistic children were able to produce correct enactive gestures, at least in a rudimentary and abridged form. But overall, they took significantly less time over miming how to use an object than did the other subjects, and their gestures were also significantly less elaborate. However with increasing IQ, elaboration also increased and these more intelligent autistic children also took more time to perform the gestures. Autistic children gave fewer indications than IQ-matched controls of pretending to "hold" the imagined object in their hands. With increased IQ, their performance in this respect still only equaled that of the less intelligent Down's syndrome children. This result may indicate that autistic chldren do not use "symbolic representations" of objects in their gestures, such as were observed by Overton and Jackson (1977) to occur with increasing frequency in the course of normal development.

## Instrumental Gestures

The same subjects were required to respond with actions of their own to gestures made by the experimenter. The autistic children with low IQs responded as adequately as those with higher IQs, and they could produce appropriate responses with the same competence as normal 5-year-olds.

Children who had responded correctly to the experimenter's gestures were also examined to see whether they could, when requested to do so, produce these gestures themselves. Autistic children with mental ages below 5 years

*Dr. Uta Frith, Cognitive Development Unit, Medical Research Council, London, was also associated with Attwood's studies on gestures.

responded similarly to the 4-year-old normal children. However, when compared with normal children of 5 and 6 years, who were able to perform the gestures more adequately, no corresponding improvement in the autistic children of equivalent mental age was evident. In contrast, children with Down's syndrome performed much better than would have been expected on the basis of their low IQs, and Down's syndrome children with IQs at or below 40 did as well as those autistic children with IQs between 60 and 90. Within the autistic groups, the ability to perform these gestures correlated with their IQs. One might thus conclude that although the Down's syndrome children's ability for this type of gestural communication was relatively IQ independent, that of the autistic children was not.

## Spontaneous Production of Gestures

It is important to differentiate between an individual's behavior in controlled situations that make specific task demands and behavior that is spontaneous and self-initiated. The series of studies on gestures reported above (Attwood, 1984) demonstrated some differences in gestural competence of children with autism, which could, at least partially, be attributed to attentional, cognitive, and perceptual factors. However, this does not necessarily imply that the differences between autistic and other children that are observable in natural settings are fully explained by such factors. The capacity to understand and produce certain behaviors does not mean that such behaviors are indeed used spontaneously. As with verbal language, we have also to consider the pragmatics of nonverbal communication.

Attwood (1984) recorded the frequency of interpersonal interactions, and the occurrence of gesturing as part of such interactions, by autistic, retarded, and normal children in natural settings, that is, during meals and playtime.

The results showed that the Down's syndrome children made contact with others to a greater and the autistic children to a lesser extent than the normals. There were a mean number of 2.35 interactions between autistic chldren compared with a mean of 10.38 interactions between the Down's syndrome children. However, when interactions took place, all subjects used the same amount of gestures. What needs to be stressed is that the autistic children with higher IQs and mental ages interacted as rarely as autistic children functioning at a lower cognitive level, and also used gestures with the same frequency. It thus seems that neither their frequency of interaction with another person nor the use of gestures during such interactions can be regarded as dependent upon cognitive level of development.

The most interesting difference between the groups was in regard to the types of gestures used. Fifty percent of the gestures used by the Down's syndrome children were expressive and communicated emotions; 25% of the Down's syndrome children's gestures were instrumental and 25% deictic; and 26% of the normal children's gestures were expressive (26% instrumental and 48% deictic). Of the few gestures the autistic children produced, 66% were instrumental and 34% deictic. Thus, the autistic children produced the largest proportion of instrumental gestures, aimed to influence the behavior of other people, but not once was an expressive gesture produced by any autistic child.

Another interesting point is that on the occasions when instrumental gestures were used by autistic children, 72% of these indicated "go away" and the remaining 28% "be quiet" (finger on lips). Both these gestures indicate a wish to terminate the interaction. However, instrumental gestures used by the other children indicated requests to "come here" and "sit down," and a few waved "goodbye."

# THE INTEGRATION OF EMOTIONAL INDICATORS

## About Relationships

In the previous section, we discussed data suggesting that autistic children used gestures as frequently as others. However, their gestures did not include those that communicate feeling states. This, of course, does not imply that autistic children do not have feelings. Indeed, both clinical impression and the observations of Ricks and Wing (1976) indicate that autistic children's spontaneous facial expressions can register strong emotions. But feeling an emotion must be distinguished from feeling or expressing it in what would normally be regarded as appropriate circumstances and from being able to recognize and respond to emotions expressed by others. An example of a failure to do this is cited by Hobson (1985), who carried out the series of studies reported in this section. An autistic boy began to laugh on entering a room in which another child was crying. On being asked why he did so, he answered "because John is making a funny noise."

A specific impairment in expressing feelings for, and toward, others had originally been posited by Kanner (1943), who concluded that in autism there is an innate defect in the biological mechanisms that enable an individual to have affective contact with other people. Hobson's approach to this issue draws upon the views of the philosophers Wittgenstein (1953) and Hamlyn (1974). The argument is that expressions of feeling by another person lead directly and without requiring inferential judgments to an emotional response in the observer. It is this empathic emotional response that enables us to establish affective contact with others. Even 7-month-old infants seem able to appreciate the relationship between the facial and vocal expressions of a particular feeling (Walker, 1982). Normal 1-year-olds react emotionally and behaviorally to their mother's facial expression (Klinnert, Campos, Sorce, Emde, & Svejda, 1982). However, Hobson suggests that autistic children may lack the capacity to "recognize" emotional states in others and may fail to react accordingly. If this is so, such impairment may undermine the autistic child's knowledge about the kind of "things" that people are.

## People and Things

Usually there are a number of nonverbal behavioral indicators signaling emotions, and these include facial expressions, nonverbal vocalizations, posture, movement, and gestures. These signs normally correspond to each other as well as to the feeling state that is expressed, and the emotion is communicated through the total pattern formed by these signs. Hobson's (1985) main contribution lies in his suggestion that the normal child's knowledge of the nature of other people, including their feelings, arises from an experience of a specific quality of relatedness to other people. He proposes that the autistic child's inability to form biologically based affective contact with others may thus be due to a lack of appreciation of the indicators that communicate the integrated expressions of emotion. His studies also aim to test whether the abnormal feature of the autistic children's development is distinct from and relatively independent of the cognitive deficits that characterize the syndrome. Hobson's (1985) investigation is thus concerned with the autistic child's ability to relate different emotional indicators to each other and to their appropriate context.

Eleven autistic children took part in the experiment. They were aged between 10 and 19 years, with a mean age of 14. They were individually matched with a group of retarded children for age and for scores obtained on the Raven's Progressive Matrices Test of Cognitive Ability. There was also a group of normal children whose chronological ages were matched with the mental ages of the other subjects. Their ages ranged from 5 to 9 years, mean age 7 years 4 months. Each child was tested individually, and was presented with a short film sequence or sound recording. His task was to select which of the five picture cards placed in front of him was the appropriate one to go with each sequence.

In the main experimental condition, the pictures were of five schematically drawn faces, sad, happy, angry, fearful, or neutral in expression. To ensure that all children could correctly identify these schematic drawings, they were first taught to select which drawn face corresponded to a filmed moving face expressing each emotion. The child was then presented with a 10-second film or sound sequences on videotape. In one film, the experimenter appeared with a covered face, and expressed in posture and gesture each of the four emotions, one by one. In another, he was seen to be involved in events for which one of the depicted facial expressions would be an appropriate response. The sounds, again presented separately, were of a person laughing and humming happily or crying and sighing or expressing vocally (but nonverbally) fear or anger. While the films or soundtrack were being presented, the experimenter said to the child: "There is the person. Listen to [or look at] him. What face goes with *that* person?" When each film sequence came to an end, the child was given an artist's drawing of a faceless figure that depicted how the experimenter had appeared in the final moment of the videotape, and he was asked to choose the drawing of a face to go with the figure. In another condition, pictures of objects or animals were used, and these again had to be matched to noises, movements, or contexts. For instance, out of five drawings the child had to choose one of a bird when he heard chirping sounds, saw a blurred image of a bird hopping on the ground, or was shown a bird's nest. Thus in this experiment, the child's ability to integrate the meaning of different emotional signs in people was compared with his capacity to integrate aspects of nonpersonal stimuli.

It was found that for the "nonperson" condition, autistic children were as able as other children to select the appropriate drawing to represent an object whose corresponding movement, noise, or context had been presented. In fact, all subjects did very well on this task, responding correctly in over 90% of trials. This indicated that there was no particular difficulty for the autistic children to relate different stimulus aspects to each other.

When having to select a face with a particular expression to correspond with the emotion demonstrated through nonverbal vocalization, gesture, or context, the results were very different. The autistic children made significantly more errors than children from the other two groups. An autistic child who had been quite able to select the picture of a train when he saw a blurred image of its moving form, heard its noise, or was shown a railway station, was often incapable of selecting an unhappy face to accompany a corresponding gesture, vocalization, or context.

## Knowledge about People

The conclusions from Hobson's (1985) studies is that autistic children seem impaired in recognizing and integrating attributes that are characteristic of people and their emotions. However, they were not impaired in comparison with subjects of a similar level of cognitive development, when they were required to relate different characteristics of objects to each other. In attempting to interpret these findings, it is, of course, necessary to keep in mind the difficult methodological problem of stimulus equivalence. Human attributes, whether referring to emotions or other person characteristics, are probably more complex and varied than characteristics of nonhuman stimuli. Nevertheless, nonautistic children found it easy to match such human attributes with each other—it was only the autistic children who encountered difficulty in the tasks involving feelings expressed by people. Hobson (1985) emphasizes that a normal child's knowledge of other people arises from the child's experience of a special quality of "personal relatedness" with others, one that involves reciprocal feeling between individuals. Kanner (1943) had proposed that autistic children lack this innate ability to form biologically provided affective contact with others, and Hobson suggests that a consequence of this is that they acquire only a partial and distorted knowledge of persons. Whether or not one accepts this interpretation, Hobson's experiments clearly demonstrated a marked lack of competence in the autistic subject's attempts to recognize and integrate the different nonverbal signs that serve to communicate feelings and emotions.

## AN ATTEMPT AT AN INTERPRETATION

### A Logico-Affective Impairment

The debate about autism has centered on whether the syndrome can best be explained in psychological terms by assuming a failure of normal, biologically determined, affective "bonding," as was asserted by Kanner (1943). Alternatively, an explanation could be sought in a profound cognitive abnormality that might cause much of the deviant behavior of autistic children (Hermelin & O'Connor, 1970; O'Connor & Hermelin, 1978; Rutter, 1978, 1983). One way of resolving this conflict has been to assume two basic but independent impairments in autistic children, one responsible for the dysfunctions in the intellectual and linguistic and the other in the interpersonal–affective areas of behavior. However, apart from the inherent lack of elegance and aesthetic appeal of such a dual-deficit hypothesis, its factual support is not too convincing. One objection to it is that, when compared with IQ-matched controls, and in spite of a similar intellectual level, there are differences in the cognitive as well as the communicative processes of autistic children that distinguish them from other children at a similar stage of intellectual development (Hermelin & O'Connor, 1970; O'Connor & Hermelin, 1978). Also cases with Asperger (1944) syndrome show characteristic impairment in affective functioning and in interpersonal relations, although they operate at a normal or even high intellectual level. Perhaps as a consequence of the affective impairment, their cognitive and, in particular, their linguistic processing, retains many abnormal and peculiar characteristics despite a relatively high functional level. What we will propose here is that such observations, as well as the findings obtained in the studies we reviewed in this chapter, enable us to deduce, in the case of autism, the existence of a logico-affective dysfunction that gives the syndrome its particular quality. Before this argument is developed further, we will reconsider the pattern of results that seem to us to justify such a conclusion.

## Group Differences and Similarities in Attentional Processes

The studies investigating the autistic children's competence in the area of nonverbal communication first concern attentional and orienting functions. Although these functions are based on subcortical arousal mechanisms located in the reticular activating system, they nevertheless come under cortical control. This cortically mediated direction of attention is rarely determined exclusively by cognition or feeling, but rather is usually the result of some combination of these two processes leading to an emotional–cognitive or logico-affective state, that determines interest, orientation, and attention. The two most notable findings referring to these functions in the series of experiments we reported here were that the autistic children's orientation toward, and attention to, people, were less frequent, more intermittent, and briefer than that of others of the same age and IQ. This conclusion is based on results using very different response measures, which all show these characteristics. These included the children's approach to both objects and people, their visual inspection of both things and human faces, and their observation and production of enactive gestures. The other aspect of these results, which should be stressed, is that within the range of stimuli used here, autistic, normal, and retarded children alike showed the same hierarchical structure of orienting behavior that allotted more attention to people than to other stimuli.

A related finding of overall reduced frequency of occurrence of certain behaviors, and yet a comparable structure within each behavioral category, was shown by the autistic children's spontaneous use of gestures during interpersonal interactions. Thus, the often-reported observation that gestures are rarely used by autistic children is not accounted for by their inability to produce them, but instead is a function of the reduced frequency of social interactions in which they engage.

## Intelligence-Dependent Functions

The results can be further described in terms of those that could be related to the level of cognitive functioning obtained by the autistic children, in contrast with other findings that could not be so accounted for. Thus in the face recognition studies, the autistic children were equal to normal and retarded mental age-matched controls in their ability to recognize photographs of partially masked faces and to put these into categories according to facial expression. Autistic children could also enact, through gestures, the use of objects, and there was no difference between them and children from the control groups in their communicative competence in regard to active responses to instrumental gestures. Finally, they were as able as other children to relate various characteristics of objects and animals to each other and to recognize the objects to which such attributes referred.

## Intelligence-Independent Strategies

Although there was a relatively wide range of nonverbal communicative indicators that autistic children could use in accordance with their intellectual level of development, there were also important qualitative differences between them and other children. It was found that although the autistic children were as able as the IQ-matched controls to relate different aspects of objects to each other, this was not the case when different indicators of a person's emotional state had to be interpreted. These autistic children were matched with the retarded for level of cognitive development and had been as competent as the controls when performing a similar integration task with different aspects of objects. It would thus be difficult to attribute their incapacity in respect to characteristics of people solely to an impaired cognitive ability in regard to the features common to both tasks, such as discrimination, salience, and the integration of different stimulus attributes. Also, as their performance level, although low, was nevertheless significantly above what would have been expected by chance alone, the autistic children obviously understood the task requirements. Consequently, their low level of competence in the comprehension of emotional indicators points to a specific difficulty with those nonverbal signals that communicate feeling states. This conclusion is supported by the absence of gestures expressing emotions in their spontaneous behavior.

It was also established that the ability of autistic children to initiate instrumental gestures was only equal to that of Down's syndrome children with much lower IQs. Similarly, although their gestural competence improved and their gestures became increasingly elaborate with increasing mental age, the performance level of even the most intelligent autistic chldren only matched that of the Down's syndrome children, who had much less intellectual ability.

One must conclude that such impairments in the autistic children's performance cannot be regarded as solely a consequence of their cognitive deficits. This raises the issue of intelligence-dependent versus at least partially intelligence-independent processing routes that could be taken in order to achieve the same level of competence in communicative skills. The present results indicate that Down's syndrome children seem to have a capacity for nonverbal communication that is above what would be expected from their IQs alone. In the identification of human faces, they had a tendency to achieve this by using mainly the upper facial features, particularly the eyes, and one might assume that this arose because normally they tended to concentrate on other people's eyes in order to establish reciprocal contact. They were also more able than autistic children matched for cognitive development to initiate instrumental gestures, and they used predominantly expressive gestures in spontaneous interactions with others. One might thus propose that the socially effective behavior commonly found in Down's syndrome children is due to an interaction of a low intellectual capacity with a high social competence for interpersonal, nonverbal communication. However, autistic children without such communicative competence have to depend much more on a purely cognitive route, and therefore only the more intelligent children can bring their increased intellectual ability to bear on the comprehension and production of nonverbal language. Thus, the balance of emphasis within the state of the logico-affective system clearly differentiates the two groups of children.

## Neuropsychological Implications

These group differences, strongly indicated by the results described above, are in accord with a variety of neuropsychological findings and speculations. Thus, for instance, Buck and Duffi (1980) found that right and left hemisphere damage, respectively, leads to differential effects on the expression of feelings or on the communication of facts and ideas. Differing levels of intellectual or interpersonal social deficits in autism could thus be consistent with a varying degree of right and left hemisphere damage in different combinations. The interpretation and integration of facial expressions, gestures, and vocalization needs some neuropsychological underpinning involving both cognitive and affective components, and although obviously oversimplified in its present form, a model involving a right and left hemisphere filtering of subcortical activation is likely to form some part of a more sophisticated interpretation. The neurological model developed by Damasio and Maurer (1978) is also of interest. It bears some relationship to Ploog's (1979) observations, but otherwise still lacks precision by implicating vast neurological structures.

## CONCLUSIONS

The set of experiments we have described here does not, of course, account for all aspects of the language performance or social behavior of autistic children. However, it is clear from such critical examples as the superior non-verbal communicative competence of the Down's syndrome children, in comparison with the autistic child of higher IQ, that the level of general cognitive functioning alone does not explain the group differences observed. However, as psychological experiments have by now extensively demonstrated, the cognitive ability of autistic children does correlate closely with their level of performance in many language-related operations. It seems justified to argue, as we have done here in regard to the communication and language skills of autistic children, that differentially impaired cognitive and affective processes interact and thus produce an abnormally functioning logico-affective state. The resulting anomalies in such a state are, in our view, largely responsible for much of the characteristically deviant behavior of autistic children, particularly in those areas that depend most on the interactions of cognitive with affective functions. These interacting functions play a particularly crucial role in the determination of attention and in the selection of salient stimulus features. They also determine competence in verbal as well as nonverbal language and the comprehension and expression of thought as well as of feeling.

## REFERENCES

Ahrens, R. (1954). Beitrag zur Entwicklung der Physignomie und des Mimikerkennens. *Zeitschrift für Emperimentelle und Angewandte Psychologie, 2,* 412–454.

Andrew, R. J. (1972). The information potentially available in mammalian displays. In R. Hinde (Ed.), *Nonverbal communications.* London: Cambridge University Press.

Argyle, M. (1975). *Bodily communication.* London: Methuen.

Attwood, A. (1984). *The gestures of autistic children.* Ph.D. thesis, London University, University College, London.

Asperger, H. (1944). Die autistischen Psychopathen im Kindesalter. *Archiv für Psychiatrie und Nervenkrankheiten, 117,* 76–136.

Baltaxe, C. A. M. (1977). Pragmatic deficits in the language of autistic adolescents. *Journal of Pediatric Psychology, 4,* 176–180.

Bartak, L., Rutter, M., & Cox, A. (1975). A comparative study of infantile autism and specific developmental receptive language disorder. I. The children. *British Journal of Psychology, 126,* 127–145.

Barton, S. (1979). Development of gesture. In N. Smith & M. Franklin (Eds.), *Symbolic function in childhood.* New York: Wiley.

Bates, E., Benigni, L., Bretherton, I., Camaioni, L., & Volterra, V. (1979). Cognition and communication from nine to thirteen months: Correlational findings. In E. Bates (Ed.), *The emergence of symbols: Cognition and communication in infancy.* New York: Academic Press.

Buck, R. (1982). Spontaneous and symbolic nonverbal behavior and the ontogeny of communication. In R. S. Feldman (Ed.), *Development of nonverbal behavior in children.* New York: Springer-Verlag.

Buck, R., & Duffi, R. (1980). Nonverbal communication of affect in brain-damaged patients. *Cortex, 16,* 351–362.

Caron, A. J., Caron, R. F., Caldwell, R. C., & Weiss, S. J. (1973). Infant perception of the structural properties of faces. *Developmental Psychology, 9,* 385–399.

Carver, J. (1975). *An observational study of a two-year-old child's nonverbal methods of communication.* Unpublished senior thesis, State University of New York at Purchase.

Charlesworth, W. R. (1970). *Surprise reactions in congenitally blind and sighted children. NIMH Progress Report.*

Chevalier-Skolnikov, S. (1973). Facial expression of emotion in nonhuman primates. In P. Ekman (Ed.), *Darwin and facial expression.* New York: Academic Press.

Churchill, D. W., & Bryson, C. Q. (1972). Looking and approach behaviour of psychotic and normal children as a function of adult attention and pre-occupation. *Comparative Psychology, 13,* 171-177.

Clark, R. A. (1978). The transition from action to gesture. In A. Lock (Ed.), *Action, gesture and symbol: The Emergence of language.* London: Academic Press.

Curcio, F., & Piserchia, E. (1978). Pantomimic representation in psychotic children. *Journal of Autism and Childhood Schizophrenia, 8,* 181-189.

Damasio, A. R., & Maurer, R. G. (1978). A neurological model for childhood autism. *Archives of Neurology, 35,* 777-786.

Darwin, C. (1872). *Expression of emotions in man and animals.* London: John Murray.

De Paulo, B. M., Jordan, A. (1982). Age change in deceiving and detecting deceit. In R. S. Feldman (Ed), *Development of non-verbal behavior in children.* New York: Springer-Verlag.

Dodd, B. (1977). The role of vision in the perception of speech. *Perception, 6,* 31-40.

Duffi, R. J., & Duffi, J. R. (1981). Three studies of deficits in pantomime expression and pantomime recognition in aphasia. *Journal of Speech and Hearing Research, 24,* 70-84.

Dumas, G. (1932). La mimique aveugles. *Bulletin de L'Académie de Medicine, 107,* 607-610.

Eibl-Eibesfeldt, I. (1973). The expressive behaviour of the deaf-and-blind born. In M. von Cranach & I. Vine (Eds.), *Social communication and movement.* London: Academic Press.

Ekman, P. (1972). Universal and cultural differences in facial expressions of emotion. In J. Cole (Ed.), *Nebraska Symposium on Motivation.* Lincoln, NE: University of Nebraska Press.

Ekman, P. (1977). Biological and cultural contributions to body and facial movements. In J. Blacking (Ed.), *Autropology of the body.* London: Academic Press.

Ekman, P., & Friesen, W. (1975). *Unmasking the face.* Englewood Cliffs, NJ: Prentice-Hall.

Evans, D. (1977). The development of language abilities in mongols: A correlational study. *Journal of Mental Deficiency Research, 21,* 103-117.

Fantz, R. L. (1963). Pattern vision in the newborn. *Science, 40,* 296-297.

Field, T. (1982). Individual differences in the expressivity of neonates and young infants. In R. S. Feldman (Ed.), *Development of nonverbal behavior in children.* New York: Springer-Verlag.

Fraiberg, S. (1968). Parallel and divergent patterns in blind and sighted infants. *Psychological Study of the Child, 23,* 264-300.

Freedman, D. G. (1964). Smiling in blind infants and the issue of innate versus acquired. *Journal of Child Psychology and psychiatry, 5,* 171-184.

Frith, U. (1970a). Studies in pattern perception in normal and autistic children: Reproduction and production of colour sequences. *Journal of Experimental Child Psychology, 10,* 120-132.

Frith, U. (1970b). Studies in pattern perception in normal and autistic children: Immediate recall of auditory sequences. *Journal of Subnormal Psychology, 76,* 413-424.

Fulcher, J. S. (1942). Voluntary facial expressions in blind and seeing children. *Archives Psychology, 38,* 1-49.

Geschwind, N. (1975). The apraxias: Neural mechanisms of disorders of learned movement. *American Scientist, 63,* 188-195.

Gibson, E. J. (1969). *Principles of perceptual learning and development.* New York: Appleton-Century-Crofts.

Goodenough, F. L. (1932). Expression of the emotions in a blind-deaf child. *Journal of Abnormal and Social Psychology, 27,* 328-333.

Goodglass, H. & Kaplan, E. (1963). Disturbances in gesture and pantomime in aphasia. *Brain, 86,* 703-720.

Greenman, G. W. (1963). Visual behavior in newborn infants. In A. Solnit & S. Provence (Eds.), *Modern perspectives in child development*. New York: International University Press.

Greenwald, C. A., & Leonard, L. B. (1979). Communicative and sensorimotor development of Down's syndrome children. *American Journal of Mental Deficiency, 84*, 296-303.

Haggard, M. P., & Parkinson, A. M. (1971). Stimulus and task factors as determinants of ear advantages. *Quarterly Journal of Experimental psychology, 23*, 168-177.

Haith, M. M., Bergman, T., & Moore, M. J. (1977). Eye contact and face scanning in early infancy. *Science, 198*, 853-855.

Hamlyn, D. W. (1974). Person-perception and our understanding of others. In T. Mischel (Ed.), *Understanding other persons*. Oxford: Basil Blackwell.

Harlow, H. F. (1962). The development of affectional patterns in infant monkeys. In B. M. Foss (Ed.), *Determinants of infant behaviour*. London: Methuen.

Heilman, K. M., Scholes, R., & Watson, R. T. (1975). Auditory affective agnosia. *Journal of Neurology, Neurosurgery and Psychiatry, 38*, 69-72.

Hermelin, B., & O'Connor, N. (1963). The response and self-generated behaviour of severely disturbed children and severely subnormal controls. *British Journal of Social and Clinical Psychology, 2*, 37-43.

Hermelin, B., & O'Connor, N. (1970). *Psychological experiments with autistic children*. London: Pergamon Press.

Herschenson, M. (1964). Visual discrimination in the human newborn. *Journal of Comparative Physiology and Psychology, 58*, 270-276.

Hobson, R. P. (1985). On people and things: The enigma of autism. *Journal of Child Psychology and Psychiatry and Allied Disciplines, 26.*

Hutt, C., & Ounsted, C. (1966). The biological significance of gaze diversion with particular reference to the syndrome of infantile autism. *Behavioural Sciences, 11*, 346-356.

Kanner, L. (1943). Autistic distrubances of affective contact. *Nervous Child, 2*, 217-250.

Kimura, D. (1979). Neuromotor mechanisms in the evolution of human communication. In H. D. Steklis, & M. J. Raleigh, (Eds.), *Neurobiology of social communication in primates*. New York: Academic Press.

Kirk, S. A., & Kirk, W. D. (1971). Psycholinguistic learning disabilities. In S. A. Kirk (Ed.), *Diagnosis and remediation*. Champaign, IL: University of Illinois Press.

Klinnert, M. P., Campos, J. J., Sorce, J. F., Emde, R. N., & Svejda, M. (1982). Emotions as behavior regulators; social referencing in infancy. In R. Plutchik & H. Kellerman (Eds.), *The Emotions, Vol 2: The emotions of early development*, New York: Academic Press.

Koopman, P., & Ames, E. (1968). Infants preferences for facial arrangements. A failure to replicate. *Child Development, 39*, 481-487.

Langdell, T. (1978). Recognition of faces: An approach to the study of autism. *Journal of Child Psychology and Psychiatry, 19*, 255-268.

Langdell, T. 1981. *Face perception: An approach to the study of autism*. Ph.D. thesis, London University College, London.

Lewis, D. (1978). *The secret language of your child. How children talk before they can speak*. London: Souvenir Press.

Lobato, D., Barrera, R., & Feldman, R. (1981). Sensorimotor functioning and pre-linguistic communication of severely and profoundly retarded individuals. *American Journal of Mental Deficiency, 85*, 489-496.

Luria, A. R. (1959). The directive function of speech in development and dissolution. *Word, 15*, 453-464.

Luria, A. R. (1961). The role of speech in the regulation of normal behaviour. London: Pergamon Press.

Michael, G., & Willis, F. (1968). Development of gestures as a function of social class, education and sex. *Psychological Record, 18*, 515-519.

Nepomnyashchaya, N.I. (1956). Some conditions of derangement of the regulating role of speech in oligophrenic children. In A. R. Luria, (Ed.), *Problems of higher nervous activity.* Moscow: Academy of Pedagogical Sciences.

O'Connor, N., & Hermelin, B. (1963). Measures of distance and mobility in psychotic children and severely subnormal controls. *British Journal of Social and Clinical Psychology, 3,* 29–33.

O'Connor, N., & Hermelin, B. (1967). The selective visual attention of psychotic children. *Journal of Child Psychology and Psychiatry, 8,* 167–179.

O'Connor, N., & Hermelin, B. (1978). *Seeing and hearing and space and time.* London: Academic Press.

Overton, W. F., & Jackson, J. P. (1977). The representation of imagined objects in action sequences: A developmental study. *Child Development, 44,* 303–319.

Pavlov, I. P. (1927). *Conditioned reflexes.* Oxford: Clarendon Press.

Piaget, J. (1952). *The origins of intelligence in children.* New York: International University Press.

Pickett, L. W. (1974). An assessment of gestural and pantomimic deficit in aphasix patients. *Acta Symbolica, 5,* 69–86.

Ploog, D. (1979). Phonotion, emotion, cognition with reference to the brain mechanisms involved. In *Brain and Mind, 6,* 79–98.

Ricks, D. M., & Wing, L. (1976). Language, communication and the use of symbols. In L. Wing (Ed.), *Early childhood autism.* Oxford: pergamon press.

Riseborough, M. G. (1982). Meaning in movement. An investigation into the inter-relationship of physiographic gestures and speech, in seven-year-olds. *British Journal of Psychology, 73,* 497–503.

Rutter, M. (1978). Language disorder and infantile autism. In M. Rutter & E. Schopler (Eds.), *Autism: A reappraisal of concepts and treatment* (pp. 85–104). New York: Plenum Press.

Rutter, M., Bartak, L., & Newman, S. (1971). Autism—a central disorder of cognition and language? In M. Rutter (Ed.), *Autism: Concepts, characteristics and treatment.* London: Churchill Livingstone.

Rutter, M. (1983). Cognitive deficits in the pathogenesis of autism. *Journal of Child Psychology and Psychiatry, 4,* 513–531.

Saarni, C. (1982). Social and affective functions of non-verbal behavior: Developmental concerns. In R. S. Feldman (Ed.), *Development in nonverbal behavior in children.* New York: Springer-Verlag.

Safer, M. A., & Leventhal, H. (1977). Ear differences in experimental psychology. *Human Perception and Performance, 3,* 75–82.

Shennun, W. A., & Bugenthal, D. B. (1982). The development of control over affective expression in nonverbal behavior. In R. S. Feldman (Ed.), *Development of nonverbal behavior in children.* New York: Springer-Verlag.

Sorce, J. F., & Emde. (1982). The meaning of infant emotional expressions: Regularities in caregiving responses in normal and Down's syndrome infants. *Journal of Child Psychiatry, 23,* 145–158.

Snyder, L. (1978). Communicative and cognitive abilities and disabilities in the sensorimotor period. *Merril-Palmer Quarterly, 24,* 161–180.

Thompson, J. (1941). Development of facial expression in blind and seeing children. *Archives of Psychology, 264,* 1–47.

Tikhomirova, O. K. (1956). Verbal regulation of movements in oligoprenic children under conflicts between verbal and direct signals. In A. R. Luria (Ed.), *Problems of higher nervous activity.* Moscow: Academy of Pedagogical Sciences.

Tubbs, V. K. (1966). Types of linguistic disability in psychotic children. *Journal of Mental Deficiency Research, 10,* 230–240.

Tucker, D. M., Roth, R. S., Arneson, B. A., & Buckinham, V. Right hemisphere activation during stress. *Neuropsychologia, 15,* 697–700.

Varney, N. R. (1978). Linguistic correlates of pantomime recognition in aphasic patients. *Journal of Neurology, Neurosurgery, and Psychiatry, 41,* 564–568.

Vigotsky, L. S. (1939). Thought and speech. *Psychiatry, 2,* 29–54.

Volkmar, F. R., & Cohen, D. J. (1982). A hierarchical analysis of pattern of noncompliance in autistic and behaviour distrubed children. *Journal of Autism and Developmental Disroders, 12,* 35–42.

Walker, A. S. (1982). Intermodel perception of expressive behaviour of human infants. *Journal of Experimental Child Psychology, 33,* 514–535.

Wittgenstein, L. (1953). Philosophical Investigations. Oxford: Basil Blackwell.

Wolff, P. H. (1963). Observations on the early development of smiling. In B. M. Foss (Ed.), *Determinants of infant behavior.* New York: Wiley.

# 14

# Social Aspects of Communication in Children with Autism

## J. GREGORY OLLEY

We sophisticated adults have long held communication to be one of the marks of our uniqueness. That belief has suffered a bit in recent years as researchers continue to document the complex communication skills of even very young infants (Kaye, 1981). Our self-esteem took a particularly strong blow when scientists at the University of Washington and Dartmouth College recently revealed a communication system among willows, maples, and poplars (Begley, 1983). In fact, it appears that communication is more prevalent than anyone had believed just a few years ago.

If we can accept the communication of babies and trees, it should come as no shock that autistic children communicate too. To be sure, problems in communication and related social deficits continue to be regarded as cardinal signs of autism (NSAC, 1978), but our understanding of communication and social abilities and disabilities in autism has grown considerably in recent years. One of the clear conclusions of this expanded knowledge is that communication and social behavior are closely intertwined.

Communication is, of course, by definition a social act. This relationship is so readily apparent that we might take it for granted or, at least, assume that it has been thoroughly researched. This assumption turns out to be only partially true. The overlap of communication and social skills in autism is widely recognized, and the social difficulties that characterize communication in people with autism have been well described in some classic books and papers (Baltaxe, 1977; Baltaxe & Simmons, 1975, 1977; Fay & Schuler, 1980; Ricks

J. GREGORY OLLEY • Division TEACCH, University of North Carolina, Chapel Hill, North Carolina 27514.

& Wing, 1981; Wing & Gould, 1979). In short, we are strong in describing the nature of the problem. Our knowledge of remediation in these areas is, however, far weaker, and the possibilities for applied research are still broad and exciting.

This chapter begins with consideration of what is meant by communication and how that concept is applied to the study of autism. It continues with a brief review of the social and communication problems that have been described in children and adults with autism. These problems have been explained in several ways and have led to some assumptions upon which treatment is usually based. Are these assumptions valid, and do they consider all of the social and communication possibilities for autistic people? The latter half of the chapter considers the application of current knowledge to improve assessment and treatment by making fuller use of social context and social consequences when teaching communication.

## WHAT IS COMMUNICATION?

The nature of communication and language has been well examined in the earlier chapters of this volume. These writers have made it clear that communication is broadly conceived, taking in the verbal and nonverbal, the explicit and the subtle. We are now accustomed to finding communication in such uncustomary places as the dress of adolescents, the backgrounds of Bergman movies, and the bumpers of cars. We accept the fact that virtually everything that we do has the potential to communicate (or miscommunicate). We adjust our attention to take in the social context of messages, and we frequently make readjustments to account for the rapidly changing social scene. If we begin to take for granted the importance of the social and cultural context of communication, a quick trip to another country or even to another region of our own country quickly forces us to re-examine the impact of every gesture and nuance.

Virtually all individuals with autism do communicate, but the subtleties of communication based on social factors present them with, perhaps, their greatest difficulty. In what sense, then, do people with autism communicate?

Current definitions of communication are quite broad (Fay & Schuler, 1980). The broadest definitions include any actions that influence the behavior of another, but Fay and Schuler (1980) and others have added the stipulation that such actions must be goal directed or have communicative intent in order to be considered communication. The intentions of another (particularly an autistic other) can be, at best, elusive to measure. But some measures of communicative intent have been suggested, and they are primarily social. Wilbur (1983) reviewed some of these measures, which include nonverbal areas such as gestures, nodding, and eye contact. Fay and Schuler (1980) suggested observing the extent to which communications are altered or *repaired* when they do not result in anticipated consequences. Such repairs would indicate intent to communicate.

The addition of intent to a definition of communication makes the act even more clearly social. Regardless of our choice of definition, however, communication can only exist in a social context, and the accuracy and effectiveness of communication often depend upon social factors.

## THE SOCIAL DEFICIT IN AUTISM

There has been wide agreement that both social and communication difficulties must be present in order to classify an individual as autistic. There has been less agreement on which problem is primary and on the relationship between the two characteristics. Perhaps Rutter's (1983) view on this matter best represents current viewpoints. He stated the position that "the cognitive deficit constitutes the core of autism; that it is an integral part of the disorder...; and that it is likely to underly [sic] many of the autistic features" (p. 516). The two most important autistic features to which Rutter referred are language and social difficulties. This basic cognitive deficit is one that affects not only speech production, but also the broader social aspects of language. Rutter's (1983) paper deftly describes the interplay among cognitive, language, and social skills and reviews the literature on these characteristics as they change over time and as they predict later abilities.

For instance, Rutter (1983) reviewed the literature on the stability of IQ over time and noted the extent to which IQ and early language abilities predict later social skills. The diversity in language and social skills among autistic people is great, but the two characteristics are linked in a complex way. Language is a prerequisite in our culture for good social skills, but even autistic adults who develop good speech by adolescence are likely to have serious social impairments (Rutter, 1983). More knowledge is needed about the ways people with autism can communicate.

The range of communication skills and problems in autism is, indeed, wide. At the lower functioning extreme, people with autism use tantrums, noises, or physical activity in some of the same ways that infants do. These actions may signal discomfort, desire for an object, an attempt to establish proximity with another, or an initiation of an interaction (McLean & Snyder-McLean, 1978). More complex forms of communication include standing in the area of a desired material, grabbing an adult's hand and taking the adult to a desired material or activity, using an object to represent another object or activity, and using pictures, typing, writing (without necessarily being able to speak), signs, symbols, or speech (Foster, 1983).

## Pragmatic Approach

Regardless of the form of communication, it has quite unusual qualities in autistic people. The earliest descriptions of autistic communication focused on deviant syntax. Recently, the emphasis has swung sharply toward a pragmatic (Bates, 1976) or functional approach (Bates & MacWhinney, 1982). From this viewpoint, communication must be examined in context and that context is, of course, social. Partly as a result of this emphasis on pragmatics, some excellent clinical descriptions of the social aspects of language and communication problems can now be found (Baltaxe, 1977; Baltaxe & Simmons, 1975, 1977; Bernard-Opitz, 1982; Fay & Schuler, 1980; Ricks & Wing, 1975).

These writers have helped us to understand communication problems in autism by stressing several points. First, there is not one autistic pattern of communication disorder. The problems are variable, as are most problems for this group. We must look at each communication characteristic or error in context to understand the social implications. One stimulus will not affect all autistic people in the same way. Also, two communicative acts that are topographically identical may have different communicative functions for different people, and their meaning may depend upon the social context. The context also helps to make it clear that very different words can have the same social purpose. The patron of a singles bar who asks "Do you come here often?" wants more than a literal answer to his question. The person with autism who asks "Do you eat French fries?" is probably less interested in culinary preferences and more interested in initiating social interaction. Individual and contextual differences abound.

This pragmatic emphasis helps us better to understand the relationship between language and the way that social deviance is identified and classified. When we consider social context, it is easy to find examples of behaviors that might be deviant in a small town, but not in a city, unacceptable in a grocery store, but acceptable at home, rude in the presence of strangers, but tolerated by friends or family. Further, a close examination of context shows how a child's speech or other modes of communication may be understood in some situations, but not in others and how one child's ability to rely on nonverbal or contextual signals may make him or her better understood.

## Social Communication Problems in Autism

Kanner's (1943) original description of autism included some very useful information about communication problems. He referred to flatness of affect, bizarre voice characteristics, speaking in a monotone, and the monotonous repetition of noises. Several later writers, such as Ricks and Wing (1975), described the "wooden and expressionless" quality of speech, the restricted range of conversation, the limited interests, and persistence on favorite subjects with no variation in topic or manner. These problems of expression, such as speaking too loudly or too softly, are usually accompanied by problems of comprehension, such as a very literal use and understanding of words and failure to recognize nonverbal signals by the listeners that might indicate lack of interest.

Many of these characteristics can, of course, be identified in nonautistic people with mental retardation or other handicaps, but Needleman, Ritvo, and Freeman (1980) found that a pattern of language problems existed for the autistic children they studied. This pattern included "imprecise articulation, echolalia, perseveration on question type, atypical intonation and atypical stress, and stereotypical expressions" (p. 395). The clinical picture that emerges from these studies of verbal autistic subjects is one of people who have learned some rigid rules about the use of words, but even when they are motivated to be social, they lack the social skills to speak or to listen effectively. Their cognitive rigidity, their preoccupation with idiosyncratic topics, and their difficulty in using more subtle aspects of communication, such as nonverbal messages, make them very odd and ineffective communicators.

The use of nonverbal means of communication combined with speech allows us to convey and receive very precise nuances and messages, but nonverbal cues also make communication quite complex and confusing for the person with autism. Argyle (1969, 1972) has conducted extensive research on nonverbal communication and the ways that these cues are used in certain cultures. They are features of communication that we often use without explicit planning, but they are essential to clear communication. We can, perhaps, understand the plight of the higher functioning person with autism better if we think of a foreign-language student who has mastered the spoken language, but not its social context. The student may communicate poorly, because he or she stands too close to the listener or brings up a topic at an inappropriate time.

The categories of nonverbal communication cited by Argyle (1969, 1972) are bodily contact, proximity, orientation, appearance, posture, head-nods, facial expression, gestures, and looking. These are the very aspects of communication that even the most highly verbal people with autism fail to master. Fay and Schuler (1980) pointed out that good social skills require combining and integrating verbal and nonverbal messages. The failure of integration results in the *robot speech* and many other social oddities commonly associated with autism. When these problems are treated by traditional speech therapy, the best one can hope for is clearer speech that is still socially inappropriate. More recent approaches to treatment emphasize remediating the social problems in communication.

## Cognitive Factors

The cognitive problems that Rutter (1983) referred to may also contribute to this failure to integrate the formal and the pragmatic aspects of communication. Baltaxe (1977) illustrated patterns of impairment in pragmatic competence. They included problems in assuming an appropriate speaker–hearer role due to inability to take the perspective of the partner, inability to speak in the proper mood (e.g., always formal), and rudeness.

Another cognitive skill that autistic people have difficulty with and leads to serious social and communication problems is *thematization*. This is a term that Duchan and Palermo (1982) defined as "the process of making sense of things" (p. 10). They described four types of problems in the use of themes. People with autism may have difficulty initiating an appropriate theme because of a lack of representational thinking and an accompanying inattentiveness to the social environment. Self-stimulatory behaviors may also interfere with initiating themes. Problems in terminating themes may be due to perseveration on one theme or a general "difficulty in shifting from one task to another" (p. 12).

A third type of problem noted by Duchan and Palermo (1982) is creating appropriate thematic contents. The contents may be too narrow with all attention focused on one aspect of a topic. In discrimination learning studies, this narrowness has been called stimulus overselectivity. Themes may also be too widely focused, with a failure to identify unique features, or so idiosyncratic that the person shares few interests with others. The result is difficulty attending to and responding to what our culture holds to be relevant.

Finally, there is a difficulty relating multiple themes—a problem that makes it hard to compare, contrast, or see incongruity among ideas. Another result of problems in dealing with two themes may be distractibility, which Duchan and Palermo (1982) presented as an inability to drop one theme in favor of a more relevant one.

These problems in four areas of using themes are congruent with Rutter's (1983) description of autism as a cognitive disorder of language, sequencing, and abstraction. These deficits are severe, even in higher functioning, verbal autistic adults who appear to be socially odd and have great difficulty in interpersonal relationships. In lower functioning people with autism, the cognitive difficulty in making sense of the world is so severe that spontaneous communication may be virtually absent.

## IMPLICATIONS OF CURRENT ASSUMPTIONS

Research and treatment in autism have grown remarkably in the last decade. Our better understanding of the nature of the social and communication handicaps of autism has brought with it some assumptions. Like all assumptions, these should be examined closely from time to time.

1. In everyday discourse among adults, we assume that speech is always social. Upon visiting an autistic child who repeats television commercials or engages in some other form of ritualized speech, one quickly learns that speech may or may not be social. Prizant's (1983) recent research has helped us to look carefully at the context of speech before assuming that it is or is not social. However, people with autism engage in many social and communicative acts that do not involve speech. The lesson is that we must not equate communication or sociability with speech. Opportunities for communication and social exchange must not be cut off or assumed to be useless for autistic people who do not speak.

2. The validity of some other assumptions is more difficult to establish. Autistic children often appear to be oblivious to social cues, or they may be distracted by them and respond inappropriately. Although few writers address this point directly, it is implicit in the work of Lovaas (1977, 1981) and others that social cues should be minimized in initial phases of communication training. The result of this assumption has been teaching in socially sterile surroundings. Although Lovaas has been an advocate of teaching in well-controlled settings, it should not be implied that he has ignored the importance of social factors. Over a decade ago, he argued for the importance of parents as teachers for their own children (Lovaas, Koegel, Simmons, & Long, 1973). Despite this suggestion, however, a recent review of behavioral research in autism revealed that most training studies have been carried out in socially sterile settings (Olley, 1981). Social variables are, apparently, still seen primarily as confounding or distracting stimuli. More research is needed in order to use the social setting effectively in teaching.

3. A related assumption states that the lack of social interest among autistic children makes social reinforcers ineffective. This assumption has led us to rely heavily on food or other tangible reinforcers when teaching.

4. We have further assumed that expression of appropriate social or affective messages will be too hard to learn; hence these skills have received little emphasis in our curricula. The other side of that assumption is to assume also that people with autism do not notice and do not respond to the social cues and messages given by others.

Of course, some evidence exists to support each of these assumptions, but the evidence is not so convincing nor so universally applicable that it should discourage us from further applied research on these topics. Research on the remediation of social withdrawal or inappropriate social/communication acts could have a large impact on the adult adjustment of many people with autism. In the following pages, a selected review of some existing research is intended to give direction to new efforts.

## REMEDIATING PROBLEMS IN SOCIAL SKILLS

Research on remediation must consider (a) social behaviors that must be changed in order to improve communication; (b) social factors as setting or contextual variables; and (c) the effectiveness of communication as it leads to social consequences. However, these are not mutually exclusive categories of research. For instance, asocial or antisocial behaviors (category a) are frequently approached as targets for behavior change, but the behavior problems may be a result of a failure to communicate (category c). For instance, some children who have communicative intent but ineffective communication skills have frequent temper tantrums. One common approach to this problem is to try to eliminate the temper tantrums directly. However, an assessment of the social context would indicate that the problem could be reduced by teaching the child to communicate a few simple messages. Current approaches sometimes fail to acknowledge this complex interplay of social factors.

Some promising lines of research do exist, however. Although our previous assumptions have limited the study of social variables, current research often recognizes that language is normally acquired in a social context. For instance, Bronfenbrenner's (1977, 1979) emphasis upon "ecological validity" in developmental psychology has been followed by some research and clinical approaches that take into consideration natural social factors in the assessment of children with autism, social factors as antecedents of communication, and social variables as consequences for communication.

### Social Factors in Assessment

Psychometric assessment of the language of children and adults has, in some ways, borrowed from experimental research. The testing environment, including social influences and consequences, has been kept consistent and somewhat barren in order that it not affect performance. The result is that we have good measures of language and other skills as they are exhibited in clinics, small testing rooms, and other atypical environments, but we know less about the way that autistic children communicate in real social settings where the motivation to communicate is likely to be much greater.

Some recently devised systems of assessment emphasize observation of social and communication skills in the natural environment. The TEACCH curricula in social and communication skills (see Watson, Chapter 9; Watson & Lord, 1982) begin with assessment in the natural social environment of school or other settings and use this information to build individualized activities.

Prizant and Duchan (1980) developed a method for assessing "interaction competence" that strongly emphasizes such social factors as the methods used to initiate interaction; responses to initiations by others; turn-taking; gaze, body posture, and orientation; proximity; and linguistic strategies. The method also is used to determine how natural social interactions break down. Assessment strategies such as these yield "ecologically valid" information that is quite useful in planning remediation.

## The Potential for Learning Social Skills

In a sense, all approaches to the treatment of autism have had, as a central goal, the remediation of problems in social skills or relating to others. Yet the research literature on social skills is surprisingly small (Rutter, 1983). Studies in which children with autism have been followed into adulthood confirm that social and communication problems are major obstacles to adult adjustment (Mesibov, 1983).

Despite these problems, researchers should not consider social skills an untreatable area. In fact, Mesibov's (1983) review indicated that adolescents and adults with autism often show an interest in social behavior that was absent in their younger years. Unfortunately, without early training, autistic adolescents lack the skills to make appropriate social exchanges, even if they are motivated to do so. The answer to this problem surely lies in research and treatment of social/communication problems in young children.

## Influence of Antecedent Social Factors

The prevailing stereotype of autistic people is that they do not respond or respond inappropriately to the natural social cues that are so easily recognized by others. This characteristic is essential to a diagnosis of autism (see for example, Schopler, Reichler, DeVellis, & Daly, 1980), and it is often apparent even in infancy. As important as this characteristic is, we should not conclude that the social environment has no effect on people with autism.

*Origins of social interaction.* Social interaction between mother and neonate is a well-established phenomenon (Brazelton, Koslowski, & Main, 1974; Kaye, 1981). When the infant has a developmental problem, this communication system is changed (Fraiberg, 1974, 1975). Adults, however, are adaptive in altering their responses to handicapped infants and young children who do not give the usual social cues or responses.

Several naturalistic observation studies have shown that people respond socially to infants and young children whose social repertoires are obviously limited. Further, adults and even children have been found to simplify their speech to young children, presumably in an effort to maintain social interaction

(Shatz & Gelman, 1973; Snow, 1972). Similar modifications in linguistic style have been observed when children interact with mentally retarded peers (Guralnick & Paul-Brown, 1977) and when mothers and teachers communicate with autistic children (Cantwell, Baker, & Rutter, 1977; Lord, Merrin, Vest, & Kelly, 1983). In parallel studies McHale, Olley, Marcus, and Simeonsson (1984) and Strain (1984) found that nonhandicapped children simplified their level of play when interacting with autistic children. These naturally occurring alterations in communication and social behaviors are antecedent events intended to facilitate interaction. They are also elements of successful programs in which peers are used to elicit social behavior and communication from autistic children (McHale, 1983).

Because language is normally acquired in a social context, the reciprocity that is part of games and other adult–child and child–child interactions must be considered as an approach to teaching. How important is this for autistic children who show little interest in others and who seem to learn poorly from modeling or observational learning?

One of the earliest forms of reciprocity is imitation. Dawson and Adams (1984) recently confirmed the earlier finding of DeMyer, Alpern, Barton, DeMyer, Churchill, Hingtgen, Bryson, Pontius, and Kimberlin (1972). Both studies indicated not only that autistic children as a group are poor imitators of motor acts, but also that those with the most impairment in imitation are the most socially withdrawn. Since imitation has an important early role in development of both communication and social skills, Dawson's current research includes efforts to facilitate imitation as an approach to improved social responsiveness.

These studies suggest that autistic and other handicapped children do respond to social stimuli. They also provide social cues to others, although these cues are often inappropriate. The result is that social messages are often misunderstood, but nonhandicapped children and adults can make adaptations that result in better communication.

*Research on social antecedents.* Examples of studies of the effects of specific social variables on language are few. Clark and Rutter (1981) compared the effects of four social conditions on several child behaviors, including *meaningless vocalizations* and *relevant speech*. One of the conditions, called *high interpersonal demands*, did result in higher measures of relevant speech, although none of the conditions affected meaningless vocalizations. The high interpersonal demand condition was an intrusive style in which the adult attempted to "impose himself upon the activity of the child," using "physical and verbal contact in attempts to get the child to respond" (p. 204).

Such a strongly intrusive style may be effective, but it is not common in classrooms for autistic children. McHale, Simeonsson, Marcus, and Olley (1980) observed the quantity and social quality of autistic children's communication in a naturally occurring classroom program. Two social conditions existed. In the first, two teachers and all six autistic children were present with the teachers taking a directive role. In the second condition, the two teachers were absent, and only the autistic children were present. The presence of the teachers resulted in communication that was more frequent and of higher social quality, although most of it was directed to the teachers rather than to other children. Both studies show that a teacher who takes a structured and direct teaching role is an effective social antecedent event that affects language.

The role of the adult is surely an important and complex social influence on language, and more research is needed both in carefully controlled settings such as that used by Clark and Rutter (1981) and in natural settings such as that observed by McHale et al. (1980). Duchan (1983) also stressed the importance of the adult as an antecedent in eliciting communication. Although she did not empirically compare or evaluate different adult roles, she developed an evaluation system to measure interaction between adults and autistic children and suggested ways in which adults might change their role in order to aid communication.

There is a growing interest in the effects of the social environment upon language and a strong move away from language training in distraction-free but socially barren environments (Halle, 1982; Prizant, 1982a,b). As remediation moves more toward natural settings, social variables may be seen as assets to training and generalization, rather than as nuisances, and studies of the effects of broad environmental variables on language will be more common (e.g., Bailey, Clifford, & Harms, 1982).

## Influence of Social Consequences

The primary consequence of language or communication is social. When we speak others respond. We receive help, understanding, information, cooperation, or perhaps a negative reply, but we affect the actions of others. Yet the world of autistic people works differently. When the social consequences of their language do not make sense to them, when they are not responsive to social consequences, one of the primary motives to communicate is missing or ineffective (Goetz, Schuler, & Sailor, 1981).

One obvious approach to language remediation is to make the social consequences of communication clearer and more meaningful to autistic people. This strategy is promising, but it has been limited by the long-standing view that most of the verbal and other behavior in autism is noncommunicative and unrelated to social antecedents and consequences. This view has led us to a strong reliance on tangible, rather than social reinforcers, and a tendency to try to eliminate any sound or gesture that is odd.

Early behavioral approaches to language instruction (e.g., McReynolds, 1970) demonstrated the use of food reinforcers in early stages of speech training and the later use of social reinforcement to maintain and generalize speech. Lovaas (1977) used this approach for many children, justifying the use of *artificial* reinforcers as essential for gaining control of *unmotivated* children. The use of artificial reinforcers was never seen as a long-term strategy. Lovaas (1977) emphasized the lack of spontaneity in speech developed in this way. He urged therapists to move to "natural daily-life reinforcers" (p. 32) as soon as possible, but offered cautions about the ineffectiveness of starting training with this approach.

The work of Lovaas (1977) and Lovaas *et al.* (1973) probably contributed strongly to the view that the odd behaviors of children with autism are noncommunicative and asocial, and such behaviors should be eliminated as a first step in training. Like many of the assumptions about autism, this one has some validity, but merits closer examination. For instance, echolalia, the tendency to repeat the words or phrases of others, is one characteristic of autism that has been widely regarded as noncommunicative, yet Prizant's (1983) analysis of echolalia revealed that it exists in many forms, some of which are social or communicative. For instance, Prizant identified seven functional categories of immediate echolalia, four of which are *interactive*. One such category is the *yes-answer*, which is similar to what Kanner (1943) called *affirmation by repetition*. In such cases, instead of saying yes, the autistic person expresses agreement by repeating the statement just given. For example, in response to the question "Do you want to go outside?" instead of saying "yes," the reply would be "Do you want to go outside?"

Much of echolalia is delayed; it is a repetition of something heard in the past. Prizant (1983); and Prizant and Rydell (1984) also identified fourteen functional categories of delayed echolalia and noted six others previously identified by Dyer and Hadden (1981). Of these twenty types of delayed echolalia, nine are *interactive* or social. An example is *protest*. This is an utterance, perhaps a standard phrase, used to protest the actions of another or to prohibit others' actions. Instead of saying "no" or "I don't want that," the child may use a standard (although irrelevant) expression to express protest. Such uses of echolalia are socially and semantically inappropriate, but they are social, and they may be quite consistent for the individual.

This realization that some forms of echolalia are, indeed, attempts to communicate should drastically change our approaches to language remediation and give us a new view toward earlier research. For instance, Lovaas, Varni, Koegel, and Lorsch (1977) manipulated social consequences and found that they had very little effect on rate of production of speech in children with delayed echolalia. However, if Lovaas and his colleagues had taken into consideration Prizant's (1983) types of echolalia, they might have found social consequences to be more effective.

Echolalia is not, however, the only form of inappropriate speech that is used to elicit and maintain social consequences. Hurtig, Ensrud, and Tomblin (1982) studied question-asking in six higher functioning autistic children who were 5 to 12 years old. They found that as many as one-half of the questions asked were inappropriate, because the children already knew the answers. In these cases, questions were not used to gain information, but rather to initiate a social exchange. Of course, the social/communication skills of such children are poor, and they were often unsuccessful in responding to their listeners' replies with comments that continued the conversation. It is important to note, however, that the autistic children did make verbal social initiations, and they were affected by their listeners' replies. When the listener gave a *minimal* reply (providing "only the information asked for," Hurtig *et al.*, 1982; p. 63) the autistic children were able to continue the conversation appropriately in an average of 53% of cases. When the listeners gave one of three types of more elaborate and social replies to the initial questions, the autistic children were far more successful in maintaining the conversation. In other words, the initiations may have been socially inappropriate or awkward, but they were attempts at social interchange, and they were responsive to social statements.

*Functional consequences.* Another source of encouragement about the potential value of social consequences comes from the growing literature on the effectiveness of "functional" consequences for handicapped learners. This is a term in need of clarification in this context, because the reader of current special education journals can easily find him or herself in a semantic *Alice in Wonderland* in which *functional* is an adjective describing speech, curricula, and/or reinforcers. The term *functional consequence* is actually the same as Ferster's (1967) and Ferster & Simons, (1966) notion of *natural reinforcement*. This view holds that consequences that naturally follow certain actions or are logically or *functionally* related to those actions are more likely to be reinforcing than are *arbitrary* consequences.

Goetz *et al.* (1981) summarized several studies in which natural or functional reinforcers proved effective for handicapped children. One example with autistic children is Koegel and Williams's (1980) study in which verbal and nonverbal communicative acts were learned faster when they led to consequences logically linked to the action (e.g., reaching for a jar, opening it, taking out a food reward). Unfortunately, Koegel and Williams's reinforcers were natural or functional, but not social. Further research is needed on natural social consequences of communication for autistic children.

Although there is little empirical research on the topic, social consequences are a major consideration when choosing a form of communication for an autistic child. One reason that speech is the preferred form of communication is that it leads to natural, functional consequences. If people with autism learn to use speech appropriately, their listeners will respond to them readily and comply with their requests. Other forms of communication, such as pic-

tures or written words, may be easily understood by others, but viewed as socially odd. Other methods, such as signing, may be understood by so few people that the social consequences of their use are very limited.

## Combining Social Antecedents and Consequences

The move away from language teaching in an isolated therapy room and
toward teaching functional communication skills in natural settings is a recent
one (Prizant, 1982a,b; Watson & Lord, 1982), and, therefore, there are few
empirical studies of its effectiveness with autistic people. Related studies with
other populations do offer promise for application to autism. The approach of
teaching language in natural settings and using natural opportunities to teach
that capitalize on children's interests has been called incidental teaching, and it
has been shown to be effective for disadvantaged children (Hart & Risley,
1975) and for a severely language-delayed child (Cavallaro & Bambara, 1982).
It is also a component of the TEACCH communication curriculum for autistic
students (See Watson, Chapter 9; Watson & Lord, 1982). Incidental teaching
combines the use of natural, highly motivating, social settings with natural social reinforcers. Two recent studies have demonstrated the value of this approach for acquisition and generalization of sign language (Carr & Kologinsky,
1983) and receptive object labels (McGee, Krantz, Mason, & McClannahan,
1983) for autistic children.

These two studies are very important advances. They demonstrate clearly
the value of natural and diverse social settings and consequences instead of
rigid, arbitrary, nonsocial conditions for teaching language. The children in
these studies not only learned useful communication skills; they also generalized their skills to new people, places, and activities. The use of social factors
in an incidental teaching approach appears to be the best solution to the problems of lack of spontaneity and generalization that Lovaas (1977; Lovaas *et
al.*, 1973) and others found in earlier behavioral methods.

Studies of incidental teaching have retained adults as the primary therapists, but a next step in capitalizing on natural antecedents and consequences
is to involve nonhandicapped peers as tutors or playmates for autistic children.
This approach has been used widely with socially withdrawn and other handicapped children (Strain, 1981), and some research exists with autistic children
(McHale, 1983; Ragland, Kerr, & Strain, 1978; Strain, 1983; Strain, Kerr, &
Ragland, 1979), but more research is needed on the value of peers in eliciting
language.

## CONCLUSION

The social and communication deficits in autism are central aspects of the
disorder, and the research and clinical literature describes these characteristics

well. Although people with autism have serious problems in those areas, they are neither asocial nor noncommunicative. Recent research that has emphasized natural, social settings and consequences has given encouragement to the view that people with autism can learn to be social and to communicate in ways that are both spontaneous and effective. The results of these efforts could lead to significant improvements in the quality of life for people with autism.

## REFERENCES

Argyle, M. (1969). *Social interaction.* New York: Atherton.

Argyle, M. (1972). Nonverbal communication in human social interaction. In R. Hinde (Ed.), *Nonverbal communication* (pp. 243–269). Cambridge, England: Cambridge University Press.

Bailey, D. B., Clifford, R. M., & Harms, T. (1982). Comparison of preschool environments for handicapped and nonhandicapped children. *Topics in Early Childhood Special Education, 2* (1), 9–20.

Baltaxe, C. A. M. (1977). Pragmatic deficits in the language of autistic adolescents. *Journal of Pediatric Psychology, 2,* 176–180.

Baltaxe, C. A. M., & Simmons, J. Q. (1975). Language in childhood psychosis: A review. *Journal of Speech and Hearing Disorders, 40,* 439–458.

Baltaxe, C. A. M., & Simmons, J. Q. (1977). Bedtime soliloquies and linguistic competence in autism. *Journal of Speech and Hearing Disorders, 42,* 376–393.

Bates, E. (1976). *Language and context: The acquisition of pragmatics.* New York: Academic Press.

Bates, E., & MacWhinney, B. (1982). Functionalist approaches to grammar. In E. Warner & L. R. Gleitman (Eds.), *Language acquisition: The state of the art* (pp. 173–218). Cambridge, England: Cambridge University Press.

Begley, S. (1983, June 20). What the trees really say. *Newsweek,* p. 72.

Bernard-Opitz, V. (1982). Pragmatic analysis of the communication behavior of an autistic child. *Journal of Speech and Hearing Disorders, 47,* 99–109.

Brazelton, T. B., Koslowski, B., & Main, M. (1974). The origins of reciprocity: The early mother–infant interaction. In M. Lewis & L. A. Rosenblum (Eds.), *The effect of the infant on its caregiver* (pp. 49–76). New York: Wiley.

Bronfenbrenner, U. (1977). Toward an experimental ecology of human development. *American Psychologist, 32,* 513–531.

Bronfenbrenner, U. (1979). *The ecology of human development: Experiments by nature and design.* Cambridge, MA: Harvard University Press.

Cantwell, D. P., Baker, L., & Rutter, M. (1977). Families of autistic and dysphasic children. II. Mother's speech to the children. *Journal of Autism and Childhood Schizophrenia, 7,* 313–327.

Carr, E. G., & Kologinsky, E. (1983). Acquisition of sign language by autistic children II: Spontaneity and generalization effects. *Journal of Applied Behavior Analysis, 16,* 297–314.

Cavallero, C. C., & Bambara, L. M. (1982). Two strategies for teaching language during free play. *Journal of the Association for the Severely Handicapped, 7,* 80–92.

Clark, P., & Rutter, M. (1981). Autistic children's responses to structure and to interpersonal demands. *Journal of Autism and Developmental Disorders, 11,* 201–217.

Dawson, G., & Adams, A. (1984). Imitation and social responsiveness in autistic children. *Journal of Abnormal Child Psychology, 12,* 209–226.

DeMyer, M. K., Alpern, G. D., Barton, S., DeMyer, W. E., Churchill, D. W., Hingtgen, J. N., Bryson, C. Q., Pontius, W., & Kimberlin, C. (1972). Imitation in autistic, early schizophrenic, and non-psychotic subnormal children. *Journal of Autism and Childhood Schizophrenia, 2,* 264–287.

Duchan, J. F. (1983). Autistic children are noninteractive: Or so we say. *Seminars in Speech and Language, 4,* 53–61.

Duchan, J. F., & Palermo, J. (1982). How autistic children view the world. *Topics in Language Disorders, 3* (1), 10–15.

Dyer, C., & Hadden, A. (1981). Delayed ecolalia in autism: Some observations on differences within the term. *Child: Care, Health, and Development, 7,* 331–345.

Fay, W. H., & Schuler, A. L. (1980). *Emerging language in autistic children.* Baltimore, MD: University Park Press.

Ferster, C. B. (1967). Arbitrary and natural reinforcement. *The Psychological Record, 17,* 341–347.

Ferster, C. B., & Simons, J. (1966). An evaluation of behavior therapy with children. *Psychological Record, 16,* 65–71.

Foster, R. E. (1983, May). *Teaching language in the classroom.* Paper presented at the TEACCH Conference on Communication Problems in Autism, Chapel Hill, NC.

Fraiberg, S. (1974). Blind infants and their mothers: An examination of the sign system: In M. Lewis & L. Rosenblum (Eds.), *The effect of the infant on its caregiver* (pp. 215–232). New York: Wiley.

Fraiberg, S. (1975). The development of human attachments in infants blind from birth. *Merrill-Palmer Quarterly, 21,* 315–334.

Goetz, L., Schuler, A. L., & Sailor, W. (1981). Functional competence as a factor in communication instruction. *Exceptional Education Quarterly, 2* (1), 51–60.

Guralnick, M., & Paul-Brown, D. (1977). The nature of verbal interaction among handicapped and nonhandicapped preschool children. *Child Development, 48,* 254–260.

Halle, J. W. (1982). Teaching functional language to the handicapped: An integrative model of natural environment teaching. *Journal of the Association for the Severely handicapped, 7,* 29–37.

Hart, B. M., & Risley, T. R. (1975). Incidental teaching of language in the preschool. *Journal of Applied Behavior Analysis, 8,* 411–420.

Hurtig, R., Ensrud, S., & Tomblin, J. B. (1982). The communication function of question production in autistic children. *Journal of Autism and Developmental Disorders, 12,* 57–69.

Kaye, K. (1981). *The mental and social life of babies.* Chicago: University of Chicago Press.

Kanner, L. (1943). Autistic disturbances of affective contact. *Nervous Child, 2,* 217–250.

Koegel, R. L., & Williams, J. A. (1980). Direct versus indirect response-reinforcer relationships in teaching autistic children. *Journal of Abnormal Child Psychology, 8,* 537–547.

Lord, C., Merrin, D. J., Vest, L. O., & Kelly, K. M. (1983). Communicative behavior of adults with an autistic four-year-old boy and his nonhandicapped twin brother. *Journal of Autism and Developmental Disorders, 13,* 1–17.

Lovaas, O. I. (1977). *The autistic child: Language development through behavior modification.* New York: Irvington.

Lovaas, O. I. (1981). *Teaching developmentally disabled children: The ME book.* Baltimore, MD: University Park Press.

Lovaas, O. I., Koegel, R., Simmons, J. Q., & Long, J. S. (1973). Some generalization and follow-up measures on autistic children in behavior therapy. *Journal of Applied Behavior Analysis, 6,* 131–166.

Lovaas, O. I., Varni, J. W., Koegel, R. L., & Lorsch, N. (1977). Some observations on the nonextinguishability of children's speech. *Child Development, 48,* 1121–1127.

McGee, G. G., Krantz, P. J., Mason, D., & McClannahan, L. E. (1983). A modified incidental-teaching procedure for autistic youth: Acquisition and generalization of receptive object labels. *Journal of Applied Behavior Analysis, 16,* 329–338.

McHale, S. M. (1983). Social interactions of autistic and nonhandicapped children during free play. *American Journal of Orthopsychiatry, 53,* 81–91.

McHale, S. M., Olley, J. G., Marcus, L. M., & Simeonsson, R. J. (1984). *Children's play and communication during interactions with autistic and with nonhandicapped peers.* Manuscript submitted for publication.

McHale, S. M., Simeonsson, R. J., Marcus, L. M., & Olley, J. G. (1980). The social and symbolic quality of autistic children's communication. *Journal of Autism and Developmental Disorders, 10,* 299–310.

McLean, J. E., & Snyder-Mclean, L. (1978). *A transactional approach to early language training.* Columbus, OH: Merrill.

McReynolds, L. V. (1970). Reinforcement procedures for establishing and maintaining echoic speech by a nonverbal child. In F. L. Girardeau & J. E. Spradlin (Eds.), *A functional analysis approach to speech and language* (pp. 60–66). ASHA Monographs (Whole No. 14).

Mesibov, G. B. (1983). Current perspectives and issues in autism and adolescence. In E. Schopler & G. B. Mesibov (Eds.), *Autism in adolescents and adults* (pp. 37–53). New York: Plenum Press.

NSAC. (1978). National Society for Autistic Children definition of the syndrome of autism. *Journal of Autism and Childhood Schizophrenia, 8,* 162–167.

Needleman, R., Ritvo, E. R., & Freeman, B. J. (1980). Objectively defined linguistic parameters in children with autism and other developmental disabilities. *Journal of Autism and Developmental Disorders, 10,* 389–398.

Olley, J. G. (1981, May). *A behavioral approach to childhood autism: Have we overlooked some things?* Paper presented at the meeting of the Association for Behavior Analysis, Milwaukee, WI.

Prizant, B. M. (1982a). Speech-language pathologists and autistic children: What is our role? *Asha, 24,* 463–468.

Prizant, B. M. (1982b). Speech-language pathologists and autistic children: What is our role? Part II. *Asha, 24,* 531–537.

Prizant, B. M. (1983). Echolalia in autism: Assessment and intervention. *Seminars in Speech and Language, 4,* 63–77.

Prizant, B. M., & Duchan, J. F. (1980, November). *Interaction competence: How to assess it and improve it.* Seminar presented at the meeting of the American Speech-Language-Hearing Association, Detroit, MI.

Prizant, B. M., & Rydell, P. J. (1984). An analysis of the functions of delayed echolalia in autistic children. *Journal of Speech and Hearing Research, 27,* 183–192.

Ragland, E. U., Kerr, M. M., & Strain, P. S. (1978). Behavior of withdrawn autistic children: Effects of peer social initiations. *Behavior Modification, 2,* 565–578.

Ricks, D. M., & Wing, L. (1975). Language communication and the use of symbols in normal and autistic children. *Journal of Autism and Childhood Schizophrenia, 5,* 191–220.

Rutter, M. (1978). Diagnosis and definition of childhood autism. *Journal of Autism and Childhood Schizophrenia, 8,* 139–161.

Rutter, M. (1983). Cognitive deficits in the pathogenesis of autism. *Journal of Child Psychology and Psychiatry, 24,* 513–531.

Schopler, E., Reichler, R. J., DeVellis, R. F., & Daly, K. (1980). Toward objective classification of childhood autism: Childhood Autism Rating Scale (CARS). *Journal of Autism and Developmental Disorders, 10,* 91–103.

Shatz, M., & Gelman, R. (1973). The development of communication skills: Modifications in the speech of young children as a function of listener. *Monographs of the Society for Research in Child Development, 38* (5, Serial No. 152).

Snow, C. E. (1972). Mother's speech to children learning language. *Child Development, 43,* 549–565.

Strain, P. S. (Ed.). (1981). *The utilization of classroom peers as behavior change agents.* New York: Plenum Press.

Strain, P. S. (1983). Generalization of autistic children's social behavior change: Effects of developmentally integrated and segregated settings. *Analysis and Intervention in Developmental Disabilities, 3*, 23–34.

Strain, P. S. (1984). *Social behavior patterns of nonhandicapped and developmentally disabled friend pairs in mainstream preschools. Analysis and Intervention in Developmental Disabilities, 4*, 15–28.

Strain, P. S., Kerr, M. M., & Ragland, E. U. (1979). Effects of peer-mediated social interactions and promoting/reinforcement on the social behavior of autistic children. *Journal of Autism and Developmental Disorders, 9*, 41–54.

Watson, L. R., & Lord, C. (1982). Developing a social communication curriculum for autistic students. *Topics in Language Disorders, 3* (1), 1–9.

Wilbur, R. B. (1983). Where do we go from here? In J. Miller, D. E. Yoder, & R. Schiefelbusch (Eds.), *Contemporary issues in language intervention. ASHA Reports 12* (pp. 137–145). Rockville, MD: The American Speech-Language-Hearing Association.

Wing, L. (1981). Language, social and cognitive impairments in autism and severe mental retardation. *Journal of Autism and Developmental Disorders, 11*, 31–44.

Wing, L., & Gould, J. (1979). Severe impairments of social interaction and associated abnormalities in children: Epidemiology and classification. *Journal of Autism and Developmental Disorders, 9*, 11–29.

# Index